THE

EVERYTHING®

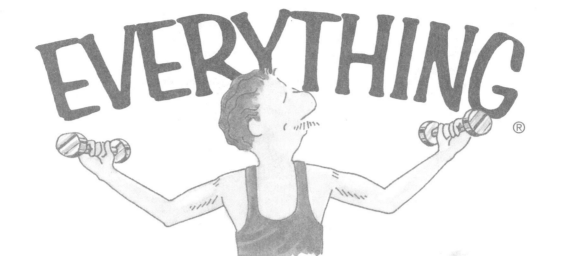

TOTAL FITNESS BOOK

A complete program to help
you look—and feel—great

Ellen Karpay

Adams Media Corporation
Avon, Massachusetts

An Everything® Series Book.
Everything® and everything.com® are registered trademarks of F+W Publications, Inc.

Published by Adams Media, an F+W Publications Company
57 Littlefield Street, Avon, MA 02322. U.S.A.
www.adamsmedia.com

ISBN: 1-58062-318-2

Printed in the United States of America.

J I H G F E

Library of Congress Cataloging-in-Publication Data
Karpay, Ellen.
The everything total fitness book / Ellen Karpay.
p.   cm.
ISBN 1-58062-318-2
Includes index.
1. Physical fitness. 2. Exercise I. Title.
GV481 .K374   2000
613.7—dc21   99-086414
CIP

Illustrations by Barry Littmann and Joel Snyder.

This book is available at quantity discounts for bulk purchases.
For information, call 1-800-872-5627.

Visit the entire Everything® Series at everything.com

Dedication

To my anima cara, for everything.

To my mom and dad, Bobbe and George Karpay,
for helping me cross another finish line.
I love you.

In Memoriam:
To Grandpa Nate Denenberg, whose love affair
with books inspired me. "A promise made is . . . "
This one's for you.

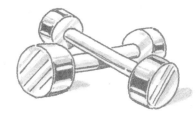

Special Acknowledgments

Thank you to all who contributed, supported, and helped to make this possible. To my pets, HollyHobo, Cally, and Sonny, for love and comic relief. To the rest of my loving family and friends, too numerous to mention, whose love and support was invaluable—thank you. Special thanks to Sally Edwards of Heart Zones, to my agent, Nancy Crossman of Crossman Literary Agency, Chicago, Illinois, and to Sarah Larson, assistant editor, and Pam Liflander, executive editor, of Adams Media Corp.

For immeasurable contributions:
Linda Lazar Allen, Sacramento, CA
Ardis J. Bow, Ardis Bow Graphics, Masters Swim
    Coach, Sacramento, CA
Sharron Brockman, Health Is Wealth Fitness &
    Food Consulting, Sacramento, CA
Laurine Brusati, C.M.T., Body Kneads,
    Sacramento, CA
Christel Cranston, M.D., Sacramento, CA
Vince J. Catalano, Ph.D. associate professor of
    Chemistry, University of Nevada, Reno
Sesi McCullough Catalano, Ph.D. University of
    Nevada, Reno
The Cooper Clinic, Dallas, Texas: Kenneth H.
    Cooper, M.D.; Cynthia Grantham, Georgia
    Kostas, M.P.H., R.D., L.D.
Lisa Downey, Sacramento, CA
Barry Karpay, Tampa, FL
Kenny Karpay, Baltimore, MD
Virginia A. McConnell, "the human search
    engine," English Instructor Walla Walla
    Community College, WA
James Mahoney, Oak Ridge, NC
Bill Nilva, Sacramento, CA
Erik Revai, Esq., San Francisco, CA
Angela Schrimp, Esq., Knox, Lemmon &
    Anapolsky, Sacramento, CA
Karen K.B. Waksman, Tampa, FL

For technical and other contributions:
Alhambra Athletic Club, Sacramento, CA
Jeanette Areia, City of Sacramento Police Officer
Catherine Cram, M.S., Comprehensive Fitness
    Consulting, Pre/Postnatal Specialist,
    Middleton, WI
Michele Canny Gilles, MPA, R.D. Nutrition
    Director Wenmat Fitness, Carmichael, CA
Mike and Meta Newhouse, Dallas, Texas
Cameron Pauly, Exercise Equipment Co.,
    Sacramento, CA
Rick Reynolds, Truckee, CA
Larry Robinson, The Rest Stop Bicycle
    Accessories, Sacramento, CA
Greig St. Clair of Paco's Bike & Ski, Truckee, CA

And for special inspiration:
Towanda!, Yanni, Andreas Vollenweider, Ellen
    Nowlin, and Daniel Rudd.

Contents

CONTENTS

CHAPTER 10: BODY FAT, BODY WEIGHT, AND YOUR HEALTH 221

CHAPTER 11: STRESS REDUCTION AND RELAXATION 235

CHAPTER 12: SPECIAL POPULATIONS AND CONSIDERATIONS . . 243

CONTENTS

CHAPTER 13: INJURIES AND ILLNESS— PREVENTION AND TREATMENT 267

CHAPTER 14: REWARDS OF BEING FIT—INSPIRATION, EDUCATION, DEDICATION, CELEBRATION, AND GIVING BACK . . 279

Introduction

Try to name something more important than your health. Did you have a hard time coming up with anything? Some people are well aware of the gift of good health and appreciate it. Others develop an appreciation for health only when, as Joni Mitchell sings, "you don't know what you've got 'til it's gone." Ask those who suffer from poor health, and they will tell you they would trade just about anything to have their health back. Are you willing to trade in your good health for income, cars, status, a job, or family responsibilities? Or are you doing it now? In effect, many people do every day. You may not have noticed yet, but without good health, life is extra-challenging, complicated, and laborious. It does not have to be that way. You have a choice, and you know it. That is why you are reading this book.

This book is for everyone who cares about health and wants to take an active role in improving it through fitness. "Active role" means you must do your part. It does not matter what type of health you have right now; you can improve it and feel better through fitness. As Ellen Nowlin, my two-time state championship volleyball coach said, "It's not what you've got; it's what you do with it."

The scientific facts and benefits of being fit have been around for a long time and continue to pour in almost daily. Exercise, nutritious eating, managing your stress, and rest will improve the quality of your health, your life. And if science does not convince you, look at all the walking, talking evidence of fit people who feel great and are doing great things with their lives. People who are fit have energy; they say yes to life; they have an "I can" attitude.

The Everything Total Fitness Book contains everything you need to become or stay fit. It will get starters started, and it will help already fit persons stay fit and motivated. It is intended to be your coach, to guide you slowly and steadily, without overwhelming you. If you are just beginning to add fitness into your life, take one bit of information at a time and "try it on" for a week or more. Once you integrate it into your life and make it routine, it is likely that you will be hungry for more. If what you first pick does not stick, then try something different. Remember that it took a long time for you to become unfit. Luckily, it will not take as long to start feeling better.

Has your doctor or loved one said to you, "I wish you would exercise, eat better, and lose weight"? Did you say to yourself, "I know they

The first wealth is health.

—Ralph Waldo Emerson

are right, but . . . " and go on without making any changes? I am hopeful that perhaps something you read here will stir you to action. *The Everything Total Fitness Book* gives you thoughts for motivation, scientifically proven concepts, and great details and fun facts to know about being fit.

Many shy away from learning about fitness and the body because they think it is complicated; it doesn't have to be. As a teacher and fitness consultant, I have been successful in helping others by sharing the facts of the matter in a way so that people can identify with them personally. You are more than capable of understanding what happens to your body when you exercise (and when you don't). With a basic understanding, you can be more successful in your fitness. So don't be surprised while reading this book that you find yourself saying, "So *that's* what that means" or "so *that's* what I'm supposed to do" or "*now* I understand why." It only takes a moment to be inspired for a lifetime. May you find many of those moments in these pages. Here's to the most important wealth, your health.

—Ellen Karpay
Sacramento, California

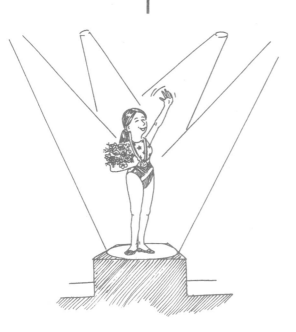

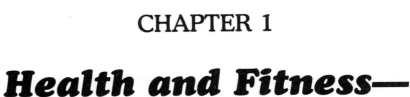

CHAPTER 1

Health and Fitness— A Case for Fitness

You don't have to be a fantastic hero to do certain things—to compete. You can be just an ordinary chap, sufficiently motivated to reach challenging goals.

—SIR EDMUND HILLARY

Technological advances over the past 40 years have drastically changed our lifestyles and our bodies. In our quest to save time and energy, to do faster, more efficiently, more conveniently, we have lost something valuable: physical movement. Households now have more automobiles, computers, televisions, and telephones than ever before. These modern technologies and conveniences have replaced everyday activities that formerly kept our bodies in use. We are less active than before. Think about the physical activity that has been "lost" through the following modern conveniences:

Automobile
Fax machine, computer/e-mail
Food processor
Cellular telephone, television and videos
Leaf blower, lawn edger, riding lawn mower, power tools
Drive-through restaurants
Moving sidewalks, shuttle cars, elevators, escalators
Golf carts
Drive-through car washes

Because we have lost even simple activities that used more of our arms, legs, back, heart, and lungs, our bodies have become flaccid, fat, and weak. This rise in inactivity alone has been devastating to our health. Truly, we have witnessed the meaning of the "use it or lose it" phenomenon. When we don't use our bodies, we lose the ability to use them. This grim reality is described by Dr. Kenneth Cooper in his revolutionary book *Aerobics*: "A body that isn't used deteriorates. The lungs become inefficient, the heart grows weaker, the blood vessels less pliable, the muscles lose tone and the body generally weakens throughout, leaving it vulnerable for a whole catalog of illness and disease. Your whole system for delivering oxygen almost literally shrivels up." The bottom line is this: We are meant to be active, and our health depends upon it. When the body is used, it thrives; when it isn't, it survives.

Historical Pushes

Because of his personal interest and concern for the physical fitness and conditioning of Americans, President John F. Kennedy enacted the President's Council on Physical Fitness in 1960. The PCOPF was his response to the declining state of physical fitness and conditioning showing up in our population. America was headed toward a sedentary, unfit direction, and the president did his part to correct it.

Then in 1968, Dr. Kenneth Cooper's *Aerobics* was published. In *Aerobics*, Dr. Cooper shared his new aerobic exercise program, one that had been tested upon more than fifteen thousand Air Force men and women. It was the foundation and springboard for an entirely new way of looking at fitness. Suddenly, Americans were armed with specifics about the benefits and methods of exercise. In the years that followed, the aerobics concept spread, manifesting in many forms. There was a boom in two fitness activities: jogging/running and an exercise phenomenon called aerobics. Since the early 1970s, fitness professionals and enthusiasts have created many new varieties of activity, all with the intention of keeping Americans active and fit. Look at the activities that sprouted between the 1970s and up into 2000: step aerobics, water aerobics, par courses (exercise stations on trails), ultimate frisbee, disc (frisbee) golf, spin cycling, and, of course, walking, running, bicycling, and swimming.

Since those significant occurrences, many Americans have gotten the message that health and fitness are important components to a quality filled life. Unfortunately, statistics show that we still need to get moving and fit.

Commitment for Life

Fitness is not a "destination" that you visit occasionally in your life. Rather, fitness is a "road trip," or excursion, and an ongoing state of health. Participating in fitness activities consistently and regularly is what ensures your best chances for improved quality and quantity of life. Fitness is the process, and fitness is the reward.

So how do you go about becoming fit? As with any project, when you utilize the right tools, the job is much more productive, efficient, and even fun. The tools for fitness include exercise, nutrition, and rest/recovery. We will be covering these in greater detail in upcoming chapters. But to get started, we need to begin where all activity originates: in your mind.

Dr. Kenneth H. Cooper and The Cooper Clinic

Kenneth H. Cooper, M.D., M.P.H., founded the Cooper Clinic in 1970. His first book, *Aerobics*, published in 1968 gained worldwide attention and inspired the aerobic fitness boom. Dr. Cooper left the United States Air Force to pursue his growing interest in exercise and preventive medicine. "The father of aerobics" has continued to be on the cutting edge of preventive medicine and health as evidenced by his books, *Controlling Cholesterol* and *Dr. Kenneth H. Cooper's Antioxidant Revolution* and development of the famed treadmill stress test. The Cooper Clinic and Cooper Institute for Aerobics Research are part of a 30-acre complex in Dallas, Texas, where private and corporate patients come from all over the world.

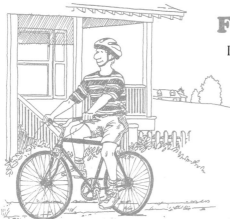

Fitness Begins in the Mind

It may sound funny, but fitness starts in your mind. In order to get your body moving, it is helpful to get your mind ready and receptive to the idea. So relax and take a slow, deep breath. Here we go!

Common Reasons Not to Exercise

There is a good chance that you have experienced at least one of the following reasons for not exercising. And if you have, you have a lot of company. Even the most highly motivated people confront these same issues. If you want to be successful, consider these healthy responses.

1. I don't have time. *Response*: You have a choice about how to spend your time.
2. I don't like to sweat. *Response*: Sweating is a natural bodily function. Be glad your cooling system is working.
3. I'll look silly exercising. *Response*: Would you rather look silly or unhealthy?
4. I don't know what to do specifically. *Response*: That's why you're reading this book. You will learn what to do specifically.
5. I'm afraid I'll hurt myself. *Response*: Read on. You'll learn what to do safely—and learn how to achieve a level of fitness that is far better than a "safe," unfit lifestyle.
6. With all my sweaty gym clothes, I'll have more laundry to do. *Response*: So you're lazy; get over it.
7. Exercise is expensive. *Response*: Being unhealthy is more expensive than being healthy.
8. It's uncomfortable; it hurts me. *Response*: Exercise done properly doesn't hurt.
9. I can't do what I used to be able to do. *Response*: The past is history. Start today.
10. It's not important. *Response*: If taking good care of your health and feeling good isn't important, ask yourself the following: What is important to me? What do I make time for? Is my health important to me? Do I take it for granted that it's just there for me? Am I happy?

From Past to Present

The good news is that you can hurdle over these reasons and successfully add regular exercise to your life. Try a new approach/perspective about exercise in your life with the suggestions that follow. Carly Simon's "new attitude" could be just the tune you want to start singing.

1. Let go of the past. Acknowledge and release old and negative attitudes. They can be unhealthy roadblocks. They are not useful to you anymore, and you have a choice about what you think about. So let go of them and start anew.

2. Think daily, non-negotiable. Do you think about whether or not you're going to brush your teeth each day? Probably you include it in your routine, and it is non-negotiable; you wouldn't think of not brushing your teeth. This is how you can think about your exercise. It is something you fit into your day; it is non-negotiable, and you just do it.

3. Adventurous spirit. When was the last time you tried something new and healthy? Challenge yourself; be a "risk taker." Do a new fitness activity or pick up a familiar but not recent one.

4. Short-term commitment. Did you commit to marriage after the first several dates? No. When you exercise, don't worry about the whole future of your exercise routine. Add exercise to your life as you would a long-term relationship: day by day. Start out "dating," go slowly, and take some time to get to know yourself through activity. Build a solid relationship. Do a 2-week exercise trial (stay with it). You have nothing to lose and a lot to gain. This will be a very healthy marriage!

5. Make peace to make health/find the appreciation. Maybe you think that you will never enjoy exercising. If that is the case, then "make peace" with exercise and find the good in it. Learn to appreciate what it does for you (improved energy, better mood, etc.). With time, you may come to love it.

6. Turn your vanity inside out. How much time do you spend on your exterior appearance such as your clothes, hair, nails, skin, and eyes? Many people spend more time attending to their exterior appearance than their interior health. The truth is that without your interior

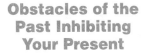

Obstacles of the Past Inhibiting Your Present

"I didn't like my gym teacher or gym class."

"I was a klutz. I was always teased, picked last for teams."

"My parents said sweating wasn't 'lady-like.'"

"I was small, and the macho guys picked on me."

Being fat hurts more than just your appearance. It can hurt your life.

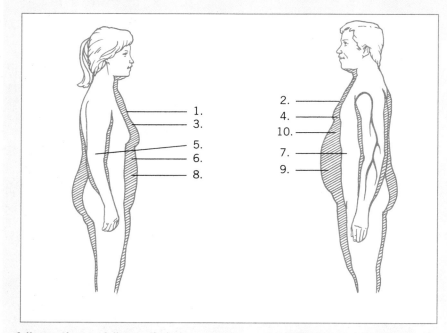

1.
3.
5.
6.
8.

2.
4.
10.
7.
9.

Adipose tissue: Adipose (fat) tissue is composed of cells which are highly elastic and contain varying amounts of fatty deposits acquired through the bloodstream. The tissue is situated throughout the body including under the skin in protective pads covering vital organs. The degree of overweight depends upon the number of fat cells present and the amount of fat they contain. In over-fat people excessive fat deposits are found in virtually all soft tissues and organs. In the course of weight reduction, fat cell volume is decreased, but the number of fat cells remains constant.

When excess weight is gained during childhood, the number of fat cells in the body increases. Since the fat cells developed in childhood remain throughout life, it becomes more difficult to lose weight as an adult.

1. Heart: Excessive fat means the heart must work harder to supply nutrients to all tissues of the body. The greater the body mass, the greater the strain on the heart. There is a higher incidence of heart disease in people who are overweight.

2. Lungs: In over-fat people, an increased body volume must be supplied with oxygen by lungs that have not correspondingly increased in their size. In addition, the presence of thick pads of fat in the abdomen restricts breathing.

3. Blood pressure: High blood pressure (hypertension) occurs more frequently in overweight people. Since hypertension can result in varying degrees of damage to the brain (stroke) and kidneys (degeneration) as well as the heart, it is essential that hypertensive overweight patients lose weight.

4. Atherosclerosis: Atherosclerosis is the deposit of fatty material in the lining of the arterial wall. It can result in narrowing and/or rupture of the blood vessel, which may lead to stroke or heart attack. The incidence of atherosclerosis is high in overweight people.

5. Joint disease: A vicious cycle is set up in overweight patients with arthritis of the hip, knees, or feet or in those who suffer from a ruptured intervertebral disc. Increased weight leads to greater wear and tear on these joints, which may become more irritated and painful. The discomfort can lead the patient to become less and less active, thereby causing further gain in weight and discomfort.

6. Diabetes: Diabetes is more common in overweight persons than in persons of normal weight. When an overweight diabetic loses weight, his diabetes often improves.

7. Gallbladder: A significantly higher incidence of gallbladder disease is observed in overweight patients than in those of normal weight.

8. Pregnancy and surgery: Excessive fat can be a factor in producing difficult and prolonged labor due to abnormal positioning of the fetus. This can cause fetal distress, which in turn may complicate labor and delivery. Surgical procedures are more difficult in overweight individuals due to the very bulk of the adipose tissues.

9. The omentum: The "pot-belly" is from accumulations of fat under the skin and from fat within the abdominal cavity, in the omentum. Fat accumulations in the abdominal area have been associated with putting one at increased risk for heart disease.

10. Hernia: Certain types of hernias, involving displacement of the upper part of the stomach into the chest cavity, are more prevalent in overweight people than in people of normal weight.

health, your exterior appearance of health is meaningless. Turn your view of your health "inside out." Next time you look in the mirror, look deeper into your body. Imagine the interior of your body and know that regular exercise will improve it.

7. Great investment. For only 2 percent of the time in your day (2 percent of 24 hours equals 28.8 minutes) you can reap tremendous returns on that small investment of time. And you, not other market considerations, control the investment. Think of your exercise time as an investment in your health that will yield invaluable returns.

8. Practical approach. Use exercise as transportation: walk, jog, run, skate, roller blade, ski, and bicycle for errands, to work, for visits. You will get fitter and so will the environment as you "spare the air." Include your family members too.

9. Military approach. So, none of the mind-sets above meant anything to you? If that's the case, then take the exercise order . . . "Just Do It" (reference Nike). It's good for you and your loved ones.

10. Real health appointments. If you had a serious life-challenging illness and through regular "treatments" you could reclaim your health, wouldn't you plan your day/week with respect to keeping and going to those appointments? Exercise sessions are also lifesaving. They are advanced lifesaving because they save your life before there's a problem.

11. Life insurance. Regular exercise is vital to achieving good health and protecting you from many preventable or lifestyle diseases. It can be less expensive than what you pay for most life insurance policies, and the benefits are realized while you are alive!

What Do Fit People Say?

Have you ever noticed people after they have exercised? Have you ever seen runners or walkers after their runs or walks, swimmers after their swims, cyclists after their rides? Very often, their eyes and skin have a radiant glow, they have an energetic "bounce" in their step, their posture is more erect than that of others, their movements reflect better than average balance, and they move with confidence. You will probably notice how confident and relaxed they appear.

A Life Without Fitness

The leading causes of deaths in the United States in 1900 and 1990*:

1900
Pneumonia
Tuberculosis
Gastroenteritis
Influenza

1990
Heart Disease
Stroke
Cancer
Accidents

As you can see, the leading causes of death and dying in 1900 were biological in nature and could be reduced through vaccines and treatments. The leading causes of death in 1990, on the other hand, were related to lifestyle and could be reduced through fitness. Fitness as prevention is effective, simple, and inexpensive compared to cost of the medical treatment for those diseases.

*Dr. Pamela Peeke, Fit & Stressed, ACSM Healthy Learning Video Series

ACSM

The American College of Sports Medicine is the largest and most respected sports medicine and exercise science organization in the world. It has more than 15,000 members in over 72 countries. They promote and integrate scientific research, education, and practical applications of sports medicine and exercise science to maintain and enhance physical performance, fitness, health, and quality of life. Members include doctors, educators, scientists, and other health fitness professionals. It is headquartered in Indianapolis, Indiana.

If you were to ask these exercising people how they feel since including regular exercise in their lives, what would you expect to hear them say?

- Exercise made me feel lethargic, grouchy, stressed.
- Exercise made me feel worse about myself.
- Exercise made me look pale and pasty.
- Exercise made me feel and look terrible in my clothes.
- Exercise made me fatter.
- Exercise made my sleep patterns poor.
- Exercise made me start smoking, start drinking.
- Exercise made my (nonexercising) blood pressure go up.

Of course not! You probably know that people who exercise regularly claim just the opposite. They boast of renewed energy, a better outlook on life, a tendency to eat healthier foods, a better quality of sleep, and more. What is it about exercise that produces all these effects?

Oxygen Feed

Aerobic exercise does for the body what no other activity can do because of one major event: utilization of oxygen. Sure, we all take in oxygen just by breathing. But when we exercise, we take in greater amounts of oxygen, and we deliver it more deeply in the body. This is good for us and makes us feel good. Your body welcomes additional oxygen and makes good use of it—like it was extra income. Your body says, "Oh oxygen, I'm so glad you're here. I know just what to do with you. I'm going to send some of you down to the toes, some up to the brain. Let's spread the wealth and send more of you everywhere throughout the body. And since you're here, let me clean out some space; let's start with those arteries, and then we'll go to . . . " The body loves regular bouts of oxygen-rich exercise and, like a welcomed houseguest, makes accommodations for it. These accommodations are the training effect benefits. Training effects from regular exercise show up in the body not only during exercise but also while *the body is at rest.*

When you consider the physiological benefits of exercise, it is not hard to figure out why exercise makes us feel better. But because "feeling is believing," try these two very short simulations for feeling better.

Simulation #1: To simulate what feeling better is, try this simple exercise: First, take your left hand and place it over your mouth. Breathe. Second, take your right hand and pinch your nose closed. Try to breathe. Wait just a few moments. Now release hands from your face.

If you are like most people, you were quick to remove your hands from your nose and mouth and wanted to resume breathing normally, right? Why? Because your breathing became labored; it became uncomfortable to be without your normal supply of oxygen.

That simulates how a body that does not regularly exercise has to labor for basic bodily functions as compared to a body that is regularly exercised and basic bodily functions (in this case breathing) are performed with ease.

In an unfit person, the heart and lungs have to work harder to provide and deliver oxygen to all the tissues and organs of the body. And if this body has low muscle mass (muscles are body tools; they do the work for you), there is additional stress from carrying around extra, nonproductive mass (fat). Now try the second simulation.

Simulation #2: Find a 5- or 10-pound weight and carry it around with you for 10 minutes. Is it pleasurable to do this, or is it tiring?

Wearing even a few extra pounds of fat can be tiring because of the extra load the heart, lungs, and muscles are carrying. Regular exercise can help you shed unwanted fat weight and can strengthen your muscles so that movement is easier. So, the bottom line is . . . do you want to feel better? Do you want to be able to perform basic daily deeds with greater ease and with less fatigue? Do you want to avoid the lifestyle diseases? Do you want to be able to participate in activities with your family, keep up with your children and grandchildren, nephews, nieces? Do you want to bounce back quicker from colds and flu when they do occur? If you say yes, then keep an open mind and keep on reading. You are on the right path.

Benefits of Exercise

It is easy to focus on the external benefit of exercise such as appearance and looking good. But that is a limited view. In fact, it is highly motivating to know what you are doing to yourself internally when you exercise. Following are some of the more common and well-documented training effects. Notice the *efficiency* theme. You will

It's not whether you get knocked down, it's whether you get up. Once you learn to quit, it becomes a habit. The good Lord gave you a body that can stand most anything. It's your mind you have to convince.

—BENJAMIN FRANKLIN

improve your appearance through regular exercise, but more importantly, you will improve your body's ability to do more with less effort, and that *feels* great! Look what awaits you:

1. Improved respiration. You will be an easy-breather. When you exercise, your body needs more oxygen to "fund" the activity. Your lungs work harder (than when they are at rest) to supply the extra demand for oxygen to the body. With repetition and time, your lungs adapt to the extra work and become more efficient at providing the extra oxygen needed for the activity. The training effect of this extra work is that you will experience better and easier breathing at rest as well as when you are active.

2. Improved cardiac output. Just as an assembly line measures its success in terms of productivity or output, cardiac output refers to the productivity or output of the heart. The heart rate and volume of blood that is pumped out with each beat are cardiac output. When you exercise, your heart beats fast so that your muscles will receive more blood. The heart gets stronger and more efficient from these exercise sessions. The training effect upon cardiac output is that the heart rate at rest is slow yet able to pump out large amounts of blood with each stroke/beat. You get more for less. This is improved efficiency.

3. Improved vascular system. Movement of blood and oxygen happens within your body's highway system, the vascular system. The training effect upon veins and arteries is that they become cleaner from a reduction of fatty deposits. It's as if blood and oxygen come burning through during the exercise session and say, "Hey fatty deposits, clear out. Here we come." The training effect also increases the number and size of blood vessels, which is the equivalent of having more paved streets in your neighborhood. Travel becomes less congested and laborious. Your circulation and blood pressure are improved.

4. Increased muscular strength and endurance. When you exercise, you use the body's tools, your muscles. You must have muscular strength in order to do or perform some activity or work. Muscular endurance is your ability to maintain that activity or work over time. The training effect of exercise is that it keeps your muscles functional.

5. Increased bone density. Muscles are attached to bone, so when you move your muscles during exercise, it is as if the muscles are massaging the bones. The training effect upon your bones is growth. Think of muscular movement like a bone massage that stimulates bone growth. Bone growth helps to keep bones dense, firm, and healthy.

6. Improved flexibility. A joint is the place where bones meet. When you have movement of your joints, it feels good; when you cannot move your joints, it feels bad. The training effect of exercise on your joints is that it helps maintain and improve the mobility or range of motion within a joint.

7. Bowel function. You may not have thought of this as a training effect, but exercise helps to stimulate the wavelike movement in the bowel called peristalsis. How does it do this? It can be related to several factors: pressure changes inside the body as a result of increased breathing (oxygen), the neighboring muscular movement, increased gravitational pull of some activities, or any combination. In addition to having enough fiber and fluid in your dietary intake, movement will help your ability to eliminate. Regular and easy elimination helps prevent hemorrhoids and constipation.

8. Improves sensory skills. As babies and youngsters, we learn how to use our sensory abilities. We learn about balance and movement in space through activity. In order to keep these sensory skills sharp, we have to use them. A training effect of exercise is maintenance and improvement of sensory skills, like balance and movement through space or from place to place.

9. Improved psychological effect. A well-known training effect of exercise is the production of endorphins. Endorphins are natural morphine-like hormones that produce a sense of well-being and reduce stress. They make you feel good and improve your mood. You may have heard of them associated with long-distance runners, but they don't have the exclusive rights to endorphin production. You too can produce your own endorphins, without being a distance runner. Regular exercise will trigger their release. The effect of endorphins can last for hours or even a few days, but beyond that, you have to re-produce them. If you could bottle them up and save them for a gloomy mood, you would be rich. But until then, you have to produce your own endorphins on a regular basis.

Thriving or Surviving?

One day at the bank, the regular customer greeted the familiar young teller. "How are you?" she asked him. With a grim, listless look in his eyes, he replied, "I'm surviving." Is this the best way to feel about your life? No! And yet plenty of us accept it.

Exercise Pays

A young woman interviewed with a large advertising agency for an entry level job. She had never worked in advertising before but felt that her credentials and background as a teacher were suitable enough to try breaking into the new field. When she walked into the vice president's office, she noticed the framed New York City Marathon poster on his wall. Being a runner herself, she immediately commented on the poster, which led to enthusiastic conversation about running, exercise, and health. An instant rapport was created, and she was hired on the spot.

10. Social experiences, direct or indirect. We are social animals who enjoy and need human interaction. Exercise helps you to build self-confidence that spills into other areas of your life. Don't be surprised that you feel a bit more outgoing and social; it is another training effect of exercise. The opportunities for social experiences can be either direct or indirect. You may choose the direct experience of exercising with others. Or if you prefer exercise to be time for yourself, you can indirectly use exercise as a conversation piece in other professional or social situations.

In either case you have the opportunity for social experiences you would otherwise not have. If you want to strike up a conversation, ask people what they do for exercise. People love to talk about what they do for exercise. And when you listen to the responses, you might learn a few new tricks that will help you enjoy yours or of an upcoming event in which you would like to participate. If you're ever at a loss for words at a party, ask a stranger what they do for exercise. It is a great ice-breaker for conversation.

11. Your loved ones will love you for it. Suppose a loved one says to you, "I started an exercise program a month ago." How do you respond? Do you reply, "Oh no, how could you do such a thing?" or "Oh, I'm so sorry"? Of course not! Most likely you will be glad, give congratulations, and offer support. This is the same reaction others will have toward you. Support from loved ones is a valuable training effect that reinforces your stick-to-it-ness.

12. You will feel better. Absolutely! That is a very impressive list, is it not? What is also impressive is that if you tried to get those benefits through "nonexercising means," that is, through medical and therapeutic services, you would have to spend numerous hours and numerous dollars, take numerous types of medications, and deal with the negative side effects. In addition, you would not have much fun in the process, and there are no guarantees that the medical and therapeutic means would work.

By now you are convinced that fitness is something you want to include in your life, that you want to begin feeling better, and that you are worth the time, the investment, and the benefits. So let's discuss what to include in your fitness program.

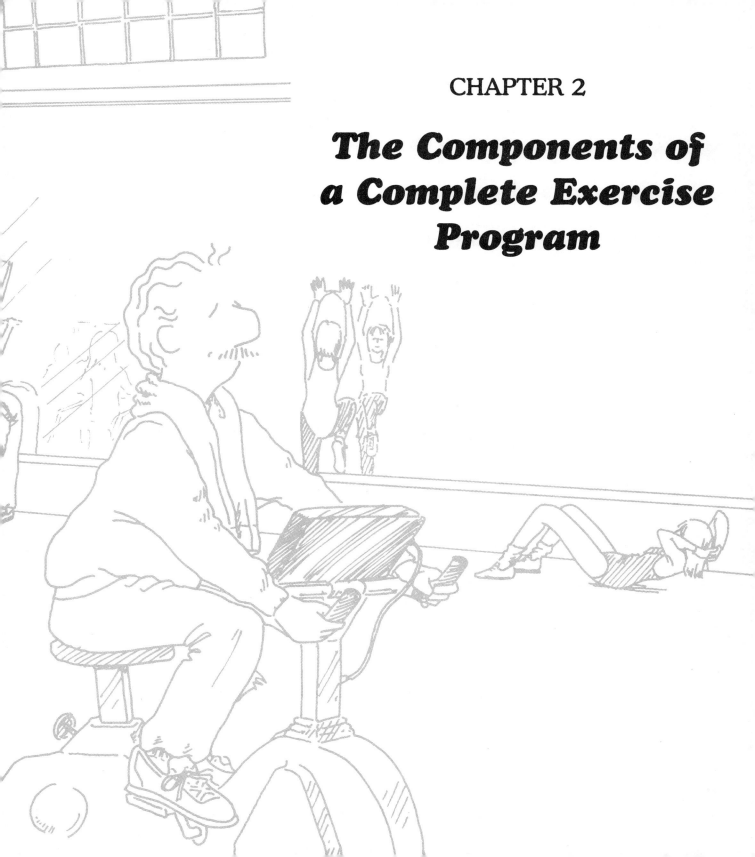

CHAPTER 2

The Components of a Complete Exercise Program

The four elements, cardiorespiratory fitness, muscular strength and endurance, flexibility, and rest are what will make you fit and your exercise program balanced and complete. Each area of fitness needs your attention regardless of your natural abilities. A good question to ask yourself is, How would I feel without any of the four? The answer is, Not too good.

Cardiorespiratory Fitness and Aerobic Exercise

Also known as cardiovascular fitness, cardiorespiratory fitness refers to the capability or fitness level of your heart, blood vessels, lungs, and breathing mechanisms. Here is a simplified version of how they work and why they are important:

Cardio = heart
Vascular, vessel = hollow receptacle for liquid
Respire = breathe

The heart is a muscle that pumps blood throughout the body. Blood, which carries oxygen, is transported by the vascular system, better known as your veins and arteries. Your lungs are responsible for processing oxygen by extracting it from the air you breathe and sending it into the blood for distribution throughout the body.

Cardiorespiratory fitness refers to the ability and efficiency of your heart, lungs, and vascular system to process and transport oxygen to your muscles. Aerobic exercise is the type of activity we use to build cardiorespiratory fitness. *Aerobic* means "with oxygen," and aerobic exercises are those that utilize oxygen during the activity. Aerobic exercise trains the body to utilize oxygen more efficiently and improves your overall cardiorespiratory fitness, that is your heart, vessels, and lungs.

The importance of cardiorespiratory fitness is that without the efficient workings of your heart, lungs, and vascular system, even light physical activity can feel labored, thus limiting your functional abilities and independence. Aerobic exercise is any activity that involves movement of your big muscle groups (hips, legs, chest, and back), is performed continuously, is (usually) rhythmic or repetitive, and is performed at an intensity level that causes your heart, lungs, and vascular system to work somewhat harder than when they are at rest.

Examples of aerobic exercise include walking, jogging, running, skipping, skiing, bicycle riding, jumping rope, swimming, and rowing. Chapter 5 will specifically address how to properly include aerobic exercise in your fitness program as well as provide a thorough list of activities and instruction on how to perform them.

Aerobic Exercise Training Effect: Reduced Heart Rate

At first this may sound scary, but be assured that a reduced heart rate as a training effect of exercise is a good thing. It means that your heart is not having to work as much or as hard to deliver the goods (blood, oxygen) during rest. As your heart gets stronger, it becomes more efficient. It can pump more blood volume with fewer contractions every minute. The purpose of aerobic exercise is to give the heart appropriate bouts of stress to strengthen it. The result is that at rest or during nonexercising times, the heart works less and with greater ease and efficiency.

Muscular Strength, Muscular Endurance

Muscular *strength* is the ability to do some work that produces some result. Muscular strength allows you to move. Muscular *endurance* is the ability to continue to perform that "work" over time. Each is critical to your fitness. If you watch the movements of sedentary, aged persons, you will notice their *inability* to do anything because they have very little strength. Or notice the person who can do something once but is exhausted when having to repeat that work over a short period of time. Muscles are the body's tools that perform work (or exercise). And just like tools that are left in the toolbox and forgotten, they can become rusty. Your muscles do not literally become rusty. They just shrink or atrophy, which makes movement laborious and difficult. And as muscles "fade away," so too does your ability to do things or to be functional. The

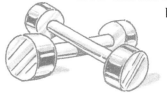

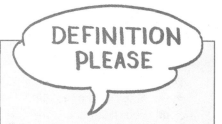

DEFINITION PLEASE

Exercise: Exercise is physical activity whose purpose is to improve components of physical fitness.

Characteristics of aerobic exercise: The activity is sustained, repetitive, or rhythmic, uses big muscle groups, and has an intensity level that is fairly light to somewhat hard.

Heartbeat Savings

The following information shows how much more efficiently your heart can work after just a few weeks of exercising. The first number refers to your heartbeats before you begin exercising, the second number is after 16 weeks of an exercise program.

Ambient HR
B: 75 beats per minute
A: 65 beats per minute

Beats per hour
B: 4500
A: 3900

Beats per day
B: 108,000
A: 93,600

Beats per month
B: 3,240,000
A: 2,808,000

Beats per year
B: 39,420,000
A: 34,164,000

The difference is +5,256,000 *more* beats per year without sustaining an aerobic exercise program. After 16 weeks, this person saved 5,256,000 heartbeats.

famous "use it or lose it" phenomenon is easily demonstrated in the body's muscular system.

Strength training exercises isolate muscles and muscle groups and build muscular strength and endurance. This keeps you functional and able to perform such simple tasks as carrying groceries, suitcases, taking out the trash, moving light boxes of papers, moving small pieces of furniture, picking up children or pets, or assisting older adults.

Improvements in muscular strength cause the body to burn more calories, even at rest. Muscle is what we call metabolically active tissue (yes, it is very busy). That means it uses many more calories (than nonmetabolically active tissue) just to keep it intact. Having more caloric-expending tissue is something most of us dream for and desire.

Another benefit of strength training exercise is that muscular movements act as a type of massage to the bony structures. When muscles are moved and used, bones (the supporting cast) are stimulated and become stronger and more dense. Strength training exercises include weight training, calisthenics, and other activity-specific exercises. Chapter 7 will address how to properly include strength training in your exercise program as well as offer specific exercises you can perform.

Flexibility

Flexibility is the ability to move a joint throughout its range of motion. A joint is the place where two or more bones meet (they are connected by ligaments/tendons). Joints allow movement, much like a door hinge, which allows the door to move. Flexibility is necessary for efficient bodily movement. Being flexible may also decrease the chances of sustaining muscular injury, soreness, and pain. Although flexibility declines somewhat after adulthood is reached, we do not know how much is due to aging and how much is due to lack of use (there it is again, "use it or lose it"). Regardless, without flexibility, movement can be limiting, painful, and disabling. Flexibility is essential to your health and a valuable component of your exercise program.

Flexibility exercises are those that *gently* stretch muscles and ligamentous tissues and keep them pliable and mobile. Flexibility exer-

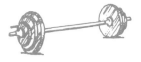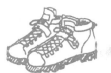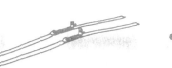

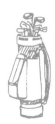

Oxygen Utilization Analogy

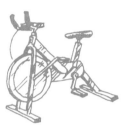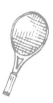

To better understand the concept of oxygen utilization, consider this analogy. You and a friend decide that you are both committed to eating better. You make an identical grocery list, go to the store, and bring home the groceries. Each of you has now stocked your individual kitchens with the identical healthy ingredients that were on the list.

Starting that day and throughout the week you prepare and eat regular and balanced meals all from that list. By the end of the week you feel very good. Your friend also started with a well-stocked kitchen, but she did not prepare meals or eat any of the groceries. In fact, your friend's kitchen is still well stocked from the items bought. By the end of the week, your friend feels no different than at the beginning. You and your friend both had the experience of taking in groceries, but only you actually used

(utilized) them. Just having groceries in the house does not mean that you are eating better than before. You have to consume and "utilize" the groceries in order for your nutrition to improve.

This is similar to what happens with oxygen utilization. A human body will take in oxygen at rest (bringing home the groceries), but during exercise, the body begins to utilize oxygen (consuming the groceries) with greater intensity and purpose. In the beginning it may be slow in knowing what to do with the extra supply and where to put it. But as the body exercises more frequently, it accommodates and adapts to this "oxygen feed." The body prefers having the oxygenating experience, and the more it gets, the more it can do. (This is the opposite of use it or lose it; rather, it is "use it and expand it!")

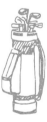

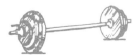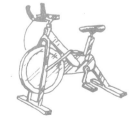

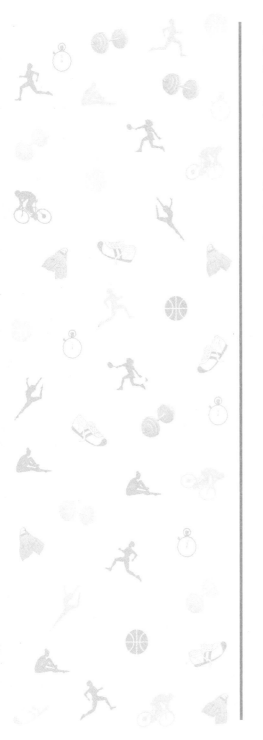

cises include stretching, ballet, yoga, and tai chi. Chapter 8 will address how to properly include flexibility in your fitness program as well as offer specific exercises you can perform.

Rest and Recovery

Rest and recovery are the last but not the least of the essential components of a regular exercise program. Too much of even a "good" thing, even exercise, is not good. Your body needs time to rest and recover. Chapter 13 will help you determine what rest is and how much of it you need to recover from exercise so that you can become stronger and stay fit and healthy. It will also discuss when and/or if you should exercise when you are sick.

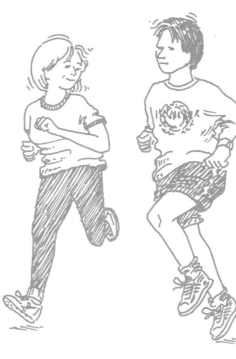

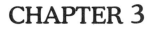

CHAPTER 3

Getting Started, Getting Organized

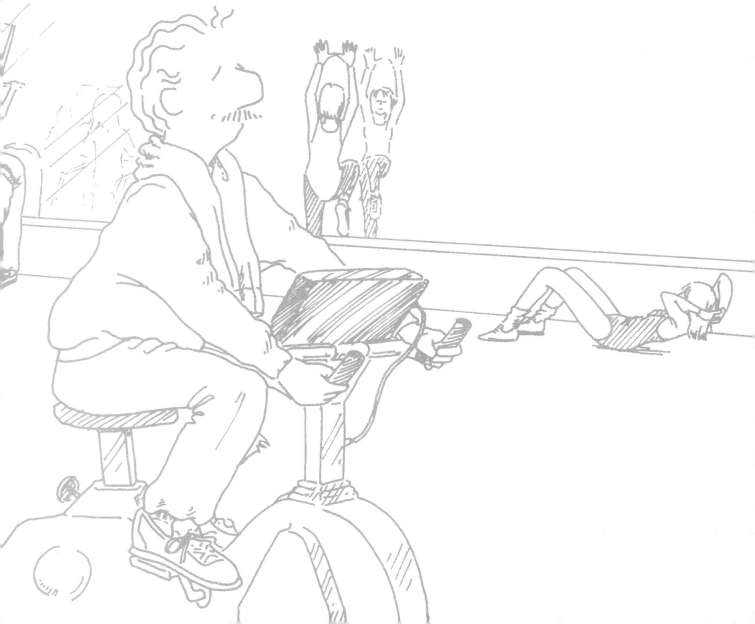

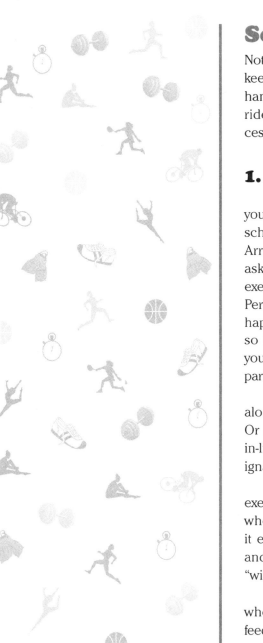

Set Yourself Up for Success

Not knowing where to start is often the most significant roadblock that keeps people from exercising. However, with the right road map in hand, you can get started, know where you are going, and enjoy the ride to your success. The following six steps will set you up for success. They are the road to your destination, Fitness-ville.

1. Plan Ahead

Pull out your daily planner/calendar and look at the week ahead of you. Schedule your exercise session into your regular, daily, busy schedule. Find the desirable time of day/evening and make it regular. Arrange for family cooperation if necessary. Have a family meeting and ask for your family's support. Share with them how important your exercise time is to you and how they can specifically support you. Perhaps a spouse can trade early morning responsibilities with you; perhaps your children can learn how to make their own breakfast/lunch so that you can exercise before taking them to school. When you use your daily planner with an opportunistic eye, you will create a small part of that busy day for your exercise time.

Think about ways to include family members if they can't be left alone. Buy a baby jogger or stroller and take the youngster with you. Or allow an older child to ride a bike with you while you walk, run, or in-line skate. A child's designated time for homework can be your designated time for body work.

A frequently asked question is, When is the best time of day to exercise—morning, afternoon, or evening? The best answer is, The time when you will do it. Some people have a regular schedule that makes it easy for them to plan their exercise time at a set/designated time and day. For others, no two days are alike, and they have to create the "window of opportunity" for exercise time.

The benefits of regular exercise (see Chapter 2) occur regardless of when you find the time to exercise. The training effects of your "oxygen feed," alias aerobic exercise session, happen to your body whenever you exercise. Two added benefits to exercising in the morning are that you will have the rest of the day to enjoy the energizing effect of your exercise session, and you will not be concerned about how to fit your exercise session into your busy day. Because exercise has an energizing effect, you might wish to avoid doing so close to bedtime. But unless you are a diabetic (see Chapter 12), it is fine to exercise anytime including late in the evening.

2. Make It Important/Make an Appointment

We manage to make time every day for the appointments we can't miss. We get to work on time, pick kids up from school, go to dentist appointments, and set aside time to read the newspaper or talk on the telephone. We make and have time for these activities because they are important to us. When you have something important in your life, you are apt to cherish it and treat it with respect. Schedule your exercise time as you would these other important appointments; keep your appointment, be punctual, and give yourself a start and a finish time. A nice side effect to being regular about your exercise time is that those around you (your spouse, partner, boss, children, coworkers, employees) will come to learn that exercise time is your "sacred time" and to be respected and not infringed upon unless absolutely necessary.

3. Make Exercise Fun and Convenient

Find activities you like to do or those that work for you. It may be something old or something new. Perhaps it is an activity that you previously enjoyed (in high school) or one you are curious about.

Create either regular or occasional workout partners by inviting a friend, neighbor, or work friend to join you. Canine companions are always happy to be included on walks or jogs. Make sure you choose someone whose company you enjoy so that you will look forward to sharing that time.

Invest in the "feel good" of exercise. What elements of exercise can make you feel good about yourself? Buy and wear exercise clothing that makes you happy. If you have been saving your worn-out T-shirts, shorts, and pants for exercise, think again. To be successful, you need to reinforce feeling good about who you are and what you are doing. When you want to make a good impression upon others, you do not put on your worst clothing. Why do anything less for yourself? In fact, wearing clothes that make you happy, give you an energetic start.

Exercise Time = Health Appointment

A breast cancer survivor shared that she never considered missing her chemotherapy appointments. Recognizing that exercise is vital to her health, she now applies the same commitment and vitality to scheduling and completing her exercise sessions. We can all learn from her appreciation!

Wearing comfortable clothing, such as fabrics that whisk away moisture and do not chafe your skin, can make the difference between you continuing to exercise or not. (See Chapter 6 for more in-depth discussion of clothing and fabric selection.)

The same "feel good" standard is true for your exercise equipment. If it feels good, you will be more apt to use it, and if it does not feel good, you will not. If you like, for example, the idea of riding an exercise bike but your bike wobbles from side to side, makes a lot of noise, and does not have a smooth pedal action, consider buying a new bike. Test ride a bike before you buy it. The right equipment (see Chapter 6) will make the difference between enjoying your exercise or dreading it, and eventually not doing it.

4. Start Incrementally/Increase Gradually

When the subject is exercise, more is *not* always better. You may not remember this, but before you learned to walk, you had to crawl. Well, the same is true for your fitness. If you want to be successful with your fitness program and want to feel good both during and after exercise, you will need to start in small increments of time and effort and then increase gradually. This is where many people set themselves up to fail. They expect their body to perform activity at levels that are neither realistic nor recommended. Afterward they feel bad and then wrongly insist that it's the exercise itself that makes them feel worse.

It is particularly important to start slowly if you have not exercised recently. When you first begin exercising, it is as if your body has been in a coma. Would you shake it and say, "Hey, come on, get going, faster, harder, more, more . . . "?

When you begin an exercise program, you should be gentle with your body. If you start slowly, your body will respond favorably, and you will reinforce the positive effects of your new exercise program. To set yourself up for success, start with small increments of time at low intensity levels until your body has had time to adjust to the new activity. Step 5 tells you how to start exercising and then how to graduate to higher levels.
Understanding and applying some basic principles of exercise will help you achieve your goals.

5. Apply the Principles of Exercise (Specificity of Training, Overload, and F-I-T-T)

The Principles of Exercise are the foundation for a solid exercise program. They help you determine the specifics of your exercise program such as frequency, intensity, time, and type. They are simple to understand, and once you do, you are equipped to apply them to any fitness activity you decide to explore. (They are explained in detail in Chapter 4.)

6. Document Your Exercise

Fitness expert, author, endurance athlete, and exercise physiologist Sally Edwards reminds us in her book *Smart Heart* that "you can only manage what you can measure and monitor." This is certainly true for exercise and health. If you want to take an active role in your fitness, keep track of what you do, how much you do, and any other interesting pieces of information that relate to your health (see calendar diagram). You can be as descriptive or nondescriptive as you like. You do not have to be obsessive about every detail but should include enough to tell a short story about your exercise and health.

Benefits of Documenting Exercise

Creates Health/Wellness Record Documenting your exercise helps you create a personal wellness record, which is useful in adjusting your F-I-T-T levels as well as pinpointing health patterns, dates, and so forth. When you feel great, it is important to pay attention to that (not to take it for granted) and to be aware of what you are doing that makes you feel that way. Are you feeling better since you have been exercising for 30 minutes four times a week, rather than for 20 minutes two times a week? Are you feeling great because you are getting 8 hours versus 7 hours of sleep? These simple notations can help you pay attention to the details that make you feel good. It will also help you evaluate when it is time to Overload or change the F-I-T-T components of your program (see Chapter 4).

The other end of the spectrum is when you feel bad. Maybe you notice that when you exercise very intensely 6 days a week, you are prone to having a sore throat. That could be a signal to adjust your

Symptoms of PMS

Premenstrual syndrome can occur 1–7 days before the onset of the menstruation period. Some of the symptoms reported by sufferers of PMS premenstrual syndrome include: moodiness, cantankerous attitude, feelings of depression, cravings for sweet, salty and high fat foods, water retention (temporary weight gain) and swelling, etc.

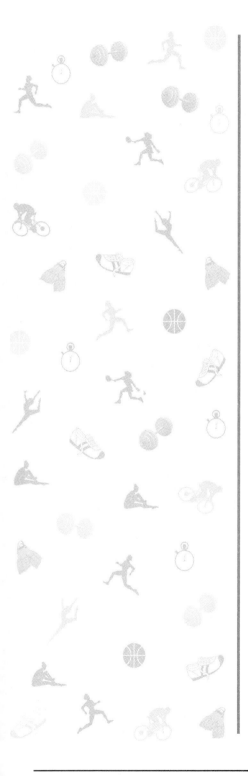

F-I-T-T. Creating your own documentation offers you an opportunity to troubleshoot your own symptoms and, it is hoped, put in a correction before they manifest into a full-blown case of something you do not want. Documenting your exercise (and rest days) and other "how you are feeling" factors on a daily basis will help you to create a personal wellness history that can be invaluable.

One concise effective method is to create symbols that represent how you feel or what you are interested in keeping track of. Let's take your energy as an example. You can use the "up" ↑ arrow to designate days when you feel energetic or the "down" ↓ arrow to designate days when you have low energy or feel lethargic. (See calendar diagram for other symbols.) What's the purpose in recording these? As we discussed earlier, fitness starts in your mind. In the few moments that it takes for you to record this (or any other area that is important to you) you become more aware of it. Bringing your attention to the issue can be just the reminder you need. And when you do so consistently (daily works the best) you begin to see patterns that either you like and want to maintain or those you want to change. By recording these few items you set up your own feedback system that can help you direct your course.

Builds Confidence and Momentum Writing down what you did validates it and you. "Seeing is believing" reminds you of your past success, which paves the way for future successes. Writing in your 20 minutes of step aerobics or one-half mile swim reminds you that "you did it." Be proud! Momentum is very important to your exercise commitment and can fuel the desire to continue.

Keeps You Honest with Yourself It is easy to lose perspective about what you have or have not done. Perhaps you have been exercising three times a week for the past 6 weeks and recently decided to exercise four times a week. But one week you exercised only twice. By having the calendar documentation, you have an objective perspective. You can see that during the other weeks you met your goal. A healthy perspective can keep you from "beating yourself up" or making yourself feel guilty about what you did not do. You can focus upon what you did do. If your goal was to exercise three times a week and you did not exercise more than three times for the entire past 3 weeks, that too will

Sample Wellness Calendar

	SUN	MON	TUES	WED	THURS	FRI	SAT
Aerobic activity	Walk outside	Rest day	Jog treadmill	Stationary bicycle	Rest day	Stairclimber	Bike outside
Time	45:00		30:00	40:00		30:00	60:00
Hours of sleep	sleep 7	sleep 8	sleep 7	sleep 6	sleep 6	sleep 7	sleep 8
Overall energy	↑	↑	→	↓	↓	↓	↑

How to set up your wellness calendar and examples of symbols and entries:

1. Record the aerobic exercise activity you performed or indicate if it was a rest day.
2. Record the amount of time you spent doing it.
3. Record any other details that interest you or patterns you suspect are affecting you.

4. At the end of the month total how many days you exercised and total exercise minutes and the other areas you recorded. Did you have more ↑ days than ↓ days? If not, why not? What can you do about it? Set realistic yet healthy goals for the next month and compare how you did. Keep a monthly comparison.

Example above: Do you get less sleep near the middle of the week and therefore have more ↓s on those days? What can you do about it? Maybe that is a good time to take your rest days.

	SUN	MON	TUES	WED	THURS	FRI	SAT
Aerobic activity							
Time							
Hours of sleep							
Overall energy							

give you an objective message that you are losing fitness and need to put in a correction soon.

Keeps You Well Are you overtraining or not training enough? If you find that you are tired frequently and not sleeping well, you could be exercising too much. Check your calendar. Did you take your rest days, or did you exercise too many days consecutively? Or have you gone an entire week or two without any exercise?

Keeps You Motivated Determine the date you began your commitment to exercise and mark it as an anniversary of which you are proud. Use that date to celebrate your good health. Reward yourself with a new workout outfit, piece of equipment, experience, or some other "reinvestment" in your fitness commitment.

Helps You Improve and Stay Balanced Are you running farther than you used to in the same amount of time, with less effort? (That means you are getting more fit.) Do you vary your activity each week? Does your program lean too heavy on weight training? Is there enough aerobic activity? Writing it down provides a total fitness story.

Helps You Set Goals At the end of each month, tally up how many days you exercised and how many minutes you exercised aerobically. Did you come close to your goal? If so, reward yourself with appreciation and confidence. If not, examine what interfered and plan how you can get closer to your goal the next month.

The six steps to success will direct and motivate you toward an appropriate exercise program. When you feel you need a dose of "direction," refer back to these steps for guidance.

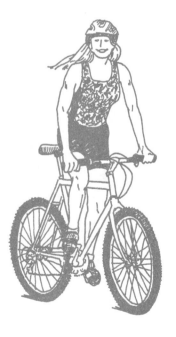

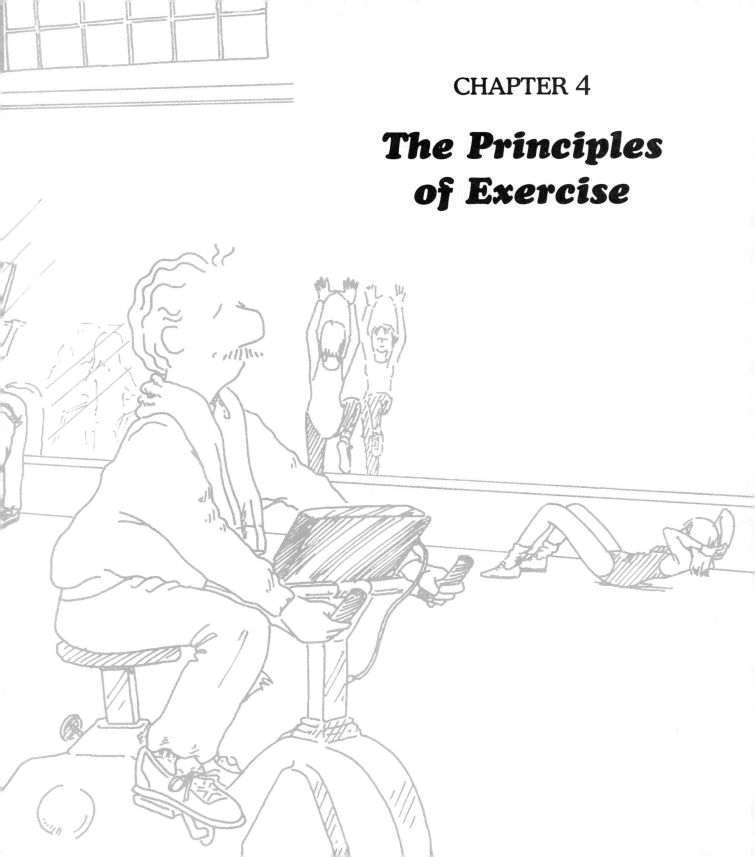

CHAPTER 4

The Principles of Exercise

The Principles of Exercise are the foundation for and what most people lack in an exercise program. They help you determine the what, the how much, the how intensely, and the how often of your exercise program. Apply them to your preferred fitness activities and you will feel and see your fitness goals realized.

The **Specificity of Training Principle** says that the body responds specifically to the type of exercise and muscle groups involved. This means that if you want improvements in flexibility, you need to perform specific flexibility exercises. For cardiorespiratory improvements, you need to perform aerobic exercise activities; to improve muscular strength and endurance, you need to perform resistance exercises. Therefore, it is important that you select appropriate **modes** or types of exercise, those that are capable of producing the results you desire.

The **Overload Principle** says that in order to improve physical fitness, the body must be taxed using loads that are greater than those to which the body is accustomed. If the word *overload* brings to mind words like *overwhelming* and *bad for you*, you can relax. This overload is good overload. Remember, our purpose is to get you fit, not kill you.

If you have recently led a sedentary lifestyle, it will not take much to overload your body and begin developing an improved level of fitness. If you have been exercising for a while and have been maintaining fitness but not improving, it may be due to a lack of overload in your activity. So, how do you overload yourself? The answer lies in the last important set of principles known as the F-I-T-T Principles.

The F-I-T-T Principles tell you specifically how to overload your body and improve your fitness. They provide the detailed plan for overloading (pushing you a bit beyond what you are accustomed to) and ensure that you are getting the results you desire from your exercise program. Once you determine your starting plan, implement it; then re-evaluate it regularly to coincide with your current circumstances.

Throughout this text you will see references to the F-I-T-T principles also as F-I-T because the "T" type or mode of activity has already been established.

As you can see from the experience of the two women walkers on page 31 in the "true story," the F-I-T-T principles work best in conjunction with each other. The women benefited from their walking program. They were maintaining a degree of fitness because they were sufficiently overloaded in three of the four F-I-T principles. However, to improve their fitness and maximize their results, they need to engage all four of the principles. The connected designation, "F-I-T-T," is a reminder to you that they are a unit and belong together. For maintaining fitness levels, you can squeak by for a while with two or three of the four but for improvements in your fitness, you must implement the four *together*.

You can apply overload and the F-I-T-T principles to each component of physical fitness—cardiovascular, muscular strength and endurance, flexibility, and rest. For now we will demonstrate how to apply the overload and F-I-T-T principles to cardiorespiratory fitness and aerobic exercise.

Frequency

Frequency refers to how often you exercise. As a general rule, ACSM recommends three to five exercise sessions per week. If you are just beginning an exercise program, you may want to start at the lower end—three sessions. If you have a level of fitness already, then five will be appropriate, depending upon your goals. Some form of daily activity is good for most everyone. If you are or have been ill (see Chapter 13), you will want to modify your exercise frequency. But for purposeful, intense aerobic fitness, the following is suggested:

Maintenance—three to four times per week
Optimum—five times per week
Maximum—six times per week
Rest days are important. Include them in your program.

Intensity

Intensity refers to how hard you exercise or your level of effort. Typically, intensity is experienced as speed, time, or resistance. The degree of intensity is critical to an exercise program because without it improvements in conditioning will be very limited. If you have become frustrated because after weeks of diligently following an exercise program you didn't get the results you expected, it very well could be attributed to the intensity level of exercise.

ACSM recommends aerobic exercise intensity to be at levels that are 60 to 90 percent of your maximum heart rate or 50 to 85 percent

F-I-T-T Goal

ACSM recommends some form of daily activity and exercise sessions 3 to 5 days a week for 20 to 60 minutes. Ideally, exercise sessions should burn 300 calories per session.

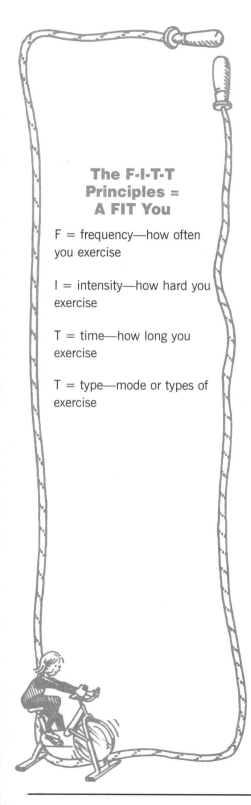

**The F-I-T-T
Principles =
A FIT You**

F = frequency—how often
you exercise

I = intensity—how hard you
exercise

T = time—how long you
exercise

T = type—mode or types of
exercise

of VO$_2$max. That may not mean anything to you right now, but it will momentarily. If your tendency is to rush past this section because it looks complicated, please don't. This is important "good stuff," and once you get it, you've got it for life. So, hang in there and take a good slow, deep breath (more oxygen to your brain!).

Heart Rate and Oxygen Utilization

From studies including thousands of human responses to exercise testing, it was shown that a linear relationship exists between oxygen utilization and heart rate response. This means that as oxygen utilization increases so does heart rate (although not equally). Put another way, exercising heart rates "mirror" or reflect the activity of oxygen utilization. This relationship is significant, opportune, and convenient. It means that we can measure and monitor the intensity level of aerobic exercise using heart rate information rather than through the impractical and costly method of measuring oxygen utilization. Heart rate, which is measured in beats per minute (bpm), is easier and more convenient to measure and monitor than oxygen utilization and can act as a speedometer for your heart during aerobic exercise. However, it is important to remember that oxygen utilization, not heart rate intensity is the actual measure or purpose of aerobic activity. Heart rate is simply an indicator for it.

Heart Rate Monitoring

Imagine if you were driving a car along the highway without a speedometer and you had to guess how fast you were traveling. Chances are you would not be exact and bets are you wouldn't want to try it if there was a highway patrol right behind you. Exercising without monitoring your heart rate is the exercise equivalent of driving without a speedometer. A speedometer helps you know how fast you are traveling so you can stay within the safe speed limits. Monitoring your heart rate tells you how hard you are exercising (in beats per minute) in measurable terms, so you don't have to guess. It ensures that you aren't wasting your time by exercising at levels that are too low and gives you confidence to push yourself more than you might without one. Heart rate information makes you more productive and efficient during your exercise time.

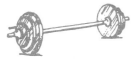 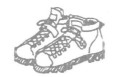 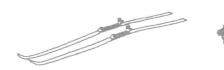

F-I-T-T in Action

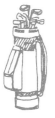

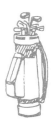

True Story: Two women walk in their neighborhood early each morning and cover a 3-mile course in an hour. They have done this diligently for an entire year, 5 days a week. They report that walking is very easy to do. In the first few months, they noticed improvements in their fitness. But they complain that since that time, they have not gotten fitter. Why is this the case and what can they do to fix it?

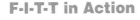

Answer: The women are not getting fitter because they never adjusted the overload and F-I-T-T of their workout. The frequency of 5 days a week is excellent; the time of an hour is also excellent. However, the intensity level (in this case their speed) at which they walk is too low and is not pushing their heart, lungs, and vascular system beyond what they are accustomed to. Also their type or mode of exercise, walking, is effective for cardiovascular fitness and muscular strength and endurance of the hips and legs but does nothing for the muscular strength, endurance and flexibility of their upper body.

Solution: They need to (1) overload the intensity component of their exercise by walking faster and (2) to include some strength training exercises for their upper body. Keep the frequency (5 days a week) and time (one hour) elements as they are. Start walking faster using the interval concept (short bouts of higher intensity interspersed with short bouts of lower intensity later in this chapter) and 3 times a week add some strength training exercises for their upper body.

  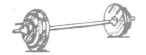

Counting Your Heart Rate

You can monitor your heart rate during exercise manually by feeling and counting your pulses or with the help of a heart rate monitor. Counting your pulses with your fingers during exercise may be the cheapest way to monitor heart rate, but it is also the most outdated, least accurate, and unreliable. It is very difficult to accurately feel and count heartbeats during exercise movement. And if you stop the activity in order to count the heart rate, it drops quickly such that you will get an inaccurate number. (See sidebar page 34).

It is also interesting and fun to see your heart rate automatically displayed. Outside of a hospital or laboratory setting can you think of another measuring device you use during exercise that tells you what is happening inside your body? Seeing your heart rate continuously displayed during exercise is motivational and gives you an opportunity to become more familiar with your body. It helps take the fear out of exercise for many who have been afraid of overexerting themselves, it motivates those who are interested in general fitness, and it helps highly motivated persons and conditioned athletes attain more precise improvements in their conditioning. The bottom line is that using a heart rate monitor properly makes you a safer, more productive, efficient exerciser who is better able to reach your fitness goals.

The Heart Rate Monitor

Heart rate technology has become as common to aerobic exercise as a pair of exercise shoes and is highly recommended for anyone involved in aerobic fitness. The heart rate monitor is a clever device that accurately tells you how many times your heart is beating per minute. For aerobic exercise it is the most practical tool that ensures you are exercising at the proper level of intensity. (It can also be used as a stress-biofeedback tool, see p. 239.) Once you establish your desired intensity level of exercise the heart rate monitor gives you the feedback about whether you are within your desired heart rate range/zone or not. It takes the guesswork out of how hard you are exercising.

For example, if you have determined that your goal is to walk with a heart rate intensity of 125 beats per minute (bpm) and your heart rate monitor shows that you are walking at 115 bpm, it means that you need to pick up the pace (intensity). Likewise, if you are walking and see that your heart rate is at 133 beats per minute, it means that you need to slow down. The benefit/concept of gauging intensity by heart rate rather than by speed or distance is that it takes into account your unique physiology on a daily basis. It can indicate when you are getting more fit, when you may be tired, or even when your immune system may be working against a cold or infection. For a list of heart rate monitoring devices, see the Appendix.

Heart Rate Lingo

Once you become familiar with a little heart rate lingo, you can best understand, in a meaningful way, the effects of aerobic exercise and why it is so important to your health. Here are some terms you should be familiar with:

- **Ambient Heart Rate**—the number of beats per minute (bpm) your heart contracts when you are awake but in a sedentary and stationary position
- **Maximum Heart Rate**—the highest number of contractions of the heart muscle in 1 minute
- **Resting Heart Rate**—the number of beats per minute (bpm) your heart contracts in a minute when you first wake up before you arise
- **Recovery Heart Rate**—the number of beats per minute (bpm) your heart rate drops immediately after exercise, usually after 1 or 2 minutes

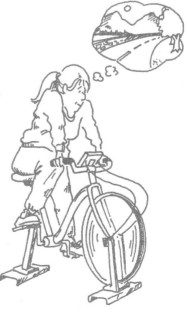

Most people use the term *resting heart rate* when they really mean their *ambient heart rate*. The difference between the two is that *resting heart rate* is the heart rate when you first awaken, before you arise, following a period when your heart truly has been resting. The ambient is the heart rate that could be taken after you have been up and about, such as during the middle of your day, but when you temporarily become still. The significance of these two heart rates is that they are the rates at which your heart works during the largest portion of your heartbeating day. So it makes sense that you want them to function with the greatest of ease and efficiency as possible.

Changes in your resting heart rate, like the exercising recovery heart rate, will tell you about your fitness progress, as well as many other aspects of your health (whether you are overtrained, stressed,

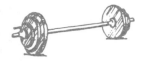
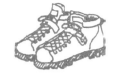
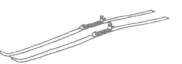

Manual Measurement of Your Pulses

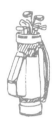

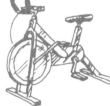

Two of the most common sites for manually measuring pulse rate are at the carotid (neck) artery and the radial (wrist) artery. The carotid pulse is located just below the angle of the jaw, high up on either side of the neck, bounded by the Adam's apple. The carotid arterial pulse can be felt by gently compressing the first two fingers (not the thumb) lightly on this area. Exerting too much pressure on this pulse can cause a slowing of the heart rate so gentle pressure is strongly advised. You should feel your pulse beating against your fingers.

The radial pulse can be found on the thumb side of the forearm just slightly above where the wrist naturally flexes/bends. As with the carotid pulse, use the first two fingers, not the thumb, to feel the pulse.

Manually counting an exercise pulse is difficult and easily subject to error*. For making the best estimate, try this:

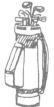

1. Locate the pulse with first two fingers, excluding the thumb.

2. A) When the heart rate is beating slowly, a longer count such as for 30 or 60 seconds is suggested for a more accurate count. For example, during your warm-up, the pulse should be relatively slow as compared to when you are engaged in the thick of your exercise session. Count the beats for either 15 seconds and multiply by 4 to estimate the number of beats per minute. Or, count the beats for 30 seconds and multiply by 2 to estimate the number of beats per minute.

Example: If pulse rate for 15 seconds is 20 beats. Multiply 20 beats by 4 to estimate the 1 minute pulse. 20 x 4 = 80 beats per minute.

Or, if pulse count is 40 beats in 30 seconds, then 40 x 2 = 80 beats in 60 seconds (bpm).

B) When the heart rate is beating quickly, it becomes more difficult to count accurately for a longer period of time, such as for 30 seconds or more. If the pulse rate is fast, count for a shorter period of time, such as for 6 or 10 seconds, and make the 1 minute mathematical estimate. Count the beats for either 10 seconds and multiply by 6 to estimate the number of beats per minute. Or, count the beats for 6 seconds and multiply by 10 (simply add a zero to the end of the number) to estimate the number of beats per minute.

3. Compare this number in beats per minute (bpm) to your desired training zone.

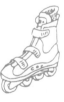

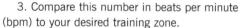

*Be aware that often the adaptation or change of position required to accommodate taking a manual pulse can increase or decrease the pulse from what it is during the true exercise position. For example on a stairclimber machine, most people hold onto the handrails to balance. However, to take a manual carotid pulse one hand must be removed from the handrail, which creates a slightly more difficult workload. Even this apparently minor change in the position of one hand can cause the heart rate to elevate higher than it was during the normal position of the activity.

Conversely, you may be walking on a treadmill and because of the motion you cannot manually feel the pulse. So you stop momentarily in order to count the pulse. The pulse rate has already dropped in that short time and will give you an inaccurate appraisal of your exercise intensity.

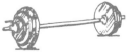
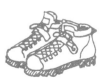
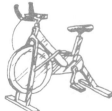

fighting a cold/flu, and so on—see Chapter 13). As you become more fit, your ambient, resting, and recovery heart rates will decrease. These are healthy signs.

Recovery heart rate is the number of beats per minute (bpm) your heart rate drops immediately after exercise, usually after 1 or 2 minutes. It is one of the best ways you can measure changes in fitness and the rate you may choose to keep track of in your fitness calendar. The significance of your recovery heart rate is that it tells how quickly your heart can respond to exercise stress. Think of a fit, conditioned heart as being a high-performance vehicle, one that can accelerate quickly and easily, yet can also return to idling quickly and easily.

The fit and conditioned heart, like the high-performance vehicle, is very responsive and can recover quickly and easily from bouts of accelerated heart rates such as during exercise. The unfit or deconditioned heart cannot control its pace (beating) as well and needs more time for it to recover. Think of the unfit heart as an eighteen-wheeler truck that is less responsive and needs more time and distance to return to idling (recover).

During the initial conditioning and improvement stages of your fitness program, you are likely to see a reduction in your recovery heart rate. This is a good sign; it means your heart is becoming stronger and more responsive.

Using Heart Rate to Gauge Exercise Intensity

Now that you know the significance of measuring your heart rate and how to measure it, you may be asking this question: How do I know what level I should be exercising at and how do I determine my correct heart rate for aerobic exercise? This is where the term *maximum heart rate* comes into the picture.

Aerobic fitness is usually expressed as *a percentage of your maximal aerobic capacity (VO_2max)*. So, first it is important to determine your maximal oxygen uptake or *maximum heart rate*. (Remember, heart rate mirrors oxygen uptake.) There are many ways to do so. The most precise method for determining your aerobic fitness, maximum oxygen and heart rate levels, is to have a maximal oxygen uptake/maximum heart rate test conducted at an exercise physiology laboratory administered by certified personnel (found at institutes of higher learning, medical facilities, or an athletic club) with a physician present.

The Birth and History of the Wireless Heart Rate Monitor

Heart rate monitors have revolutionized aerobic fitness around the world. Chinese physicians introduced the first heart rate monitoring 6,000 years ago. They manually monitored pulse rate to diagnose disease. Paul Yuen and his family, who today still own Dayton Industries, a Hong Kong company, designed the first electronic device in 1978. Dayton continues to manufacture some of the finest heart rate monitors in the world. The very first monitors were hard wired, with the monitor mounted directly on the chest strap. The first wireless wrist monitors were developed in 1982 by Dr. Seppo Saynajakangas, an electrical engineering professor at Oulu University in Finland. He later left the university and became the owner of Polar Electro Oy, the largest manufacturer of wireless, portable heart rate monitors in the world.

The next best determinant is to have a sub-maximum heart rate test, which can be administered by a certified fitness professional. Whereas the maximum test will try to have you reach your maximum heart rate, a sub-maximum test will push you to reach only 85 percent of your age predicted maximum heart rate. There are also many self-administered sub-max tests you can use, which can be found in *Sally Edwards' Heart Zone Training* book.

The next best and least expensive way to estimate maximum heart rate (Max HR) is to use documented formulas. These formulas have been derived from research on thousands of human responses to exercise testing. They provide a fairly close determination of your max heart rate, and you can calculate them yourself.

The formula "220 minus your age" is useful for those beginning an aerobic exercise program. Another formula used for those who are in fit/athletic condition is "205 minus ½ your age." Even though these formulas are not as precise as being individually tested, they are safe and good second bests for estimating maximum heart rate. Once you have determined your max heart rate, you can establish your training "zones" or percentages of your maximum heart rate.

Facts about VO$_2$max

VO$_2$max stands for maximum oxygen uptake. It is the gold standard for cardiovascular fitness testing and represents the greatest volume of oxygen that can be processed by the heart, lungs, and muscles per minute while engaged in strenuous exercise. In VO$_2$ tests, the subject's expired gases are captured and measured. Oxygen utilization is commonly measured in milliliters of oxygen per kilogram of body weight per minute (ml/kg/min). In the case of oxygen uptake, more is better; the more oxygen that can be processed by the body, the greater the person's aerobic capacity. If you have had or plan to be tested for your oxygen uptake, here are some general criteria to help you understand your results.

Fitness levels defined by VO$_2$ (oxygen uptake):

- A person with a measured VO$_2$max of less than or equal to 30 ml/kg/min would have a low level of fitness.
- A person with a measured VO$_2$max of 30 to 50 ml/kg/min would have a moderate level of fitness.

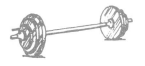
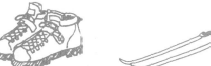
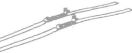

How to Get Started Using a Heart Rate Monitor

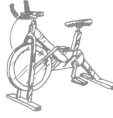

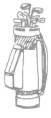

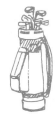

1. The sensor strap is going to fit directly on your skin upon your torso. But first you must moisten the underside of the battery/sensor strap where the sensors are positioned with either water or your saliva. The moisture helps conduct the electrical activity to the monitor.

2. Attach one end of the elastic strap to the battery/sensor strap. Next, with one hand hold the battery/sensor strap against the front of your torso just below the breast area (yes, men have a breast area and it is the same area as women's). With the other hand reach behind and around your body and grab the other end of the elastic strap. Pull it around your torso and attach it to the other end of the battery/sensor strap. It should now be secured around your torso.

3. Adjust the circumference of the elastic strap so that it is snug but not uncomfortable. If you can slide your finger easily between the battery/sensor strap and your skin or if the entire belt piece slides up and down upon your torso, it is too loose; tighten it a bit. However, it should not make a deep imprint-tattoo on your skin.

4. Hold up the wrist monitor approximately 6–10 inches directly in front of the position of one of the sensors (you moistened the back side of them in step 1) on the battery/sensor strap. This engages the communication between the sensors and the monitor and in a few moments your heart rate in beats per minute should be shown in the wrist monitor.

5. The monitor will read and display your heart rate in beats per minute as long as it stays within 1–3 feet of the sensors. Should you lose the signal in the middle of an exercise session, simply bring the wrist monitor up in front of the sensors again and it will re-engage. Bicyclists (stationary or regular) can mount the wrist monitor on the handlebars using a bike mount apparatus or by tightening the wrist strap around the bars.

Note: In some cases of electrical interference a heart rate monitor will have a blank display. Check for some of these possible sources of interference. Static electricity on your body/clothes or someone standing close to you, an electrical appliance (TV, stereo) very close to you, within 1–3 feet, or someone very close to you (1–3 feet) also wearing a heart rate monitor.

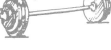

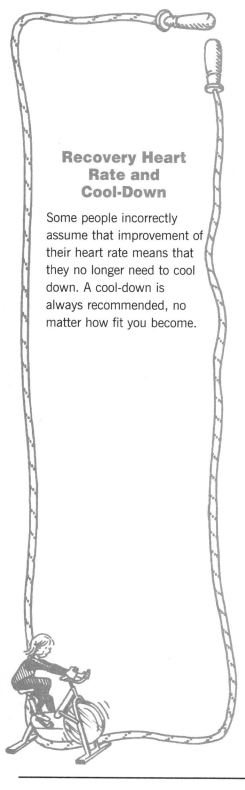

- A person with a measured VO_2max of 50 to 90 ml/kg/min would have a high level of fitness.
- A fun fact to know: The highest recorded VO_2max was a Norwegian cross-country skier who had a measured VO_2max of 94 ml/kg/min.

Training Levels and Zones

ACSM recommends that you exercise at aerobic intensity levels of 60 to 90 percent of maximum heart rate or 50 to 85 percent of VO_2max. Although these are very broad ranges, they all deliver results. Your goal is to match up your current level of fitness capabilities with the appropriate intensity levels or zones of exercise. If you are just starting an exercise program, you will begin exercising at the lower levels of heart rate or percent of VO_2max. Once your body has adapted to that level, you can then progress slowly (there's that Overload principle again) and gradually into higher levels if desired. The beauty of training with exercise intensity training zones is that you can use them to plan for and achieve specific training results.

Exercise physiologists know that certain adaptations and responses occur when we exercise at percentages relative to one's maximum heart rate or maximal oxygen uptake. We can use these percentages as general guidelines for determining the intensity level of exercise and for generating specific training goals. Applying the percentages to your estimated maximum heart rate is what creates your training zones. Each "zone" provides varying degrees of aerobic conditioning and metabolic (energy burning) benefits. Training zones act as a road map directing you toward the appropriate intensity level for your aerobic exercise.

For example, exercising at 60 percent of your maximum heart rate may seem to require very light effort, but it will still benefit your cardiovascular system. It also burns a high percentage of fat as fuel. However, it requires more time to burn the caloric equivalent of exercising at a higher intensity level. Exercising at an aerobic level of 85 percent of your maximum heart rate will require more effort and will condition your cardiovascular system more quickly than at the 60 percent level. It will also burn a higher percentage of glucose than fat, but for the same amount of time burns a higher total number of calories. It is useful to exercise for varying amounts of time in each of the zones.

Create Your Own Zone Chart

You can make your own training zone chart. If you already know your maximum heart rate or estimated heart rate, use that number. But for now, let's use the formula "220 minus your age" to estimate maximum heart rate.

1. What is your age? _____
2. Subtract your age from 220: "220 minus your age" = _____
   Example: If you are 40 years old, then the answer to #2 above is 180.
   Age 40 – Estimated Maximum Heart Rate = 180 bpm.
3. Use the answer of #2 above (i.e., 180) as your estimated maximum heart rate.
4. Multiply each percent of the training zone times (x) your estimated maximum heart rate to create your training zones. In this example we are using the 180 bpm for Max HR.

Example: Zone 1 is when you exercise with your heart rate at 50 to 60 percent of your estimated Max HR; so you want to multiply your Max HR by .50 and .60 respectively. These two heart rates in beats per minute (bpm) comprise the Zone 1 training level. It means when you exercise with your heart rate between 90 and 108, you are in Zone 1, a low intensity training level of aerobic exercise.

50 percent x 180 = 90. 60 percent x 180 = 108.

Fill out the chart using the estimated maximum heart rate (i.e., 180 bpm).

Zone 1—Healthy Heart Zone Easy does it/very low aerobic fitness happens at 50 to 60 percent of your maximum heart rate.

Multiply your maximum heart rate times 50 percent (.50) and 60 percent (.60).

These two numbers make the low and high end, respectively, of Zone 1.

Pros: Activity is easy to sustain. You can easily talk. Intensity is low. Risk of injury is low. Good overall health benefits. Burns high percentage of fat but small number of total calories.

Comment/Advice: Great zone for starting your program and for warming up, but don't stay here exclusively forever. It requires more time and frequency for attaining significant weight loss goals but gets the job done if your nutrition is balanced.

Facts about Maximum Heart Rate (also called Max HR or HRmax)

- HRmax is the highest number of heart beats in one minute (bpm = beats per minute).

- It is the highest number of bpm no matter how intense or prolonged the exercise stress.

- It does *not* necessarily mean you will have a heart attack if you reach it.

- It is used as the reference point for determining aerobic exercise intensity.

- HRmax testing should be performed by or in the presence of a physician.

- It can be estimated by sub-max (near maximum) heart rate testing.

Zone 2–Temperate Zone Building health/low aerobic happens at 60 to 70 percent of your estimated maximum heart rate.

Use the 60 percent figure from above for the low end of Zone 2. Multiply your maximum heart rate times 70 percent (.70) for the high end of Zone 2. These two numbers make the low and high end, respectively, of Zone 2.

Pros: Activity feels sustainable. You can still talk. Intensity is mild. Risk of injury is low. Basic health benefits. Burns high percentage of fat and more calories than Zone 1 but fewer overall calories than at higher levels.

Advice: A good first goal for those getting started. Good for exercising when you are tired, traveling, or just want an easy session. An appropriate warm-up for very fit folks.

Healthy outcomes happen faster here than in Zone 1.

Zone 3—Aerobic Zone Fitness and aerobic efficiency happens at 70 to 80 percent of your maximum heart rate.

Use the 70 percent (.70) figure from above for the low end of Zone 3.

Multiply your maximum heart rate times 80 percent (.80) for the high end of Zone 3.

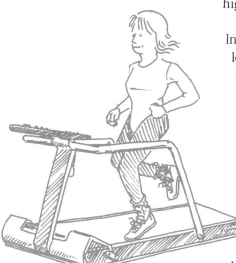

Pros: You are giving more effort but it's doable. You can still talk. Intensity is medium, somewhat hard to hard. A very efficient aerobic level where you burn fat and many total calories for less time than it takes in lower zones.

Advice: Fit happens quickly here, as does fat, glucose, and calorie burning. Make sure you include rest days. Risk of musculoskeletal injury increases slightly. In the higher zones (Zones 3, 4, and 5) each few beats of your heart will feel more intense than at the lower levels. Zone 3 feels really good especially as you get fitter, but don't get complacent. Remember to "overload." You can do so within the span of the zone (the beats per minute starting at the low and going to the high).

Zone 4–Threshold Zone Threshold training levels are what you experience in Zone 4. At 80 to 90 percent of your maximum heart rate, you span from high aerobic toward your anaerobic threshold (where you are no longer aerobic). Use the 80 percent (.80) figure from above for the low end of Zone 4. Multiply your maximum heart rate times 90 percent (.90) for the high end of Zone 4.

Pros: You are exercising at a level that builds fitness and performance. Your perceived exertion feels somewhat hard to hard and, although it is challenging, you could talk if you had to. You are still aerobic but are flirting with being anaerobic. Since fat can only burn in the presence of oxygen, you won't burn as high a percentage of fat as in the lower zones, but you are burning lots of calories and they add up fast.

Advice: Zone 4 pushes you, so it is important to heed the call for rest days and allow for adequate recovery time. At high intensities you increase the possibility of musculoskeletal injuries.

Zone 5—The Performance Zone, also known as "redline," is exercising at 90 to 100 percent of your maximum heart rate. Use the 90 percent (.90) figure from Zone 4 for the low end of Zone 5. Use your maximum heart rate number for the high end of Zone 5.

Pros: These performance-enhancing, anaerobic levels of exercise are fine for interval training (alternating high and low intensities of exercise) once or twice a week, but even at that are not recommended for very long. Zone 5 exercise helps to expand your aerobic zone so that what once seemed challenging becomes easy. It also pushes your anaerobic threshold (later in this chapter) closer toward your maximum heart rate, another high performance training effect.

Advice: Unless a doctor has given you the green light for high intensity exercise, stay away from this "redline." It causes intense, quick increases in blood pressure and heart rate. In Zone 5 you burn very little fat, mostly glucose, and it doesn't last for long. Your risk for musculoskeletal injury is the highest of all the zones. You will need recovery time from this exhausting level of exercise.

5. Plug in the numbers from Step 4 to create your target heart rate training zones chart.

TRAINING ZONE	INTENSITY RANGE (FROM LOW TO HIGH) IN BPM	
	Low	**High**
Zone 1	50 percent = 90 bpm	60 percent = 108 bpm
Zone 2	60 percent = 108 bpm	70 percent = 126 bpm
Zone 3	70 percent = 126 bpm	80 percent = 144 bpm
Zone 4	80 percent = 144 bpm	90 percent = 162 bpm
Zone 5	90 percent = 162 bpm	100 percent = 180 bpm

F-I-T-T in Action

Fitness starts with the going but results come from the doing. A single parent reorganized his busy schedule in order to make time for exercise. He woke 2 hours earlier than usual each morning 4 days a week so that he could exercise at the gym and be home in time to feed and prepare his young children for school. At the gym he rode the stationary bicycle for 10 minutes, worked out on the stairclimber for 10 minutes, and walked on the treadmill for 10 minutes. After 1 month, he noticed big improvements, but after 1 year of this routine, he became frustrated because he was not getting any fitter. Once Super Dad learned of the F-I-T-T principles, he recognized that he was not applying enough intensity to any of the aerobic activities to make continued improvements. Once he increased the intensity level of the aerobic activities he noticed improvements.

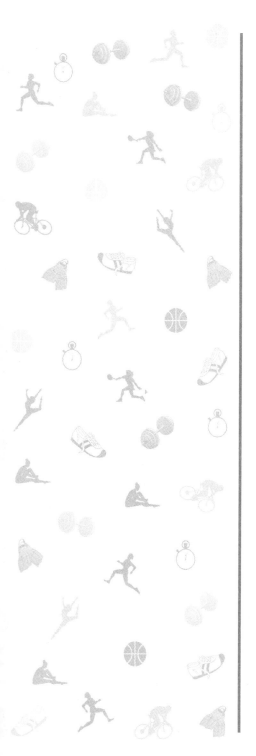

or a simplified version of your training zones looks like this:

Zone 1	90–108
Zone 2	108–126
Zone 3	126–144
Zone 4	144–162
Zone 5	162–180

6. The next step is to decide your fitness goals. Then plan your exercise sessions using these heart rate training zones by spending designated amounts of time in the desired zones. This plan enables you to pace yourself so you don't overexert but also to push yourself so you continue to overload. For general fitness you would spend most of your time in Zones 1–3. You could dabble periodically in Zone 4 if you are interested in the benefits of interval training (later in this chapter). You will also reap the benefits of exercising in the different aerobic training zones.

Here is one way to plan your exercise session. Example: For a 30-minute walk, you can plan your walking time as follows:

5-minute warm-up—heart rate gradually builds; muscles loosen as they get warm.
5 minutes in Zone 1—heart rate between 90 bpm–108 bpm
5 minutes in Zone 2—heart rate between 108 bpm–126 bpm
5 minutes in Zone 3—heart rate between 126 bpm–144 bpm
5 minutes in Zone 2—heart rate between 108 bpm–126 bpm
5 minutes cool-down—heart rate should gradually descend back to Zone 1 at 90 bpm–108 bpm or low Zone 2

If this plan is too rigorous, you can either reduce the number of minutes you spend in the higher HR levels (Zone 3) and increase the time in the lower Zone 2. Or, eliminate the higher HR levels (Zone 3) for now but with the goal of building up to including it in a period of weeks. Forming your own workout intensity is as much art as it is science.

Intensity and RPE Scale

Another less scientific yet helpful way to gauge exercise intensity is to implement the Borg Scale for Rating of Perceived Exertion (RPE). It is a subjective measure of how hard you are exercising and helps you to take into account not only your personal fitness level but also environmental conditions and general fatigue factors. The scale corresponds to the increase in VO_2 and heart rate during exercise. The cardiorespiratory training effect is best achieved at intensity levels that are "somewhat hard" to "hard," which corresponds to a rating of 12 to 16 on the scale. Even when using a heart rate monitoring device, it is helpful to keep the RPE Scale in your mind to ensure that you are exercising at a level that will Overload you yet not overly exhaust you. There is also a Revised Borg Scale, but the most commonly used is the Original, which is the one referred to in this book.

The Borg rating of perceived exertion Original Scale:

6		14	
7	Very, very light	15	Hard
8		16	
9	Very light	17	Very hard
10		18	
11	Fairly light	19	Very, very hard
12		20	
13	Somewhat hard		

The Borg RPE on the Revised Scale:

0	Nothing at all	7	Very strong
0.5	Very, very weak	8	
1	Very weak	9	
2	Weak	10	Very, very strong
3	Moderate	*	Maximal
4	Somewhat strong		
5	Strong		
6			

Aerobic versus Anaerobic

Aerobic exercise is exercise at levels of intensity at which your cardiovascular system (heart and lungs) can keep pace with the demand for oxygen. This steady supply is what allows the activity to comfortably take place. Walking, jogging, and non-sprint running, are aerobic activities whereby the heart and lungs can keep pace with the demand for

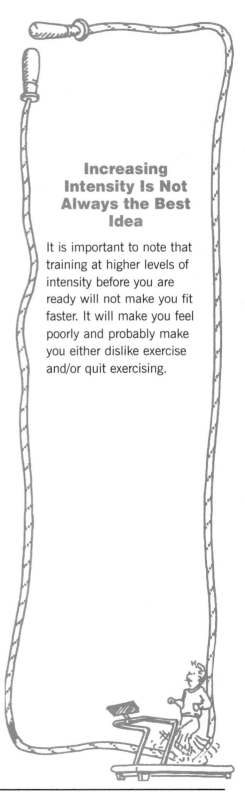

Increasing Intensity Is Not Always the Best Idea

It is important to note that training at higher levels of intensity before you are ready will not make you fit faster. It will make you feel poorly and probably make you either dislike exercise and/or quit exercising.

(continued on next page)

Checks and Balances: RPE Scale and Heart Rate Monitoring

Suppose you have determined that you feel good exercising at a heart rate range of 140–145 bpm; it feels not too hard, nor too easy. On the RPE Scale you describe this intensity as "somewhat hard to hard" or the numbers 13 to 14 and it feels normal for you. Now suppose you notice that during the last few days your overall effort still feels to be "somewhat hard to hard" (numbers 13 to 14) but your heart rate has not risen above 130 bpm. What does this mean?

It could mean many things. Your body could be telling you that it is tired, needs sleep, or a rest day. It could mean your immune system is busier than normal working against a

oxygen. Exercising at aerobic levels strengthens your heart, burns fat, and improves your overall cardiovascular strength. If you exercise harder, such that the heart and lungs cannot keep up with the demand for oxygen, as in going from jogging to running very fast, you are no longer aerobic but anaerobic.

Anaerobic means your body is working so hard that the heart and lungs cannot keep up with the demand for oxygen. At this point the method of oxygenation changes and digs deep. Exercising at anaerobic levels improves cardiovascular endurance and athletic performance. Whatever oxygen your muscles and cells have stored will be the new source. And as you may have already guessed, the stored supply doesn't last for long. This explains why you can sprint only for short distances. Sprinting is an anaerobic activity that relies upon the stored amount of oxygen deep in your tissues.

Anaerobic Threshold

The point at which the supply of oxygen changes from aerobic to anaerobic is called the anaerobic threshold. Just as the threshold of a door is a marker that you have entered a new room, crossing over the anaerobic threshold means you have entered the anaerobic oxygenating territory. Exercising at your anaerobic threshold improves your cardiovascular endurance.

Benefits of Anaerobic Exercise

Remember the Overload principle? In order to improve your fitness, you must push your body slightly beyond what it is accustomed to. Anaerobic exercise, or exercising at intensity levels above and beyond aerobic levels, can be used intermittently during an aerobic exercise session to overload the cardiovascular system. Intermingling short periods of anaerobic exercise into your aerobic exercise session is one way to overload your cardiovascular system. These "intervals" of high intensity exercise expand and increase your aerobic capacity. The result or training effect is that when you exercise or perform work at previous aerobic levels, it will feel easier.

Interval Training

This involves a repeated series of intense exercise work bouts interspersed with rest or recovery periods. Intervals are commonly used to make gains in endurance, strength, and/or speed and are used to improve both aerobic and anaerobic performance and conditioning. Their effectiveness can be likened to hitting the "fast forward" button of progress, as long as they are not overdone. Intervals are fun because of their variety, intensity, and feelings of satisfaction after completing them. Plus, when you use your heart rate monitor, you can watch your different heart rate responses.

Highly trained endurance athletes have mastered interval training such that they are able to sustain high aerobic levels, close to their anaerobic threshold, with ease.

Designing Your Own Interval Session

You can design a variety of interval sessions for any activity. Here are some key points to include when planning your interval training session.

1. Always include a thorough warm-up.
2. Remember that intervals are for limited periods of time and are not to be practiced for the entire portion of an exercise session.
3. Interval sessions should not exceed 1–2 times per week.
4. The benefits of interval training can be achieved by exercising at intensity levels that are either higher aerobic levels or by crossing the anaerobic threshold into anaerobic levels.
5. To interval train adjust your exercise session either by (1) increasing the exercise intensity or length of the intense work interval, (2) by decreasing the length of the rest/recovery phase, or (3) by increasing the number of intervals per session.

Training Effect

The training effect phenomenon is why over time your exercising heart rate and RPE (rating of perceived exertion) will change. In the beginning, you may perceive exercise to be "somewhat hard" when your heart rate is at 125 bpm. But after 4 weeks of consistent aerobic exercise and with a little interval training you may find that when your

Checks and Balances: RPE Scale and Heart Rate Monitoring

(continued from previous page)

cold or infection and that it is trying to conserve energy for the extra work.

If you were to gauge your exercise intensity strictly by heart rate number alone, you would continue to push toward the 140 bpm mark and might overexert yourself in the process.

Using the RPE Scale in conjunction with your heart rate monitor is a great checks and balances system that can keep you exercising within the appropriate degree of effort on a daily basis.

heart rate is at 125 bpm your RPE is now "fairly light." This indicates that a training effect has occurred, good job! And it also means that it is time for you to continue to apply the overload principle and to exercise at an intensity level that feels "somewhat hard," which will likely be a higher heart rate (bpm).

It is important to understand that the many positive bodily adaptations to exercise can occur with regular aerobic exercise when you apply the overload and F-I-T-T principles, with or without interval training. Interval training is simply a way to make them happen faster. The result or training effect is that when you return to exercise or perform work at the previous aerobic levels it will feel easier. This is because your cardiovascular system, through Overload, has become more efficient. You are now able to do more with less effort. This is a good sign. It means that you are getting more fit and are in better condition.

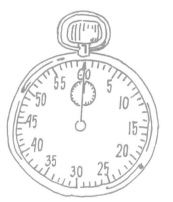

Reviewing Intensity

By now you have a better understanding of the importance of the "I" in the F-I-T-T principles, intensity. And you now know that there are several ways to gauge intensity as well as how to apply them to your exercise sessions. To clarify how these different methods relate to each other, review "The Total Intensity Picture" chart. The chart uses the example of a 40-year-old person with an estimated maximum heart rate of 180 bpm. It illustrates exercise intensity by maximum heart rate, by RPE (rating of perceived exertion), by exercise activity, and by defining aerobic, anaerobic threshold, anaerobic, and maximum heart rate levels.

Time

The duration of your exercise is the amount or length of time you spend exercising. ACSM recommends 20 to 60 minutes of continuous aerobic activity. Yet even bouts of 10 minutes can be effective in establishing the exercise habit and yielding benefit. (For severely deconditioned individuals, multiple sessions of short duration [10 minutes] may be necessary.) The most widely accepted minimum time to achieve aerobic fitness is 20 minutes. Longer periods are needed to optimize specific goals such as calorie burning, endurance, performance, and so forth.

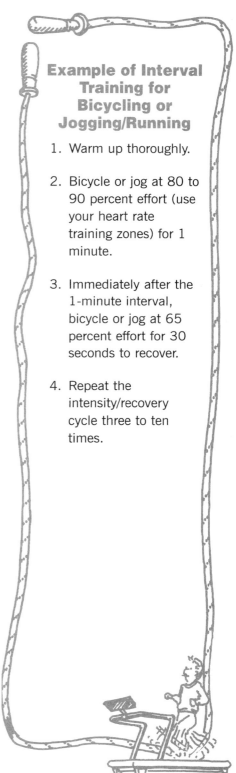

Oxygen, Time, and Calories

Even though we have been speaking of measuring and monitoring exercise by heart rate in beats per minute (bpm), you may recall that the real aerobic benefit comes from training the body to utilize oxygen. When the body is busy processing all this oxygen, a lot of energy is expended. This energy can be measured in units known as calories. A fun fact to know is that for every 1 liter of oxygen (per kilogram of body weight) processed during aerobic exercise, the body spends 5 kilocalories. The more energy you "spend" and the longer you exercise, the more oxygen is processed and the more calories you burn. If weight management is one of your exercise goals, consider exercising at moderate to lower intensity levels for longer periods of time. When planning to exercise for lengthier periods of time, be sure to balance your routine by decreasing the frequency and intensity so as not to produce an overtraining effect or overuse syndrome injury (see Chapter 13).

Time Is Flexible and Adaptable

Adapt your exercise time to work with your frequency and intensity. For instance, if you normally exercise five times per week but have a hectic week approaching that allows for only three times per week, you can adjust your exercise time for longer periods to compensate for the lower frequency. Also, if you want to exercise at a higher intensity level than normal, you should shorten your time of exercise accordingly.

Make Time for a Warm-Up and a Cool-Down

Each exercise session should begin with a warm-up and conclude with a cool-down. A **warm-up** increases blood flow to the working muscles and increases body temperature. This decreases the likelihood of muscular or joint injuries. A warm-up can be in the form of light calisthenics or performing the same exercise activity at a very low intensity. It should last 5 to 10 minutes, after which time the intensity of the activity can be increased to the higher conditioning levels. A **cool-down** should occur at the end of your exercise session to prevent blood from pooling in the legs and other extremities. Blood pooling causes a sudden drop in blood pressure and can make you feel dizzy or faint following exercise. To "cool down," reduce the intensity level of exercise gradually, spanning about 5 minutes. Using your pulse or heart

Example of Interval Training for Bicycling or Jogging/Running

1. Warm up thoroughly.

2. Bicycle or jog at 80 to 90 percent effort (use your heart rate training zones) for 1 minute.

3. Immediately after the 1-minute interval, bicycle or jog at 65 percent effort for 30 seconds to recover.

4. Repeat the intensity/recovery cycle three to ten times.

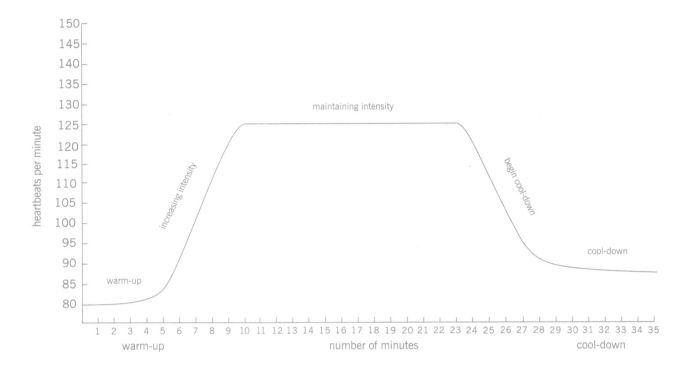

Anatomy of an Aerobic Exercise Session (without interval training)

rate monitor will serve as a guide for cooling down. Bringing your heart rate down to levels slightly above where you started would be sufficient for a cool-down (approximately 5 to 10 beats above your starting heart rate). Rarely will your heart rate decrease to preexercising levels during a cool-down, nor is it necessary. When you piece together the warm-up, the conditioning phase, and the cool-down, your exercise session may look something like the figure above (bell curve).

The Healthy Threesome

Using each of the F-I-T-T principles in conjunction with each other is critical to getting the results you want. Here is why. Suppose you exercise for 20 minutes two times per week at an appropriate intensity level. Will you get much benefit? Sure, you will feel better for that spe-

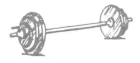
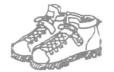

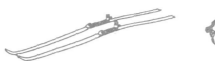

The Total Intensity Picture: Aerobic, Anaerobic Threshold, Anaerobic, and Max HR

Example: Using a person with a maximum heart rate of 180 beats per minute and degrees of walking, running, and all-out sprinting.

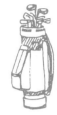

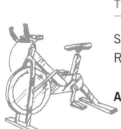

DEGREE OF THE ACTIVITY	% OF MAX HR	CORRESPONDING HEART RATE	RPE	AEROBIC OR ANAEROBIC EXERCISE
Sprinting	95%	171	19	Anaerobic exercise
Running fast	90%	162	18	Anaerobic exercise
Anaerobic Threshold		**Anaerobic Threshold**		**Anaerobic Threshold**
Running	85%	153	16–17	High aerobic
Jogging	80%	144	13–15	Aerobic
Striding	75%	135	12	Aerobic
Fast Walk	70%	126	11	Mild aerobic
Walk	65%	117	9–10	Low Aerobic
Slow Walk	50–60%	90–108	9 and under	Lowest Aerobic

Maximum heart rate—the highest number of heartbeats in 1 minute of exercise.

Anaerobic—level of exercise at which cardiovascular system cannot keep up with the demand for oxygen

Anaerobic Threshold—the point where exercise changes from aerobic to anaerobic.

Aerobic—level of exercise at which cardiovascular system can keep up with the demand for oxygen.

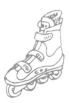

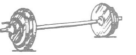

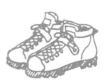

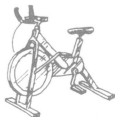

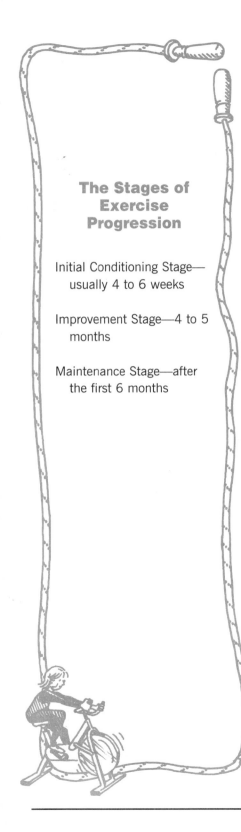

cific day or the day after. But you will not create the cumulative fitness or training effect that you desire or that is your overall goal.

Suppose you exercise five times per week for 20 minutes and your intensity level is only at 50 percent of your Max HR or at RPE (rating of perceived exertion) of 6–9, very, very light. Again, you will feel good and will be getting some important benefits to your health. But if your goal is to improve fitness, lose weight, and so on, you need to go at it with greater intensity.

And what if you regularly exercise four times per week at an appropriate intensity level (RPE 13) and you do it for 10 minutes? Will you receive some benefit? Ten minutes may be an appropriate amount to start with, but after several weeks, you need to increase the amount of time while keeping or improving the other F-I-T principles of frequency and intensity. A healthy exercise goal might be to exercise five times per week for 30 minutes at an intensity level that is 80 percent of your Max HR or an RPE of 15 (hard).

The Overload and F-I-T Principles structure your exercise program. *Paying attention* to your results will help you evaluate and decide when it may be appropriate to make a change in your overload through frequency, intensity, and/or time. The sixth step of Set Yourself Up for Success tells you how to "pay attention" to your exercise results so that you know when a change is in order.

Rates of Progression

When you apply the F-I-T Principles to your exercise plan, you will experience periodic physiological changes. The period of initial conditioning usually lasts 4 to 6 weeks and should include light muscular endurance exercises and low-level aerobic activities. Such a plan might be exercising three times per week, nonconsecutive days, for 12 to 15 minutes and progress to 20 minutes. That is followed by the improvement stage, which typically lasts 4 to 5 months, with progression in all of the F-I-T Principles. Once your exercise program has become a fixture in your life (after that 4- to 5-month period), you enter the maintenance stage. Throughout these periods, you make adjustments in your exercise program to ensure that you're both improving your level of fitness and enjoying yourself.

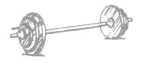
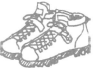
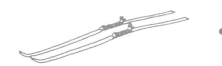

Summary Chart of Heart Rate Training Zones 1–5

NAME	% OF MAX HR	FEELS	INTENSITY	CHARACTERISTICS
Zone 1 Healthy Heart	50–60%	Easy	Low	Cardiovascular benefit Low risk of injury Burns ↑ % of fat
Zone 2 Temperate	60–70%	Still easy	Mild	Cardiovascular benefit Low risk of injury Burns fat and more calories
Zone 3 Aerobic	70–80%	Challenging	Medium	Aerobically efficient Burns fat and calories ↑ Risk of musculoskeletal* injury
Zone 4 Threshold	80–90%	Harder	Somewhat hard to hard	Fitness fast and performance Burns ↓ % of fat but many calories ↑ Risk of musculoskeletal injury
Zone 5 Performance	90–100%	All out	The most	Not for everyone! Performance enhancing ↑ Risk of musculoskeletal injury

↑ = higher or increased   ↓ = lower or decreased

* Musculoskeletal refers to the muscular and skeletal systems including muscles, connective tissues, bones, and related matter.

Adapted from *Sally Edwards' Heart Zone Training*

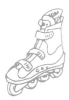

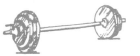
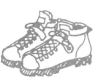

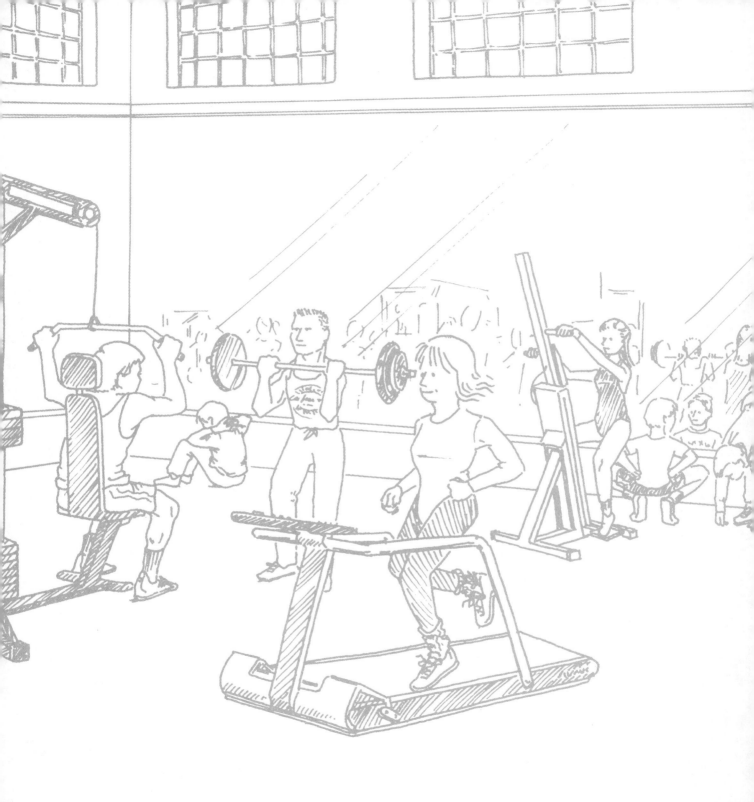

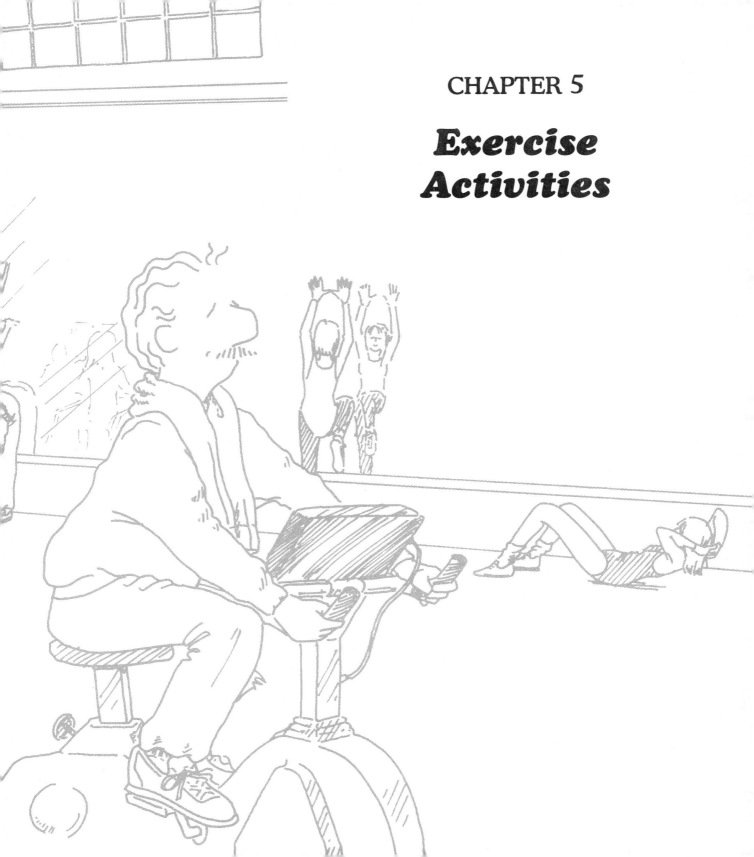

CHAPTER 5

Exercise Activities

S elect exercise activities that are fun, convenient, and familiar, or perhaps new and interesting. How do you know which are the best activities for you? *The best exercise activities for fitness are activities you will do and continue to do with some degree of enjoyment or appreciation and without injury or distress.* With all the choices of exercise activities available to you, you should let a few important considerations steer you toward selecting the right ones. Completing the personal inventory that follows will help you choose activities that will fit you. Surely there is at least one activity that will touch your fancy.

Personal Inventory: Considerations for Selecting Exercise Activities

1. Expediency. How much time will you allot for exercise? If you are really pinched for time, you may want to focus on exercising from your home, either indoors or out. Or find out if there is a gym or health club close to home or work. Is the time of day that you exercise flexible or regular and repeatable? Do you have to fit in your exercise early in the morning, before the rest of the household awakens, or do you live alone and do as you please, when you please? Do you work out on your lunch hour and have to be back in exactly 1 hour?

2. Alone versus others. Do you like exercise time to be "alone time," just for yourself? Do you need or enjoy having others around you? Do you prefer a class environment? Do you enjoy team sports and are those opportunities available to you? Do you like getting out of the house, or would you rather exercise in the privacy of your own home? Do you have a safe environment and enough space to exercise?

3. Indoor versus outdoor considerations. What do you enjoy doing indoors, and what do you enjoy doing outdoors? It is helpful to find at least one indoor and one outdoor activity for exercise. This way you can be more flexible and have more options for those times when the weather seems more challenging than your workout, when you travel, when it is dark, when your favorite machine is being used by someone else, and so on. It also allows you to have some variety.

4. Variety. Variety gives you options, which is good for you socially, physically, and mentally. Maybe you have been housebound or

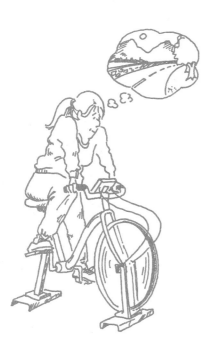

office-bound for days and are savoring even the idea of being outdoors or just being around other people. Variety keeps your body from experiencing repetitive overuse syndromes (injuries or painful conditions that result from doing the same activity with the same muscles in the same way time after time after time). Having two or three different activities that you can choose from keeps you mentally fresh and a good distance away from burnout.

5. Skill or technical training. If you have always dreamed of taking up horseback riding, fencing, or tennis, prepare yourself that first you will have to learn the skills and techniques. This is not said to discourage you at all; rather it is to mentally prepare you to be patient. The same learning curve consideration is taken into account if you decide that martial arts, rowing, sculling, kayaking, rock climbing, gymnastics, and ballet are for you. These are all wonderful fitness activities with degrees of skill that are more demanding than walking or using a stair climber. So consider how much skill is involved, be prepared, be patient, and have fun learning something new.

6. Cost. Although cost is an important consideration, try not to let cost dominate your fitness activity choices. If you truly enjoy aerobics and know that you will go to an aerobics class four or five times a week but have a hard time going out for a walk on your own, then the money spent for the class is worth it. Sure, you could put on your shoes and go for a walk, which is less expensive, but if you don't do it, then what have you accomplished? Consider too all the other benefits and joys that you get from the paid class. For many people, a financial commitment is what motivates them to continue going to the class or the gym/club. So keep cost in mind, but don't let it steer you away from an activity that you enjoy and will continue doing.

Activities

What follows is a thorough list of *aerobic* fitness activities, some with profiles with enough detailed information to get you moving. The profiles include a description of the activity, major benefits, skill level, equipment and clothing needed, and associated risks, as well as instructions and other key information. Remember, regardless of the activities you select, you will need to apply the Overload and F-I-T Principles (see Chapter 4) to ensure you get fit and receive the maximum benefit for your effort.

High impact aerobic activities are usually weight-bearing (body weight and gravity are factors) aerobic activities, repetitive in nature, that cause varying degrees of jarring, jolting, or pounding to one's musculoskeletal system. Activities include running/jogging, walking, jumping rope, high impact aerobics.

Note: Weight-bearing activities, in moderation, help stimulate the production of bone growth and improve bone density.

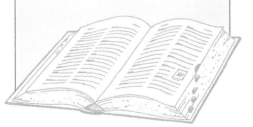

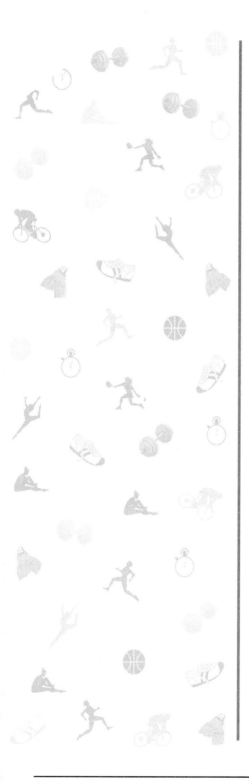

Also, you may want to check out Chapter 5 for great ideas on things to think about during exercise.

Aerobic Activities Outside

When it is a lovely sunny day, the sky is blue, and the temperature is mild, it is hard to beat a great exercise experience outdoors. And even when the weather's not perfect, it still is invigorating to be outside in the fresh air, taking in the little and big sights of the world. At the end of this chapter is a list of fitness activities. As you read through the list, mark the activities that interest you. Then go back through the list of those that interest you and mark those that meet the criteria listed in the personal inventory considerations. By then you will have a few activities to get started with.

Walking

Walking is a form of locomotion in which at least one foot is always in contact with the ground. Walking sounds too easy, and that is probably why some people do not use it for exercise. They have a pre-conceived notion that exercise has to be difficult or that it has to hurt. Neither is true. Walking can make you fit; you just have to do it with frequency, intensity, and for enough time. (There they are again, the F-I-T Principles.)

Major benefits: Walking is a low-impact aerobic activity. The big plusses about walking are that it will not forcibly jar your skeletal system, yet because it is a weight-bearing activity, it will stimulate bone growth and density. You can walk nearly anywhere, in the city, in the country, in a neighborhood, in a shopping mall, or for transportation. Walking builds muscular strength and endurance in your legs, arms (if swung properly), and the muscles of the back and abdomen that keep your trunk erect.

Skill: A low degree of skill is required, although proper technique is important.

Seasonal: You can walk through every season and really enjoy the seasonal changes by taking in the scenery around you. For wet and winter walking, invest in some wet-weather gear. When you walk on grey wet days, it may seem as though you have the outdoors all to yourself. What a treat to be out experiencing nature's medley while everyone else is cooped up inside.

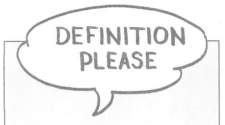

Risk: Aside from tripping or walking in a heavily trafficked area, you are at low risk for injury.

Equipment: Get a good pair of walking shoes. Your body parts are worth it, and you will enjoy feeling the support they provide in all the right places. Good walking shoes help support and protect your spine, hips, knees, ankles, and feet. One unnecessary trip to the doctor is more expensive than what it costs for a decent pair of walking shoes, so do not hesitate to buy them. Buy shoes that are truly meant for walking. Avoid aerobic or court shoes because they do not provide the type of support needed for walking. If you are a combination walker/jogger, you may choose to get running shoes instead. But if you are exclusively a walker, get a pair of walking shoes. Walking shoes offer a bit more flexibility, which you need because when you walk, you flex your feet and push off with your toes more than when you run. Because you land on your heels, you need a stable shoe that has a heel counter, the cup-like device in the heel of the shoe that helps to secure your foot from moving around. Although it's good to incorporate walking into your daily routines and errands, it is best not to walk as rigorously or for as long a period of time in your dress or street shoes as you would when walking strictly for exercise. Your feet will pay the price with pain and/or blisters.

Cost: Walking is a low-cost activity with no monthly fees/dues or hourly rates. The biggest expenses go toward a good pair of walking shoes and comfortable clothing, and, if you are adventurous, wet-weather gear. You can expect to spend $40 plus for a good pair of walking shoes, and $50 to $100 for a wet-weather suit, top and bottom.

Walking for exercise—Leg/foot action: Start by standing erect. Imagine a cord coming out of the center and top of your head that gently pulls you up straight. Lift the heel of one foot and transfer your weight forward as you roll from your heel to your arch, then to the ball of your foot until you push off with your toes. Your foot is now airborne, and the same leg moves forward until you land on your heel, whereupon you begin the process again, simultaneously alternating legs/feet. We'll save the "walk and chew gum test" for another chapter. However, you should be aware of some of the common errors walkers make.

One of the most common errors walkers make is leaning forward rather than standing erect. Keep your hips directly under your upper body. You don't want to be stiff, but you should avoid bending at your

Low impact aerobic activities are usually non-weight-bearing (body weight and gravity are not factors) aerobic activities, repetitive in nature, that generate little, if any, jarring, jolting, or pounding to one's musculoskeletal system. Activities include swimming, water aerobics, bicycling, rowing, cross-country skiing, stair-climbing, and elliptical machine exercise.

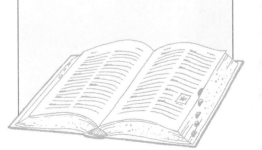

How Can You Walk Faster?

Imagine that you are using your feet to pull the ground surface underneath you as you move forward. Think about the rest of your body rotating around your spine, which should be erect. As you walk faster, your hips will take turns rolling and dropping. This allows your legs to move more freely and quickly. Quick turnover of your legs will make you faster but be careful not to exaggerate your stride so that you have sacrificed your healthy posture.

hips or hunching your shoulders. Another common error is walking with the head down, looking at the ground immediately in front of the feet. Keep your head up and look several feet *ahead* of where your feet are landing. As long as you keep your head up and remember to *pick up your feet*, you will see the divots, potholes, loose gravel, branches, curbs, bicyclists, vehicles, and other pedestrians that may be in your path.

Upper body action: Your arms should be relaxed (taking a deep breath helps) and balanced so that the actions of both arms are the same. Swing your arms counter to your legs. Keep them bent near a 90-degree angle, and hold them close to your body rather than winging out. Swinging your arms will also help you to elevate your heart rate. Your hands should swing a bit, but not across the midline of the body or above the level of your chest. Hold your hands with the thumbs up and with a loose fist.

Recommendations: Once you are comfortable with your walking technique, spice up your experience by developing several different courses with varying sights, terrain, and distance. It is fun to map them out to fit your different moods. Use a heart rate monitor to gauge your intensity level and to motivate you to move at a good clip but not to overdo it. Set some goals for time, speed, and distance and occasionally test yourself to see your progress. Check your heart rate during exercise and your recovery heart rate. When you see those numbers improving, then it is time to overload yourself, increasing at least one of the three F-I-T Principles. Vary your pace by speeding up for short intervals of time or distance. Invite others to join you only if they can keep up with you; you don't want others to impede your intensity level. Treat yourself to the fun experience of signing up for a walking or jogging event such as a 5k (kilometer = .625 of a mile) or 10k. Having such a goal will motivate you, and participating will definitely elevate you.

How to get started: If you are just getting started, go out and walk for a short period of time, maybe 10 minutes. Check in with your body the next day, and if all systems are go, then repeat the 10-minute walking period. Gradually increase the time of your walk, perhaps in 5-minute increments over a period of days or weeks if necessary. If you are feeling pretty good and pain free, you can walk on consecutive days, but if pain or soreness is a problem, then either select a different activity or rest completely for a day or so. Continue to check in with

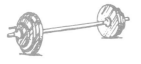
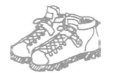
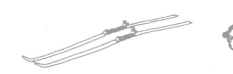

Sample 12-Week Walking Program for Beginners

Always warm up and cool down gradually.

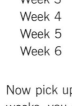

Week 1	Walk 1 mile in 24 minutes 5 days a week.
Week 2	Walk 1 mile in 22 minutes 5 days a week.
Week 3	Walk 1 mile in 20 minutes 5 days a week.
Week 4	Walk 1.5 miles in 30 minutes 5 days a week.
Week 5	Walk 1.5 miles in 29 minutes 5 days a week.
Week 6	Walk 2 miles in less than 40 minutes 5 days a week.

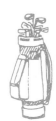

Now pick up the pace. If you have not experienced any adverse effects during the first 6 weeks, you are ready for a higher level.

Week 7	Walk 2 miles in 38 minutes 4 times a week.
Week 8	Walk 2 miles in 36 minutes 4 times a week.
Week 9	Walk 2 miles in less than 35 minutes 4 times a week.

If you are doing well with the faster pace, move up to the next level. If you are not ready for the faster pace, stay at the 6-week or 9-week level. You will still achieve major health benefits.

Week 10	Walk 2 miles in 34 minutes 4 times a week.
Week 11	Walk 2 miles in 32 minutes 4 times a week.
Week 12	Walk 2 miles in less than 30 minutes 3 times a week.

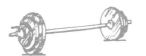

your body for any soreness, aches, or pains. Soreness is a natural outcome when you are just getting started; pain is not. When the soreness is light, you can continue to increase walking time. Over time, you can build up to 30 minutes or even an hour of walking and can increase from walking every other day to nearly every day.

Jogging/Running

The difference between jogging and running is mainly intensity. Jogging is a slower, less intense version of running. Running is moving with quick steps on alternate feet, never having both feet on the ground at the same time. Running is one of the most popular aerobic activities.

Major benefits: As compared to most aerobic activities, the act of running utilizes more liters of oxygen minute for minute. And since the body expends 5 calories for every liter of oxygen processed, running is an efficient way to burn calories and manage body fat and weight. Running is also an effective means of producing endorphins—those feel-good hormones—so much so that the term *runner's high* is often used interchangeably to describe the endorphin effect. Running is a high-impact aerobic activity that is both good and bad. It is good because it stimulates bone growth/density and bad because it jars the skeletal system. You can run nearly anywhere and cover a lot of turf in a short amount of time. You can conveniently "take running with you" when you travel. It is a great way to explore new areas, as long as you have a good enough sense of direction to get you back to where you started. Running builds muscular strength and endurance of the entire body, especially the hips, legs, and feet. These are only some of the reasons why running is such a preferred aerobic activity. Talk to runners, and they will share with you how they love running and what it does for their psyches.

Skill: Running does not require many skills, but technique is important—because of the increased gravitational force absorbed by the body, it is even more important than in walking.

Here are some running tips:

1. If your knees or hips are prone to soreness, pay attention to the camber—the slightly arched shape of the surface of the road or trail—and try to run on the flattest portion. This will reduce the angular stress that may contribute to the problem.

Heavy Hands, Yes or No?

Carrying weights in your hands while walking (heavy hands) was conceptually a good idea for helping to elevate the heart rate and build muscular strength. However, the reality is that it has caused many people joint problems in the elbows, wrists, and shoulders. If you want to elevate your heart rate, walk faster, walk on a course with some hills, or walk with a weighted backpack. If you want to strengthen your upper body, go to Chapter 7 and learn how to strength train. But mixing weights with walking is not the way to go.

2. The shortest distance between two points is a straight line. In training, it is fine to hug the wide lines. But when you are running in a road race or timed event, look for and run the shortest, but still legal, distance, especially on curves and turns. Hugging the outside border of the road can add mileage and time to your performance.

3. Especially if you are a morning runner, be sure to use the bathroom before running.

4. For hot, humid days or runs over ½ hour, carry cool fluids with you.

Seasonal: You can run through every season as long as you adequately hydrate and dress appropriately.

Risk: Any activity that sends you completely off your feet poses greater risk than those that keep your feet on the ground. Keep your head up and your eyes focused ahead of you rather than directly in front of you. If you run in the dark, make yourself visible to others with reflective clothing, decals, or tape. Carry a small flashlight so you can see where or what you are landing on. If you run on a trail, let someone know where you are going and when you left and expect to return. For safety reasons, women should consider finding companions to accompany them when running in unpopulated areas. Dogs and human companions can be fun additions to running, and they provide security against some undesired interactions.

One negative effect of running high mileage or too frequently is the possibility of musculoskeletal injuries or overuse syndromes. Common injuries to the knees, hips, and Achilles tendons are often the result of too much running. Listen to your own body and don't compare what is "too much" for you against what is "too much" for someone else. If you plan to run for your main aerobic exercise activity, make sure you stretch (see Chapter 8). It can also be helpful to alternate other aerobic activities with running and to plan for rest days.

Equipment: Shoes, shoes, shoes. Their importance cannot be overemphasized. Run in running shoes only! You can buy running shoes to fit your uniqueness; important considerations are your body weight, whether you have high arches or no arches (flat feet), your running style, whether you intend to run short or long distances, shoe stability, shoe flexibility, shoe weight, shoe breathe-ability (mixed mesh or solid uppers), and, most important of all, fit.

What's the Difference? When to Stop and When to Go!

Soreness refers to a light achy feeling that reminds you that you did something. It's okay to proceed.

Pain refers to an acute and sharp unpleasant feeling. Stop!

An *ache* is a continuous dull pain. It's a fifty/fifty call, but it's probably best to stop temporarily.

If You Run with Your Dog

Remember to carry along some water for your canine runner; they have smaller operating systems than humans and can overheat quickly. For long runs, check out the dog packs that your four-legged friend can carry on his/her back; just remember to keep it light. Also, be considerate of how much running your particular dog can handle.

Try on the shoe with the style sock or one of similar thickness to the one you will wear when running. When standing in the shoe, you should have a distance equal to the width of your thumb between your big toe and the end of the shoe. Your heels should not come out of the back of the shoe. Since you will be doing more than standing in your running shoes, you will want to run around in them. If the store has space, run around inside—and get off the carpet onto a hard surface. Don't run outside with them, unless you've asked for permission first, or you could have security running right after you. If the store won't let you run in them, make sure they have a generous return policy. Otherwise, go to another store.

The shoes should feel good on your feet and not make you feel that you cannot take them off fast enough. Unless you are a light short distance runner, stay clear of racing flats. They are great for short-distance, fast-paced running (hence the name racing flats), but for most joggers and runners, support is the more important need. Also, running shoe companies work hard to get your attention. Their designs and colors are meant to attract you so that you will buy their shoes. However, resist buying a particular style of running shoes because you want to make a fashion statement. If you think function first, you will do yourself a big favor.

Lacing your shoes may sound like a silly thing to discuss, but how you lace your shoes can make a tremendous difference in how your feet feel in the shoes. (See Chapter 6 for details on lacing your shoes.)

A general sock rule is activities that produce a lot of foot friction require a thicker sock. Sports like basketball and racquetball generate a lot of friction and warrant thicker socks. Unless you are running trails (high friction), you can be comfortable running in a thin sock but, again, go with what feels good. There are numerous fabrics being used today that make socks fit, hold up, and release moisture (so that you don't have wet feet, which can cause blisters) better than ever before. There is no need to suffer with socks that bunch and slip down into your shoes. These will only irritate you while running and produce some nasty blisters that will be popping up to say hello to you when you finish running. (See Chapter 6 for a review of athletic socks.)

Women will want to have a supportive sport bra. There are many different styles and varieties from which to choose. (See Chapter 6 for a review of sport bras.)

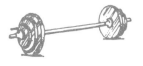
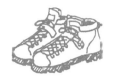
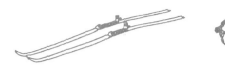

Cross-Training

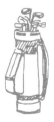

If you want to adopt a healthy training concept, this is it. You cross-train by including a variety of activities as your regular training program. It is a way to stay fit and healthy by balancing the positive and negative effects of the different activities. The sport of triathlon is a great example of cross-training in action. It involves swimming, biking, and running. The benefit is that you are getting an aerobic workout and you vary the effects upon your body. Swimming is aerobic, improves your flexibility, uses most of the muscles in your body (improving muscular strength and endurance), is not weight bearing (giving your skeletal system a rest from the pounding effect of running). Biking is aerobic, uses the hip and leg muscles as well as some of the upper body, works your balancing abilities, and, like swimming, is not weight bearing. Running is aerobic, uses the hip and leg muscles, is weight bearing but also jarring, and is calorically expensive.

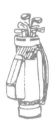

	AEROBIC	WT. BEARING	MUSCULAR STRENGTH/ENDUR.	FLEXIBILITY	CALORIC EXP.
Swimming	yes	no	many	yes	good
Biking	yes	no	lower and some upper	some	good
Running	yes	yes	lower and some upper	some	best

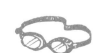
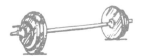
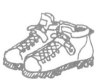

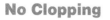

No Clopping

Clop is the sound made by horse's hooves. If your feet make a clopping sound when you run, adjust your technique.

Cost: Aside from the shoes and clothing, running is a low-cost activity. If you treat yourself to organized runs (5ks, 10ks, half marathons, marathons, ultra marathons), entry fees can range from $10 to $50. Usually you can figure that the older, more organized and longer events will have the higher entry fees. The entry fee typically includes a T-shirt, a colorful and memorable reward for your accomplishment.

Running for exercise: Your earliest running experience may have been when you were a kid, playing, chasing, or racing someone or something. And when you ran, it was fast and furious but not for long. Short sprint-type running is different from jogging/running for exercise because it involves more severe flexion of the foot, less heel landing, and more forefoot/toes push-off.

Use these running instructions to develop proper running technique:

- *Posture:* Start by standing erect and imagining a cord coming out of the center and top of your head that gently pulls you straight up.
- *Head:* Use your neck muscles to keep your head looking forward and neither buried in your chest nor cocked back.
- *Face:* Keep your face relaxed by letting your jaw drop and your cheeks "flap." Keep your eyes on the ground about 10 to 20 feet ahead of you. Looking too close to your feet can be dangerous for you and others.
- *Torso:* Pull up with your abdominal muscles and focus on running tall with your torso perpendicular to the running surface. Thinking perpendicular helps you keep your chest open (making easy access for oxygen) and better able to adjust for hills. Leaning too far forward keeps your legs from extending properly, and arching your back restricts your momentum.
- *Shoulders:* Let your shoulders hang relaxed and low, not drawn up toward your ears.
- *Arms:* Hold your arms close to your body and do not let them "chicken wing" out to the sides. They should bend at 90-degree angles to your upper arms, staying near-parallel to the ground. Your arms should swing counter to your legs. They should not cross the midline of your body or swing above the level of your chest.
- *Hands:* Hold your hands with the thumbs up (always a good sign, don't you think?) and with a loose fist. Your palms should be facing each other.

- *Hips:* Keep your hips directly under your upper body.
- *Stride:* Lifting one leg slightly in front of you as you extend the other behind you propels you forward. Each foot should land directly under the center of your body weight, not out in front of you. Long strides mean each foot stays on the ground too long, which slows you down. A short, light stride is the most efficient.
- *Feet:* Landing on the balls of your feet will cause you to waste a lot of energy going up and down rather than forward. You should land lightly on your heel or midfoot, roll forward onto the ball of your foot, then push off with the balls of your feet and toes. The running motion should be smooth, fluid, and relatively quiet. If your feet make a clop, clop, clop sound, check your technique versus how you want to be running and make the correction.

Bicycling, Biking, Cycling

Remember how free you felt on your first set of wheels? Riding a bike is just plain fun, and it is not just for kids. The increasing numbers of cyclists is proving that it is a great lifetime activity. Feeding the popularity of road biking has been the American success stories at the prestigious Tour de France bike race. First there was Greg LeMond in 1986, 1989, and 1990. And then there was the exciting, inspirational achievement in 1999 of winner and cancer survivor Lance Armstrong. If biking piques your interest, you can enjoy road or mountain biking, or both! Road biking takes place on the road and allows you to travel long distances with speed. Mountain biking is more technical, is tedious, and requires a sense of adventure and a secure sense of balance. Although the name implies it, mountain bike riding does not mean you are limited to riding only on mountains. It just means that you can. Bicycling requires that you have some basic equipment. You can get into it for a few hundred dollars, but you can spend much more. There is a direct correlation to the depth of love for the sport and the depth of money spent on it. The deeper you fall in love, the deeper you dig into your pockets. But don't let that discourage you. You are a good cause!

Major Benefits: If you slow-poke around on your bike, you will probably have a nice visual experience but miss out on the fitness benefit. When you ride with the purpose of exercise, it can be very rewarding. Riding for fitness means you ride with intensity, specifically

How to Run the Streets

Have you noticed how today's automobiles are actually masquerading as mobile homes (equipped with cell phones, cup holders, eating pads, televisions, stereos)? It means that drivers are more distracted than ever. Then there's "road rage" and the unfortunate attitude of some people who don't want runners on "their" roads. So remember to walk against traffic and stay to the far left side of the road. A life-saving piece of advice is that when you run on the streets, *assume that no one sees you* and make yourself visible as best you can. Wear bright contrasting colors and reflective tape or clothing on the front and back of you. You have a right to be on the road (as long as there is no sign restricting pedestrians), but don't let that lure you into a false sense of security.

This biomechanical invention of Steve Tamaribuchi is helping both athletes and nonathletes. The e3 grips are made from a soft yet durable plastic called Santoprene. They come in a set of two, one for each hand, and are held in the hand in an upright position with the thumb resting upon the "thumb shelf." The claim is that each e3 grip positions the hand, fingers, and thumb such that it dramatically improves balance and posture throughout the entire body. And, that they reduce stress on joints and enhance agility, speed, and strength. One size fits all (except for very small children). Along with runners, triathletes, and basketball players, hospitals and physical therapy offices are also using e3 grips for many of their patients. (See Appendix Resources www.biogrip.com.)

with speed and for time. When you ride with intensity, bicycling is an aerobic activity that uses your hips/buttocks and hips/thigh muscles. There is no pounding (as there is in running) and as long as you have a proper fit with your bike, you may feel as though you can ride forever. To ensure you have the proper frame size and fit on a bike, talk to your local bike store expert or bike club. As far as seat positioning goes, your knees should have a slight bend (15 to 20 degrees) when you are in the down phase of the pedal stroke, and your hips should not sway from side to side when you pedal.

How to get started: If you have never ridden a bike in your life and have no idea what it feels like, you need to go to a different book first. Once you can ride a bike and can balance safely, come back to this page. Now, for the rest of you, if you are riding again for the first time in a long time, do so in an area where you can relax and familiarize yourself with the gearing and braking systems. They may seem complicated at first, but once you understand how they work, you'll breeze right through them. Your body will initially have to adjust to cycling, so limit your first few rides to shorter periods of time and build up to longer rides gradually.

The pedal stroke is a smooth circular motion whereby you want to not only push on the downstroke but also pull on the upstroke. That is hard to do on a bike that does not have toe clips or clipless pedals (an explanation of these follows shortly), but that is the correct bicycling motion.

How do you know how hard to ride and which gears to use? The sport of bicycling has three major themes: efficiency, practicality, and self-sufficiency. Gearing is all about efficiency. You want to ride in the gear that will allow you to *spin* at a *cadence* that is comfortable yet taxing (here's the good ol' Overload principle again). To *spin* (or *spinning*) is a biking term that describes quick circular revolutions and, in this case, quick pedal strokes. In order to spin, the selected gear has to be at a tension that allows you to push the crank (what the pedals are attached to) without straining. Cadence refers to the rhythm and number of revolutions per minute that you turn the crank. Serious cyclists spin at 90 to 110 rpms (revolutions per minute), and it is not unrealistic for recreational riders to spin at 70 to 80 rpms. The beauty of thinking about your cadence and spinning is that it keeps you from pushing too hard a gear, and that helps you avoid straining your muscles and other injuries. Once again, more is not always better.

Seasonal: Depending upon where you live, bicycling can be a year-round or seasonal sport. With winter gear, you can ride your bike outdoors as long as you are mindful of the slick conditions. Many outdoor cyclists (usually road bikers) who feel confined to the indoors during the winter, resort to devices that simulate outdoor cycling. They are known as wind trainers and rollers, and each utilizes the bicycle's gearing system to create resistance. Although boredom can be a factor when exercising indoors (see Chapter 5), these apparatus allow for riding an outdoor bike indoors, which delivers the feel for and the aerobic effect of the outdoor bike. The other redeeming quality about wind trainers and rollers is that they keep your cycling skills sharp and require mental focus. Having to concentrate on the activity can be a stress-reducing mental getaway and will build your appreciation for riding outdoors. After a wintry season of indoor cycling, you will be physically fit, mentally sharp, and emotionally eager as spring welcomes you back on the road.

Wind Trainer: The wind trainer utilizes the bike's gearing system and the wind trainer's flywheel to create wind resistance. The bike is temporarily and securely mounted onto the trainer either from the front or the rear wheel, or hub (the central part of the wheel). Wind trainers are useful for focusing on cadence (rhythm, in this case revolutions per minute) and interval training and put less emphasis on handling and balance.

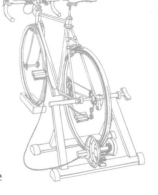

Wind Trainer
A wind trainer allows for riding your bike indoors and is a convenient and efficient fitness option. No technical bicycling skills are required.

Rollers: Rollers look like the biker's version of a logrolling contest. There is nothing that secures or mounts the bike onto the rollers. Therefore, the rollers should be situated parallel to a wall or near some other form to secure the rider's balance. The rider balances the bike on top of the front and rear rollers by pedaling. Only the rider's balance keeps the bike upright.

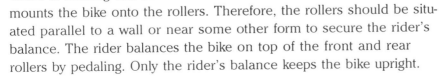

Be Prepared

Knowledge of how to remedy a flat, bike/frame pump, saddle bag, spare tubes, patch kit, tire levers, ID: In keeping with the self-sufficiency theme, these items complete the list of what you want to take along so that you can be more prepared than a Boy Scout. Most of the items you can fit inside your saddle bag, which attaches to the rear of your saddle. Having the equipment with you can make the difference between having a fun experience or a disappointing one.

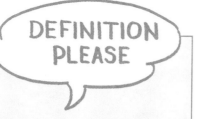

DEFINITION PLEASE

Cadence describes the number of pedal revolutions performed in one minute. Cadence will vary depending upon many conditions, such as whether you are riding on a smooth road or rugged trail, or up or down a hill.

Spinning is pedaling with quick even strokes at a comfortable and efficient cadence; this causes less fatigue in the legs than when pedaling at a lower cadence in a more strenuous gear.

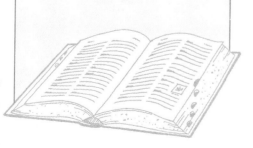

Rollers are particularly effective in improving bike handling and balancing skills because they are very challenging.

Risks: As in running, anytime you are airborne and leave the ground, you put yourself at some degree of risk. However, life is meant to be lived, not feared, and bicycling is a joyful reminder of the simple pleasures in life. Both mountain biking and road biking have inherent associated risks, which are related to their respective environments.

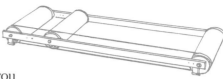

Rollers
More advanced and technical than a wind trainer, rollers also allow for indoor bicycling on your bike. In addition to keeping the rider aerobically fit, rollers help improve balance and handling skills.

Types of Bikes

- *Mountain bikes:* Mountain bikes allow you to ride on a wide variety of surfaces including grass, dirt, rock, puddles, and paved roads. Mountain bikes are bigger, heavier, and more stable than road bikes and *at rest* are more comfortable than road bikes. However, when you are riding a mountain bike up or down a dirt path, and over rocks or tree roots, comfort becomes a relative term. Mountain bikes have three chain rings (for gearing) and numerous gearing options that make it possible to ride through all types of challenges. The wheels and tires are larger than on any other bike in order to tackle the variety of terrain. Mountain bikes even come equipped with shock absorbers to help absorb some of the impact.

- *Hybrid bikes:* These are in-between upright bikes, a combination mountain-road bike. They are best for those who prefer to ride on roads (great for commuting) but want greater stability and comfort than what road bikes offer. Hybrids are slower than road bikes and not nearly sturdy enough for serious mountain biking. They are heavier than road bikes but not as bulky or as heavy as mountain bikes.

- *Road bikes:* Road bikes are made from various grades of steel, aluminum, carbon fiber, and titanium. Generally, the lighter yet stronger materials command the heavier prices. *Components* is the term used to describe everything but the frame; it includes the brakes, shifters, derailleurs (front and rear), chain, chain rings, and cogs. Higher-priced components deliver a smoother, lighter, more reliable, more efficient, and more durable riding experience than lower-priced components. If you are a novice who expects to ride occasionally, you do not need to spend the money for the top of the line frame or components. But if you anticipate being a frequent and regular rider, it will be money well spent to buy the mid- to upper-range frame and components.

- *Recumbent (lying down or reclining) and semi-recumbent bikes:* If you have seen someone riding these bikes you are unlikely to forget them. The rider appears to be either lying down or in a semi-reclined position. Their unusual look is also attributed to the frame that is generally long and thin, the seat that is bordered by a long full backrest, and the front wheel that is usually smaller than the rear wheel. Most are foot-powered but some also have hand cranks for arm power. The main appeal of recumbents and semi-recumbents is comfort. Riders boast that they experience less fatigue in their low back, neck and wrist as well as a reduction in saddle soreness as compared to upright bicycling riding. A drawback of these bikes is that they can be slower and more difficult to pedal up hills. Because the bike puts the rider in a sunken position, they are not very visible on the road. Therefore, it is a good idea to carry or attach a tall, highly visible flag/marker to the bike.

- *Softride (a brand name—as of yet there is no other in its category):* This is another "if you see one, you'll never forget it" bicycle. The distinguishing feature of the Softride is the soft comfortable ride it provides to the cyclist. It does this better than other bikes because it has no seat tube (the metal piece that runs from the crank shaft up to the seat). It appears as if the seat is floating on air, hence the floating rib image. Instead, the seat is attached to the top tube (the tube that starts at the head set/stem and runs horizontally until it reaches the seat). This reduces the road friction absorbed by the rider. Although on the high end of the price range, these are dearly appreciated by riders who ride for longer distances or periods of time.

Fun Fact to Know

American Greg Lemond won the Tour de France as a member of the French (non-American) team. American Lance Armstrong's victory was especially cherished for many reasons, one of which was that he was the first American to win the Tour on an American team.

- *Tandems:* The old bicycle-built-for-two is ever popular and just as technically savvy as its modern single companion. Usually the strongest of the two riders takes the front position and leads the charge. Yes, you can get fit riding a tandem, but there is a caveat: Because of their shared nature and the fact that one rider leads while the other follows, they have been known to cause heated discussions and the breakup of relationships. So pick your tandem partner carefully and clearly define your riding plan before you take the tandem plunge. If you survive the power play, you can have a great time.

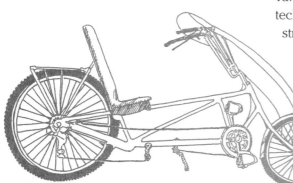

Semi-Recumbant Bike

Equipment: Bicycling is a relatively simple activity, yet the sport could win the contest for having the most toys. You can limit some of the equipment, but the one item that is absolutely essential is a helmet. In the event that you fall in love with bicycling, as have millions of others, following is a thorough rundown of the equipment:

- *Aerobars:* Necessity is the mother of invention, and that is exactly how aerobars came to be born. Since drafting (following closely behind another rider to avoid wind resistance) is not allowed in the sport of triathlon (road bikes), triathletes and bike manufacturers came up with a legal way to cut down on wind resistance. Aerobars are U-shaped handlebars (or a handlebar extension device) that positions riders more aerodynamically, with less air resistance. To use aerobars the bicyclist leans forward and rests the forearms in the aerobar pads. In this position there is less air/wind resistance than in upright riding. They are best used on flat smooth courses. In addition to reducing wind drag, aerobars offer a greater level of comfort. They give the arms, shoulders, and hands a restful feel as compared to riding down in the handlebar drops (the lower curling portion of the handlebar) or on top of the hood levers (area on top of the brake levers). What is sacrificed in the aero position is dexterity and handling ability, but because riders can move freely in and out of the aero position as needed, they are well worth the sacrifice. Aerobars can be used effectively on road, touring, and mountain bikes.

- *Cleats:* Cleats are a fitted wedge type projection that is securely screwed into the bottom of the bike shoe. The shoe/cleat then inserts into the fitted pedal.

- *Toe clips:* Toe clips are metal or plastic pieces that partially cover and help keep the foot attached to the pedal. With the foot inserted into the toe clip, the rider then tightens the toe strap to secure the foot in place. Toe clips keep the foot from coming off the pedal. They allow the rider to pedal efficiently because with the foot secured on the pedal, the rider can then pull up with forceful tension to create equal resistance through the pedal stroke through the entire circular range of motion. But toe clips have two major drawbacks. The first is that they can cause the feet to go numb when the feet are in them. The second drawback is getting out of them. To release a foot from a toe clip, the rider must loosen the toe strap first before pulling the foot up (out of the cleat) and out of the toe clip. Many riders either forget to loosen the strap or can't react fast enough and fall over to the side, still attached to the bike at the pedal! Usually these falls happen at slow speed or when just barely moving, so the greatest injury is usually to the ego and not the body.

- *Clipless pedals:* These are safer, faster, and more comfortable! Bicycling borrowed a page from the alpine skiing technology book when it came out with the clipless pedal. "Good-bye foot numbness, hello easy access and exiting ability." Clipless pedals mimic the downhill ski-boot-binding system, yet with a sleeker, lighter, bicycle-specific adaptation/application. These funny-looking devices keep the cyclist's foot firmly in place, which is actually on top of the pedal. Some even allow for wiggle room while the foot is cleated in. To get into a clipless pedal, the rider steps

Clipless Pedals

Clipless pedals provide for efficient, comfortable pedaling because the rider's foot, shoe, and cleat are securely attached to the pedal at the bottom of the shoe. The clipless system makes getting the feet in and out of the pedal easier and safer than with a traditional toe clip system. In a traditional toe clip and pedal system the foot may move about and toe clips can cause numbness from pressure on top of the foot.

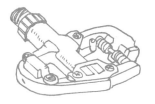

Out of the City but Not Out of the Woods

Five cyclists left behind the challenges of city street riding and met for a morning ride in the country. Riding far out on a beautiful country road, they suddenly heard what sounded like an animal chasing them. They couldn't see the animal because of the long vine-covered fence. One of the cyclists yelled a warning to the others: "Doggie on the right, behind the fence." In an instant, the spooked "doggie" changed course and jumped over the fence, crossing the road right in front of the lead riders. The lead riders, luckily, were able to avoid the fleeing animal and hold their line. After the "doggie" crossed their path, it became obvious that the "doggie" was actually Bambi (a deer). The moral of the story is that when riding in the country, you need to be aware of deer, dogs, cats, chipmunks, skunks, and squirrels who may cross your path. Always be on the lookout, whether in the city or country.

Aerodynamics or Comfort?

Remember the advertisement in which friendly bickering takes place about whether the product "tastes great" or is "less filling"? The same type of positive argument is made by those who use aerobars. Some claim the benefit is the aerodynamic advantage; others claim the improved comfort is the major benefit. They are both right.

• • •

A Dentist's Advice for Bicyclists

"Doctor, do I have to floss all of my teeth? It's so hard to get to all of them," a patient complained. The dentist replied, "Only floss those you want to keep."
Wear It Right! Wearing a helmet improperly is like saying, "I only care about protecting this little section of my head; the rest of it is expendable."
The moral of the story: Floss all your teeth and wear your helmet properly.

into the cleat until a clicking sound is made, indicating that the pedal has received the cleat. To exit a clipless pedal, the rider simply pulls the foot up and out, away from the bike. The exiting, pulling action starts with leverage from rotating the heel out and continues with pull coming from the rest of the leg. The learning curve for getting in and out of clipless pedals is short and can be easily practiced on the bike. Once mastered, cyclists enjoy the freedom and strength they get from using clipless pedals.

• *Helmet:* Absolutely, positively wear one. Since you care about being fit, you obviously already care about protecting your head. Even if you are an experienced rider, you can't control the other entities that could force you off your bike unexpectedly. Hard 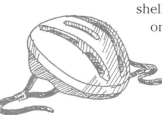 shell ANSI or Snell approved helmets are recommended, and when it comes to quality, you do not want to skimp here. Most helmets are designed as one-crash helmets. That means they have a life of one crash. Some of the reputable companies will replace your helmet if you send the cracked helmet to them along with your crash story. (Sounds odd at first, but after all, it is their business.) The biggest error made by novice cyclists is not wearing the helmet properly. It should fit snugly enough so that even before you tighten and secure the straps, it should firmly grasp your head without moving around. The helmet should rest toward the front of the forehead, NOT slanted up at an angle, and should cover the entire top of the head.

• *Shoes:* If you are going to ride, you will want to get bicycling shoes. They have a very firm, inflexible bottom and a place for a cleat. The cleat provides added resistance against the pedal and adds strength to your pedal stroke. Shoes and cleats for mountain and road bikes are different, so make sure you specify which you want.

• *Gloves:* These resemble the rough guys' knuckle covers in the old movies because the fingers are covered up only to the first set of knuckles. This allows for finger dexterity and ventilation. The padding on the inside reduces the friction that comes from prolonged riding or unexpected bouncing and jarring. Gloves help prevent blistering and reduce overall stress in your hands. They protect your skin from road rash in the event of a fall. The least publicized (until now) but much appreciated role the glove fills is that of being a convenient handkerchief. You may wish you had a real handkerchief (remember necessity IS the mother of invention), but . . . you don't. And for some reason, when people exercise, their noses have a tendency to run and/or the corners of their mouths get a residue/saliva buildup. Enter the all-too-convenient glove(s) that can easily wipe away these bodily responses and make you feel better while riding. In case you are wondering, bicycling gloves *are* washable.

- *Glasses:* Protect your eyes from the sun, wind, dirt, dust, and other airborne particles hanging around. Sport-style glasses are designed to be lightweight and somewhat flexible. This means they will be comfortable even after many hours of wearing them. They are also highly durable, and as with most glasses, they will last a long time—as long as you keep track of them.

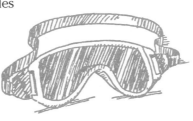

- *Biking shorts:* Once you ride in biking shorts, you won't want to ride without them. That's because of the strategically placed seams and padding. The old style shorts featured a chamois, a soft pliable leather used for padding. But with today's high-tech fabrics, the leather chamois is nearly history. Synthetic chamois, as they are now known, will delight your personal parts with added support, comfort, and durability. Aside from the chamois, the shorts are made from a stretch type of material such as Lycra, spandex, and Supplex, which offer support to the hips and leg muscles. They also help to prevent chafing along the leg and groin area.

- *Biking jerseys:* Bicycling is all about being practical and self-sufficient. The bike jersey serves that purpose with its multi-pocketed back. Riders can fit most items in their back pockets

Was Arte Wearing Toe Clips?

Most riders who have used toe clips can recall at least once how their experience in toe clips imitated art or, at least, television. Arte Johnson's character on *Laugh-In* rode his tricycle down the street and then inexplicably fell over sideways onto the ground. Ouch! Was he wearing toe clips? Suffice it to say that such accidents bruise the ego more than the body!

• • •

Just for Fun, Unicycle!

Unicycles are not just for circuses. For the ultimate challenge in balance and coordination, learn to ride one. Yes, that's uni, as in one wheel. Although you may not get aerobic riding one, the accomplishment of doing so is exhilarating and can take your breath away.

Fixing a Flat

Flat tires happen, and if you ride a bicycle enough, you will get the opportunity to change a tire.

A patch kit is used to secure a tube with a hole in it. The downside of patching a tube is that first you have to find the hole. When you are out riding, it isn't exactly the way you want to spend your time. So when time matters, just put in a new spare tube and patch the punctured tube later at a more convenient time.

Tire levers are short flat pieces of either plastic or metal that help you to prop the tire away from the rim of the wheel so that you can access the tube.

such as bananas (the cyclists' "meal in a peel"), sports foods, money, cell phones, identification, clothing, and many other items. All are within an arm's reach. Whereas experienced riders can reach behind and retrieve the desired item from their pocket while riding without losing control of the bike, novice riders may want to stop riding before retrieving these items. Bicycling jerseys are also designed for aerodynamic efficiency and safety. A proper fit is a snug, yet comfortable fit. Wearing a baggy shirt while bicycling is dysfunctional and dangerous because it can get caught in your knees and even your chain (leaning over or down)!

- *Miscellaneous clothing: Arm warmers, leg warmers, paper jacket, booties.* These items are great and worth the money if you are a regular cyclist. Arm warmers look like a long pair of thin Lycra socks with the feet removed. They keep the arms warm without encumbering or restricting movement. The same description can be given for leg warmers, except they are wider to accommodate your legs. The last time you wore *booties* you were probably too young to walk in them. Here's your chance to bootie-up again, but it is best to avoid walking in these too—because these booties were made for riding, not walking. Booties protect cyclists' feet from the cold air that can numb feet quicker than you can say "where are my toes?" They are made from soft flexible fabrics that have some "give" to them. They slip over the front of the biking shoe and, generally, zip up the back of the ankle. They also have a space to accommodate the cleat.

- *Floor pump:* This is not the pump you carry on your bike; it's the one you use before you ride away. Although you may get anaerobic using it, it is much easier to use than your bike/frame pump for inflating tires because it exerts a lot of air pressure with each pumping action.

- *Fluids:* Two options for carrying fluids (which, of course, you will remember to drink a lot of) are two water bottles held in the bicycle's water bottle cages. Most bikes have room for two cages. Or you can use a hands-free drinking system that you wear like a backpack. For really hot and/or humid days, you may want to use both bottles and a hands-free system. The advantage is that you are able to carry a variety of fluids such as water and electrolyte replacements.

- *Other miscellaneous equipment:* Other items that might prove useful include air cartridges for speedy tire inflation, sunscreen, lip balm, paper money, and coins for a pay phone.

Here are some safety tips for riding:

1. The left-handed brake lever slows the front wheel; the right-handed brake lever slows the rear wheel. When you apply the front (left) brake, do so gently to avoid the force of your weight throwing you forward and overboard (or rather, "overbike"). To slow down or stop, "feather" the brakes, which means alternating between squeezing and releasing them. It keeps you from being thrown off the bike, and it keeps your brakes from overheating and becoming less effective.

2. Be in control of your bike and speed at all times. Reckless abandon has no place on a bike and can produce some unnecessary and dangerous results.

3. When you ride on the street alongside parked cars, keep an eye out for drivers and passengers who are opening their car doors and don't see you coming.

4. When you are unsure about a vehicle's next move, look at the vehicle's wheels. If the wheels have the least bit of motion, then watch out. Even when it appears that a driver is looking right at you, it is not safe to assume that you are seen. Glare and other distractions play a large factor in drivers' inability to see a cyclist.

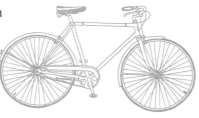

5. Know bicycling etiquette. Communicate to your fellow cyclists. Common biking jargon includes calling out "on your left" to indicate when you are passing someone. Also, if cyclists are riding close behind you, it is good biking etiquette to literally point out with your finger or hand debris on the road that they may not be able to see because they are close behind you, or "on your wheel."

The Cost of Bicycling

Following are some average costs or price ranges of bicycling equipment:

Bikes ....$300–$1000+
Aerobars ....$40+
Helmet...............$30–$150
Cleats ....$15–$25
Shoes ....$60–$200
Toe clips/ $6
   straps
Gloves ....$12–$30
Clipless pedals $50–160
   (cleats come with pedals)
Glasses ....$17–$100
Tires and tubes....$4–$50
Biking shorts ....$25–$80
Bicycle ....$15–$90
   computer
Biking jersey........$21–$70
Frame pump........$8–$30
Arm warmers $15
Floor pump ....$25–$50
Leg warmers........$25
Saddle pouch ......$6–$12
Booties ....$25–$45
Patch kit $3
Tire levers $3
Air cartridges $12
Wind trainer $105
Rollers $170

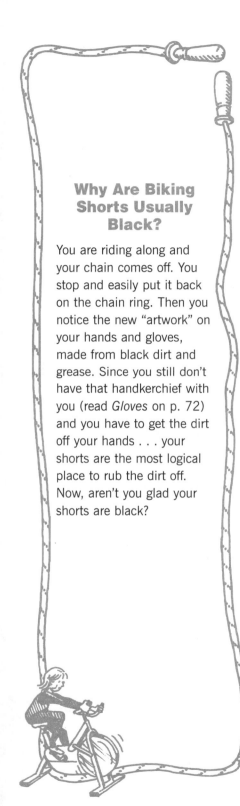

Why Are Biking Shorts Usually Black?

You are riding along and your chain comes off. You stop and easily put it back on the chain ring. Then you notice the new "artwork" on your hands and gloves, made from black dirt and grease. Since you still don't have that handkerchief with you (read *Gloves* on p. 72) and you have to get the dirt off your hands . . . your shorts are the most logical place to rub the dirt off. Now, aren't you glad your shorts are black?

6. STOP! *It's the law.* Bicyclists must observe traffic signals/signs and should use hand signals to alert others when turning or stopping.

Swimming

The gentlest of all aerobic activities is swimming. Although the motion has zero impact on your skeletal system, it makes a big impact on your fitness and health. Water is a healing medium and is especially recommended for those who want to prevent injury, use it for cross training, are pregnant, are recovering from an injury, are suffering from joint or bone conditions, or are overweight and want to exercise in a weightless environment. You can build muscular strength and endurance, as well as improve flexibility and cardiovascular fitness, through swimming. If you swim for the aerobic benefit, do not be concerned that your heart rate does not get as high as it does during other activities. The loss of gravitational force, the horizontal position, and the cooling effect of the water temperature all contribute toward keeping your heart rate low. This does not mean that your aerobic efforts are in vain. Remember, aerobic exercise is about oxygen utilization, and the heart rate is just a mirror for what is happening on an oxygen level. But in this case, the mirror is reflecting a hazy and distorted picture of what's really going on. Even though the conditions in swimming produce relatively lower heart rate numbers, your body is still processing oxygen, and that's what counts! A general rule is that the swimming heart rate is typically 10 to 20 beats per minute less than what it is for dry land activities. As long as you apply the Overload Principle of intensity (RPE of "somewhat hard" to "hard"), you will be aerobic.

Learn to swim: If you did not have the opportunity to learn to swim as a child, it is never too late to learn. Many adults who do not know how to swim have justifiable fear about water and regret how their lives have been limited because of it. For many adults, facing their fear and learning how to swim proves to be as much a psychological relief as it is an enjoyable lifetime fitness activity. They no longer fear going to the beach, to the lake, on a boat, on a cruise, being around children in water, or around other anxiety-producing, water-related circumstances. Your community recreation centers will have information on beginning swimming lessons.

If you already know how to swim but feel like you are treading water more than swimming, a few lessons can make the difference between frustration and enjoyment and continuity. Another way to enjoy and enhance your swimming experience is to swim with the Masters. Masters swim is an organized group that meets to swim structured workouts made up of intervals and technique drills. Many communities that have a public recreational pool offer a Masters swim program. Masters groups meet several times a week at many locations and offer instruction, motivation, support, social interaction, and fun. Ask your local schools, community centers, and athletic clubs/gyms about Masters programs at their pools.

Open water swimming: If you are privileged enough to live near an outdoor body of water, expand your swimming horizons to include aquatic workouts in open water. The freedom of swimming without walls, lines, and chlorine is very uplifting. Add to that swimming in a beautiful outdoor environment, and you are set for a peak experience. For safety reasons, it is best to swim accompanied either by other swimmers or watercraft enthusiasts such as canoeists, kayakers, rowboaters, or surfboard paddlers.

If you plan to be out in the water for a long time or on a hot day, your watercraft chaperone can carry drinking water or electrolyte replacement fluids. Swimming, like all other aerobic activities, causes the body to lose fluids. But because you are in a cool fluid environment, it is nearly impossible to notice the sweat you produce. Add to that fluids lost from saliva and nasal secretions, and you can understand why you need to hydrate even while surrounded in water.

Stay abreast of the current weather and water conditions that will affect your safety, such as tides, undertow, strong waves (even in big lakes), and temperature. Your local parks or recreation department may have valuable information about the water that you plan to swim in.

Wet suits: Normal body temperature is 98.6 degrees, and the colder the water you swim in, the faster your body temperature is lowered. If the water temperature feels uncomfortably cool, consider using a wet suit—not a scuba diver's wet suit but the type worn by triathletes. They are made of a thinner, lighter, sleeker neoprene than those used for diving and are designed to allow a full range of motion in the shoulders, as well as greater all-around unrestricted movement. Their effectiveness comes from capturing and reflecting your body temperature

The Cost of Swimming

Following are some average costs of swimming equipment:

Swim suit........$12–$50
Swim cap........$2–$12
Goggles ....$4–$27
Earplugs..........$2
Noseplugs $5
Kickboard........$13
Pull-buoy $13
Hand paddles..$13
Fins...............$15–$40

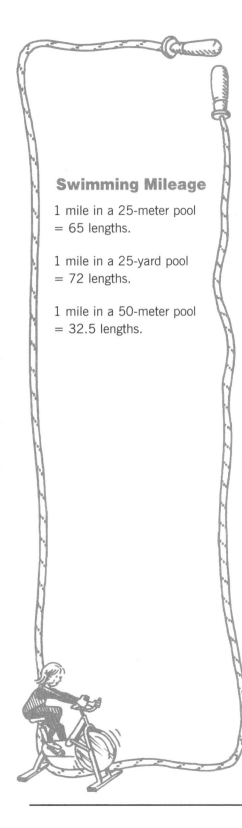

Swimming Mileage

1 mile in a 25-meter pool = 65 lengths.

1 mile in a 25-yard pool = 72 lengths.

1 mile in a 50-meter pool = 32.5 lengths.

back to you, which keeps you warm. They give you a slight feeling of buoyancy, which can be comforting.

Swimming wet suits come in many styles. The warmest style has full-length arms and legs, and the coolest version is sleeveless and runs calf length. When trying on a wet suit on dry land, it should fit very snugly; it will give just a bit once in the water. A definite must when using a wet suit is to apply a lubricant around your neck so that the turning-breathing motion doesn't cause your skin to chafe. Non-petroleum lubricants such as Body Glide are recommended, rather than petroleum-based products (petroleum jellies or gels) because of the damaging effect they have on the wet suit.

Beanies: When you want some added warmth from cool water but a wet suit is more than what you need, try a neoprene beanie. A majority of your body heat escapes from your head, even when you are swimming. In moderately cool waters, a beanie can provide enough additional heat reflection to keep you comfortable. Wet suit companies also manufacture these (see Appendix).

Dolphin and Polar Bear Clubs: In addition to Masters swim groups, there are open water swim groups that meet regularly. Appropriately named Dolphin and Polar Bear Clubs, you can locate them through your local or US Masters Swim Association (see Appendix). It is surprising, but even in cool waters, most of these swimmers do not wear wet suits. Their bodies have adapted to the temperature with a thin layer of body fat that seems to insulate them. But if you are considering swimming with the Dolphins and Polar Bears, and the no-wet suit factor is inhibiting you, don't let it. Wear it and join the swim.

Seasonal: Swim outside when possible so that you can get the therapeutic benefits of the natural air environment. However, the sun's reflection off the water is powerful, so remember to use waterproof and sweatproof sunscreen (without these two capabilities, it won't stay on for long) on your face and the back side of your body. Indoor swimming can be a year-round activity, which is a big plus because it is reliable. It is always nice to have options for those times when the weather does not cooperate with your outdoor plans.

Risk: Swimming when you are exhausted is not a good idea; neither is swimming alone, before you are a competent swimmer. If you kick too hard off the wall when swimming lengths, you can hurt your knees and even cause cramping in your legs. Training too vigorously without a proper warm-up or with swim apparatus is an easy way to injure your shoulders, hips, and knees. And swimming with your eyes closed could get you an unexpected run-in with another swimmer or even the wall. Therefore, get some goggles! Otherwise, there is not much risk involved. So become a competent swimmer, keep your eyes open, and the rest should be easy.

Swimming Pools: If you want to swim, you have to have water, and most people resort to the swimming pool. There is also a tank-style swimming device that you can set up in your home for "stationary swimming." But for most folks, the $15,000 plus price tag rules it out. Aside from home- or hotel-style swimming pools, most are either 25 meters, 25 yards, or 50 meters long. If you like to motivate yourself by counting the number of lengths (and the time it takes), you can then figure the distance swum and chart your progress. If it took you 45 minutes to swim a mile 3 months ago, and now you're doing it in 35, you know you have gotten faster and fitter.

Swimsuit: Swimsuits are functionally designed for performance and allow for comfort, reduced drag, and ease of movement in the water. With the many designs available, you can certainly find one that is attractive, supportive, and comfortable. When trying on a swimsuit, make sure the seams are comfortable around the legs (and for women, around the upper area too). If the body of the suit is made of Lycra or spandex (as most are), it should feel slightly snug when you try it on because it is designed to expand slightly in the water to a comfortable fit. However, the seams and joints will not expand, even when wet, so make sure they are comfortable when dry.

Some of the best-looking suits can be literal pains in the rear (or front) if they don't fit you properly. So go for comfort, and if it does not feel good, try a different suit. There is a big differ-

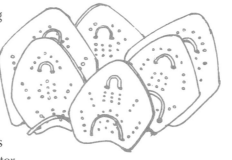

Training Paddle
Training paddles help simulate the proper feel of hand action during the stroke and build shoulder strength. The hand slips entirely through the larger rubber band, the middle finger slips under the smaller rubber band, and the paddle and the hand are as one unit.

Swim Apparatus

- *Kickboard:* You don't kick *it*; you kick *with* it. This Styrofoam board helps stabilize your body position (you grasp the sides with your hands) so that you can practice your kick.

- *Training paddles:* These thin hand-sized hard-plastic sheets with thick rubber semicircles through which you insert your fingers exaggerate awareness of the hand and shoulder positions and motions so that you get a feel for how your hands should be in the water. They keep you from slicing through the water and reinforce the correct technique of "grabbing," or "pulling and pushing," the water. They are also used to strengthen the arm and shoulder muscles by creating a larger surface area of resistance (there's that Overload Principle again).

Swim Apparatus

- *Pull-buoy:* Here's another Styrofoam device. Placed between your thighs, it keeps your legs afloat, the body in a horizontal position, and isolates the upper body so that you can practice your arm stroke technique.

- *Fins:* Your feet slip inside these. Kicking with fins will make you feel turbo-powered in the water. It is hard to kick inefficiently with fins, but it is easy to kick too hard, so be careful. They put greater resistance on the quadriceps, hamstrings, and gluteal muscles, which strengthens your legs. They also create greater flexibility in the ankles, which makes for better kicking motion.

ence between a swimming suit and a bathing suit. Unless you are open to the idea of skinny-dipping and performing a bathing-suit-recovery-exercise, save your skimpiest, least functional bathing briefs or bikini suit for leisurely water activities and swim in your swimsuit. To enhance the lifespan of your swimsuit, rinse it out thoroughly in tap water after each use and let it drip dry without wringing the life out of it. Chlorine, salt water, and lake residue can wear the fibers out prematurely. While you are at it, rinse your goggles too.

Swim cap: This little cap does more than you might think. A swim cap protects your hair from total chlorine immersion, keeps your hair from clogging up the pool filters, helps keep your goggles in place, keeps your hair out of your face, and keeps your head warm. If your regular latex swim cap likes to eat your hair, use a silicone cap. It is softer, easier to apply and remove, and your hair will stay on your head where it belongs. If regulating your temperature is a concern, use a latex cap in warmer environments and silicone in colder ones.

Goggles: Goggles are used for seeing underwater and to keep your eyes dry and out of the chlorine. The fit is very individual; however, even good goggles can fog up occasionally, so check that they are snug against your face but not so much that you get a headache or temporary tattoo. Try them on and see which ones cover your eye sockets best. Most have an adjustable head strap, and some also have an adjustable nose bridge, which you can use to tailor the goggle distance between the eyes. Occasionally, it is good to clean your goggles with soap and water. This removes the gradual buildup of facial oils that can cause the goggles to fog.

Earplugs and noseplugs: Many people do not like putting their head in the water because the water seeps into their ear holes quicker than a mosquito on a hot balmy night. If you are one of them, a cheap pair of swimmer's earplugs is a quick fix. Some are made from plastic and others from silicone, which, when warmed by your body heat, form to your ear hole. And if water up the nose and sinuses is irritating, use a noseplug. Once again, the fit and comfort is very individual.

Instruction: Swimming is an aerobic, skill-oriented, stretching activity that improves nearly everything in your body except bone density (since it is not weight bearing). The skills and ability to swim are stored in your muscle memory, which means that when you take a break from it, you don't "forget" how to swim. It also means you can make improvements at any age. The four competitive strokes are crawl (freestyle), backstroke, breaststroke, and butterfly. Two strokes that are less strenuous and can provide a type of swim-rest are the sidestroke and elementary backstroke. Each stroke has an upper shoulder/arm action and a lower hip/leg kick action with proper mechanics.

Freestyle is the most efficient of them all and the one most swimmers use for fitness. *Butterfly* is the most technically challenging and requires the most flexibility and coordination. Because it is the most physically demanding, it cannot be sustained for long periods of time. *Backstroke* also requires and improves flexibility and can feel like the greatest stretch of your life. Each arm reaches over and behind your head and then enters the water at full extension above the head and pulls down along the side of the body to your upper thigh. *Breaststroke* is fun to do and requires good timing. But if you have sore knees, you might avoid breast-stroke because of the lateral movement involved in the kick.

Swimming efficiently comes from practicing your technique. Even accomplished swimmers devote time to the basics. Swimming is considered to be 70 percent dependent on mechanical efficiency and 30 percent on fitness ability. Efficient swimmers can stroke and glide quickly across the pool using as few as twelve strokes versus the twenty or more it can take for less efficient swimmers. The power originates from the center of the body's mass, the hips. It is a gentle way to enjoy aerobic exercise because during the exercise, the muscles are elongated with less contraction than in other weight-bearing activities. This can balance out the effects of other impact activities. Regardless of the stroke you choose, you want to create a productive glide, a smooth continuous advancing motion. Your reward is the fun, the feel, and ease of swimming like Flipper (the 1970s dolphin TV star).

Freestyle—arm/hand/shoulder action: The stroke alternates between the left and right arms. Think of the hands as paddles. When the fingers are close together, the hand can pull the water more efficiently than when the fingers are spread open. Reach forward with a fully extended arm and use the hand to pull the water behind and beside your hip. As you pull, you will feel the water against the inside of your palm moving behind you, which propels you forward. Once the pulling arm is extended to the level of the upper thigh, it begins the recovery phase and repeats. This pulling action can be challenging for

Above the Neck, Very Individual

Perhaps we have discovered a theme in regard to the fit of equipment. It seems that the head area is more sensitive to individual differences—maybe because it is closer to the brain. In any case, you can usually try on goggles before you buy them. But earplugs and noseplugs are, thankfully, nonreturnable. So you will have to risk a few dollars (they are inexpensive) to find the right fit. But it's worth it.

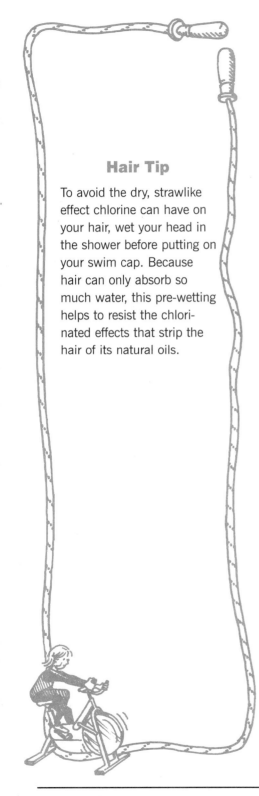

Hair Tip

To avoid the dry, strawlike effect chlorine can have on your hair, wet your head in the shower before putting on your swim cap. Because hair can only absorb so much water, this pre-wetting helps to resist the chlorinated effects that strip the hair of its natural oils.

those with weak triceps (muscle on the back of the upper arm) and shoulders. The good news is that this stroke will strengthen them.

Hips: The body rolls from side to side causing a purposeful rotation, allowing the water to slip by. During this rotation, the gluteal muscles (your buttocks) move the center of your mass from side to side. The hips roll to a rhythm. The shoulders and arms are in sync with the hip rhythm and rotation. Good freestylers (and backstrokers) spend little time on their front or back sides and a lot of time rotating from side to side.

Freestyle leg/hip/foot action: The kick motion is gentle, not forceful, and originates from your hips, not from your knees. The range of motion is shallow rather than deep. A loud thumping sound and big splash are indications that you are kicking too much air. The feet are relaxed yet extended so that the toes follow a horizontal line with the rest of your body.

The largest muscles in the body are from the waist down, and they use the most oxygen. When you see swimmers splashing vigorously, gasping for air at the end of the pool, they are usually swimming with the belief that the "engine power" comes from the kick, but that is not the case. The real purpose of the legs is to help maintain the ideal horizontal body position and to do so by kicking naturally, not forcefully.

Freestyle breathing: You have two choices to make about breathing. You can choose to breathe on the same side each time or to alternate breathing between your left and right sides, called bilateral breathing. For same-side breathing, breathe every two (or other even number of) strokes and for alternate breathing, breathe every three (or other odd number of) strokes. Most people are used to one-sided breathing and find it awkward to breathe on the opposite side. The benefits of bilateral breathing are that you can see other swimmers on either side and you will strengthen and stretch the muscles on both sides of your neck.

Let's say you decide to breathe on your right side only. As your right hand pulls and slides past your hip, your body rolls to your side so that you are facing the sidewall of the pool. Your head rolls with your body until your mouth clears the water. After you've taken your breath, roll back with your body until your head resumes its normal face-down position. Slowly release the air simultaneously through your nose and mouth until it is time to breathe again.

Swimming lengths continuously each time you swim can be boring. Work in some variety with intervals and drills using pull-buoys, paddles, fins, and a kickboard. An example would be to warm up for 5 to 10 minutes by swimming lengths and then vary the intensity level by grouping together numbers of lengths. For example, swim your warm-up and follow it with five sets of 50 meters (two lengths) at moderate speed. After each set, take a short rest period, say 15 to 30 seconds, before starting the next set. After completing those five sets, you can do a few lengths of stroke and kicking drills. Then return to length swimming in sets of varying numbers. Remember to cool down when you are finished with the intensity part of your swim. (For more on interval training, see Chapter 4.)

Pre-swimming etiquette: Most pools post signs asking you to shower before entering the pool. Removing body oils, aftershave, perfume, and sweat before getting in the water helps keep the water cleaner and may help reduce the amount of chlorine used to keep the water clean. The one sign that is not typically posted but would be a healthy reminder is the "empty your bladder before swimming" sign. Some people are so excited and/or pressed for time that they quickly change their clothes and head right into the pool when suddenly their bladder begs for attention. Don't be one of them.

Swimming etiquette—lane-sharing: Some pools have designated rules about lane-sharing. If there is no sign posted and all the lanes are occupied, wait a few moments and survey the situation. Find a lane where the swimmer or swimmers swim similarly to you. "Similarly" can mean either stroke or speed. For example, if you plan to swim freestyle, it could be risky to share a lane with someone doing backstroke or elementary backstroke. And if you are slower than the shark that is swimming in the same lane with you, it could be uncomfortable for each of you.

Unless the swimmer is swimming for time intervals, it is generally acceptable to interrupt and to ask to share the lane. If the swimmer is rigorously swimming intervals, wait until a rest/break in the workout to interrupt. Pregnant swimmers or swimmers nursing a serious injury, in which being kicked would pose a serious threat to their health, should not share lanes.

Before you share the lane, ask the swimmer how he or she prefers to share the lane. If it is just the two of you, it is acceptable and oftentimes preferred to split the lane into left and right halves, claiming one

Dog Paddle

Good ol' dog paddling will keep you afloat, but if you watch a dog swim, you will see how quickly he fatigues. And so will you. Learn the other strokes and leave the paddling to the pooch.

• • •

A Lap or a Length?

Is swimming from one side of the pool to the other considered a lap or a length? A length refers to the length of the pool, which is usually 25 yards or meters. A lap refers to a sort of circuit, which in this case means when you start at one end, reach the other end, and return to where you started. A lap is typically 50 yards or meters.

side for each swimmer. For situations in which there are multiple swimmers in one lane, you swim in a counterclockwise direction. Think of it as traveling in the flow of vehicular traffic, in the United States, by staying to the right side. In this case, stay on the right side of the black line on the bottom of the pool.

In-line Skating

This outdoor fitness activity has often been better known by the brand name that introduced it, Roller Blade or roller blading. Since the debut of Roller Blades in 1980, other manufacturers have also been producing these "ice skates on wheels." An in-line skate closely resembles an alpine ski boot, and the four-in-a-row wheel alignment resembles a wheeled ice skate.

In-line skating can be aerobic; it works the gluteal (rear end) muscles; and it refreshes the areas of the brain responsible for balance and coordination. It can also humble even the experienced skater with a single fall. Adults typically work hard to master in-line skating; kids seem to pick it up quickly and keep on going without missing a beat. Learning in-line skating is great for your sense of humor as long as you are able to laugh at yourself.

The motion: The skating motion is alternating your legs, pushing sideways against the ground, then gliding. This works the very large and powerful lateral muscles of the hips and buttocks, so it is easy to gain speed quickly. Gliding swiftly over the pavement on your feet is fun. But until you have mastered slowing and stopping, the fun can come to an unplanned and abrupt halt. So if you are mentally ready for the experience, be prepared with the right equipment and practice your stopping and slowing skills. You can consider yourself an experienced skater when you can control your skates and stop at will.

Seasonal: Whenever the ground is clear and dry, you can skate. If it is snowing, change over to your ice skates and hit the rink. In the fall months, watch for fallen leaves and debris that can interrupt a nice glide.

Equipment—In-line skates: the boots should fit snugly so that your feet do not move around inside them. This gives you better control when you are skating. The boot (or bootie) is usually a foam interior covered in hard-shell plastic, which gives you some ventilation and comfort. If you have weak ankles, this may not be the sport for you. Or maybe it could be—you will surely build ankle strength if you can stay with it long enough.

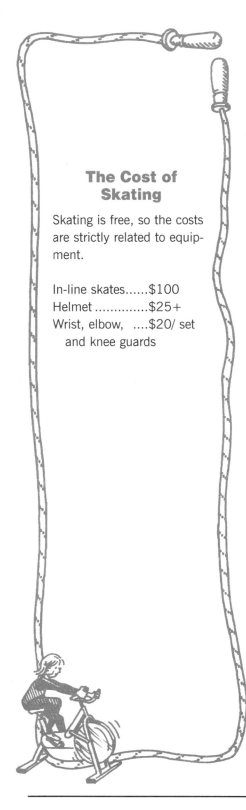

The Cost of Skating

Skating is free, so the costs are strictly related to equipment.

In-line skates......$100
Helmet ....$25+
Wrist, elbow, ...$20/ set
   and knee guards

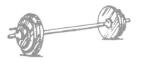
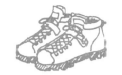
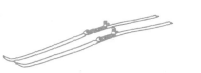

Sample Swim Workouts

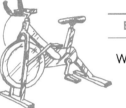

Many swim centers will have sample workouts posted on the board near the pool that you can follow for your workout. Do not be intimidated by the numbers and symbols. They are usually written in abbreviations, so if you forget what they represent, ask someone nearby to help. Note that the designations are given in either yards or meters, not in numbers of lengths. It is generally assumed that the stroke used is freestyle, unless it is specifically designated otherwise. Of course, you can apply your choice of strokes to the workout. Here are some examples:

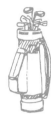

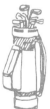

BEGINNER WORKOUT	INTERMEDIATE WORKOUT	ADVANCED WORKOUT
Warm-up 1 x 100 swim	Warm-up 1 x 300	Warm-up 1 x 500
1 x 100 P	1 x 300 P	10 x 50 K R:10
1 x 100 K	1 x 200 K	4 x 150 P R:20
4 x 50 S R:20	4 x 100 S R:15	10 x 100 (alternating
Cool-down 200 easy	8 x 25 S R:10	100 H R:20
Total 700 yards	Cool-down 100 easy	100 E R:15)
or meters	**Total 1500 yards**	8 x 25 sprint
	or meters	Cool-down 200 easy
		Total 3000 yards
		or meters

K = kick (kicking drill using kickboard)
P = pull (pulling drill with pull-buoy and/or training paddles)
H = hard (very intense effort)
E = easy (light effort)
R:20 = rest 20 seconds between each exercise
S = sprint

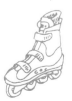

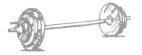
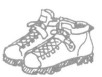
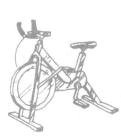

Basketball

Basketball is extremely aerobic when played with intensity by yourself, one-on-one, two-on-two, or more, as long as you are moving continuously. You do not have to play like Michael Jordan to enjoy a workout with the round ball. In fact, even if you play solitary basketball, you get a lot of exercise from shooting, dribbling, and chasing after the ball (you *will* miss sometimes). When you play with some intensity, you use just about all of your muscles when running, passing, shooting, catching, jumping, and smiling (it is fun!). Your brain will enjoy the refresher course in hand-eye coordination, agility, and the kinesthetic activities of balancing, jumping, and leaping. And if you keep score, you can even practice your mathematical skills.

(continued on next page)

Helmet: In-line skating helmets cover your head from front to rear. If you already have a bicycling helmet, that is a decent substitute, but be aware that it does not cover as much of the back of your head as the in-line skating helmet.

The guards—wrist, elbow, and knee: These are highly recommended, especially if your work is dependent upon your hands (all you computer users take note!) or legs. If you approach in-line skating with the preventive expectation that at some point (and probably many) you will fall, these protective pieces are worth wearing. Think of them as cheap insurance and less expensive than a trip to the emergency room.

Instruction: To get started, wear the skates on a thick soft surface (grass or carpet) and practice walking and balancing in them. Progress to a vacant parking lot or school yard and practice the basic movements of skating, gliding, turning, and stopping. Slowing and stopping come from the rear of the skate (for you former roller skaters, it is *opposite* of what you remember) and require you to angle the braking skate toe-up so that the heel and brake go down. It will take a little time to perfect this; be patient and have a sense of humor.

Etiquette: When skating on the road, go with the flow of traffic. You are bound by vehicular laws, signs, and signals, so act accordingly. Be considerate of runners, walkers, and bicyclists. There is a good chance that they are wary of you because out of the four of these different athletes—runners, walkers, bicyclists, and in-line skaters—you are probably the least stable on your feet, and they want to avoid you. Keep that in mind and slow down when passing or coming upon them from behind. Borrowing the bicyclists' warning motto, "on your left," before passing is a wise thing to do.

Organized Outdoor Activities

Hiking: Check out the weather forecast before heading out for a long hike. Hiking will clear your head and work your body. Wear close-toed supportive shoes or boots, carry food, water, a map, and/or compass, and you are set. Make sure you know how to get back.

Par Course: Made popular in the late 1970s and early 1980s, these trail courses are the "treasure hunt" version of exercise. Your series of clues are the exercise stations, and your *treasure* is the fun fitness experience outdoors. By design, you run/jog short distances along the numbered trail until you come to a station, where you will see instructions about exercises to perform. If the exercise calls for equipment, not to worry; it is waiting there for you. Benefits include aerobic conditioning, flexibility, muscular strength, and endurance. Remember, for it to be aerobic, you want to keep your heart rate up, so keep moving even when you are at the exercise stations. You can find par courses along designated bike trails, at university campuses, state parks, and even some housing complexes/subdivisions.

Winter/Snow-Related Exercise Activities

Just because winter brings about cold and snow does not mean you have to hibernate or lose fitness. Even for high-caliber athletes, the concept of "on season-off season" has been replaced with "fitness year-round."

Another reason to be active in the winter is to feed the brain light and produce endorphins. These appear somewhat effective in combating a condition known as seasonal affective disorder (SAD). Many people become depressed in winter from the lack of sun and light exposure. The brain not only wants its glucose (as you will learn in Chapter 9), but it also wants light. And for many people, a light-starved brain can cause depression. Two forms of treatment include physical activity (calling up those endorphins again!) and exposure to light. Exercising outdoors, even if the sun is not shining, will keep you fit and help combat SAD. Even if you do not suffer from SAD, winter sports will keep you *fit* and happy.

Snow and fitness—benefits: If you are lucky enough to be close to snow and ski areas, you have three thrills to choose from: classic cross-country skiing, skate skiing (also called diagonal striding, a form of cross-country), and snow shoeing. These superb fitness activities will keep you aerobically and muscularly fit and psychologically elevated. Classic cross-country and skate skiing involve the muscles of the upper and lower body and your cardiovascular system. In fact, it is hard to think of a muscle that they do not involve. By nature of the sport (being out on trails), you will "overload" your muscles for both strength and muscular endurance, but with special emphasis on muscular endurance.

Basketball
(continued from previous page)

If you live in the city, most playgrounds and school yards have several courts, backboards, hoops, and nets. If you live in a residential neighborhood, attach a hoop and backboard to the house or garage, roll out one of the free-standing (on wheels) pole-style setups, or use your neighbor's (another social opportunity!). Playing basketball or shooting around in your neighborhood can be a magnet for social interaction. It is unclear whether it is the sight or the sound of the bouncing ball, but basketball lures others to come out of the woodwork and offer, "Hey, wanna shoot around?" James Naismith, basketball's founder, would have been thrilled to see how his game, started with fruit baskets and a ball, has grown and matured.

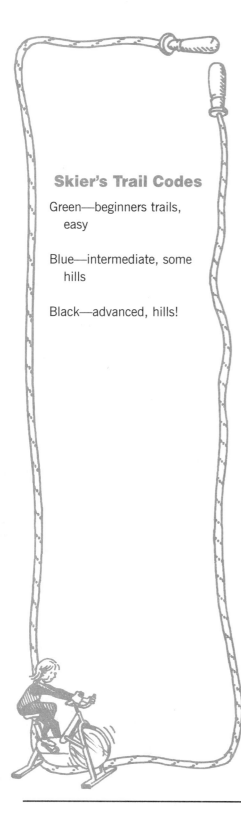

Skier's Trail Codes

Green—beginners trails, easy

Blue—intermediate, some hills

Black—advanced, hills!

Another benefit is that the whole family can go cross-country skiing; even young children learn and become very capable skiers quickly.

Risks: These activities are less risky and have fewer injuries associated with them as compared to alpine (downhill) skiing. That may be because they are not as crowded as alpine skiing runs and because they are generally performed at lower speeds as compared to downhill skiing. Of course, you can still land on your butt, but it is a lot more fun being on your butt in the snow and great outdoors than on the sofa watching another wintry day go by.

As in downhill skiing, you have a choice about the degree of difficulty for the trails you ski (see Skier's Trail Codes). Increased trail difficulty is not necessarily synonymous with fitness. Fitness can happen on green trails just as easily as it can on blue trails. Once again, it comes down to intensity. Just being suited up with skis, boots, and poles will not make you fit. You have to use them to move, and when you do, "fit happens."

If you are barely moving your upper and lower body, then oxygen utilization and heart rate are probably not at aerobic levels. But it does not take a lot of effort to be aerobic when cross-country skiing.

Equipment: You can rent skis, boots, and poles from the ski centers and, oftentimes, from retail stores that sell ski equipment. The skis and poles are both long and thin. The longer the ski, the more you will glide. The nice part about renting is that the skis have already been waxed and prepared for use. Wax is used to make the skis glide more efficiently over the snow. Skate skiing is less known, so do not assume that a retail store has skate skis to rent; make sure you ask before showing up. Renting equipment is convenient, inexpensive, and an opportunity to try out different types and sizes. If the sport grabs your soul and you decide to buy your own equipment, then you have a better idea of what to buy.

Clothing: Layering is the clothing theme for each of these activities. Get used to the idea that you may peel layers off while you are skiing or snow shoeing and be eager to put them back on when you stop for rest or a snack. You will work up a sweat, and the moisture wicking fabrics that are available are perfect for these sports (see Chapter 6). If you already have Supplex, Coolmax, or similar moisture wicking clothes that you use in other sports, you can wear them here too. These fabrics keep you warm and dry by keeping body heat close while moving moisture away from your body. The moisture evaporates and you stay dry and warm. Once you experience these fabrics you will become a moisture wicking fabric fan. It is also a good idea to wear gloves and a medium to thick sock made of either wool or the fabrics listed above. Your hands and feet will serve you well when skiing, as long as they are warm and dry enough to move normally.

Cost: Nordic skiing is significantly less expensive than its cousin, alpine skiing. There are trail fees, but they are a lot less than alpine lift tickets. If you do not live near a snowy climate, plan a trip to one. In the United States, there are plenty of places on both coasts and in between to ski. Plan a snow/fitness winter vacation by visiting relatives or friends who live near ski or snow areas. Skiing at a ski center allows you to ski on groomed trails, rest at warming huts along the way (where you can also replenish fluids), and picnic in the great outdoors. Crowds and congestion are usually not a problem in cross-country skiing (except in the bathroom and food lines at the main lodge) because there are literally miles and miles of trails. Plus, there are no lift lines, so you don't stand around getting cold in the process. The trails/runs are usually marked for difficulty and distance, but each skier should always carry at least one copy of the trail map. You do not always need groomed areas to snow shoe or ski classic. You can snow shoe and ski classic in the woods. But if you are a novice skier, it is best to wait for that until you become adept and confident.

Background: If you have experience in either alpine skiing, ice skating, roller skating, or in-line skating, you might find skate skiing easier to grasp. Alpine skiers actually skate for a few moments when they turn their ankles out to glide to the lift lines. Here is a review of the big three—classic, skating, and snow shoeing.

Classic Cross-Country Skiing

The best known of the two cross-country ski sports, classic is also referred to as diagonal striding. If you can shuffle your feet on skis, you are nearly there. Actually, there is more to it than that, so it is a good idea to take a short classic lesson before going out the very first time. But the basics are easy enough to learn that you can head out on the trail following your lesson. Mastering the technique, developing the strength to push, and having properly waxed skis for the conditions are the factors that determine the skier's speed.

One Fine Ski Day!

Imagine for a moment that you are surrounded by the pearly white snow, the aromatic pine trees, and the majestic mountains. You left your cell phone behind, you are unhurried, and you are using body power to propel yourself forward as you glide gently atop the snow. You feel the need for energy, so you stop for a picnic. You notice that everything tastes exaggeratedly good (because you are *very* hungry!). Then, when you finish eating, you get to ski again. Sounds like a pretty fine day!

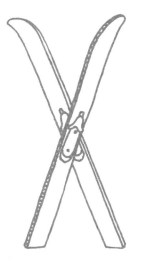

Ski centers groom their trails and carve into them snow-packed grooves the width of the skis. These are called parallel tracks and run the length of the trails. Classic skiers spend their time in the tracks. They also spend their time eating and replenishing their energy supply. The simplicity, outdoor beauty, and physical activity associated with classic skiing make it ripe for picnicking. When you prepare for cross-country skiing, put plenty of high-carbohydrate foods and snacks in your fanny pack. You will be hungry and grateful for every bite.

Cross-Country Skate Skiing

This event, born in the 1980s, grew out of the marathon skate event. During a race on the World Cup Circuit, American skater Bill Koch took one leg/ski out of the track and used it to push sideways, propelling himself forward and on to victory. This one episode triggered interest and other events that would lead to a new event known as skate skiing.

To a beginner, it may seem more physically demanding and faster moving than classic, but good classic skiers will argue that point. Skating has evolved from the "one foot in and one foot out of the track" to mostly skiing with both feet out of the tracks. Ski skating *is* what its name describes, skating on skis. Whereas classic skiing is more of a shuffle, the action in skating is alternating your legs, pushing sideways against the snow, and then gliding. The skis are long and thin, as are the poles. Your upper body gets a thorough workout because you use the poles to propel yourself by pushing off of the snow. The green trails will keep beginners pleasantly challenged yet smiling. For those who enjoy speed and varying terrain, follow the blue markers; when you are really secure on your skate skis, you can head for the black diamond expert trails.

It is a good idea to take a short skating lesson so you can learn the basics, before going out the very first time. Aside from learning how to stop, which is very important, you will learn how to ski in the grooves and out of the grooves, as well as the all-important herringbone technique for climbing hills.

Snow Shoeing

Originally used for functional tasks (hunting, hiking) in the snow, the design of the formerly webbed-foot extensions known as snow shoes have come a long way. The modern snow shoe entered the fitness scene in the mid-1980s. The lightweight, aluminum frames make walking and even running on the snow possible. The foot slips into each snow shoe and is secured with either a bungee style cord or other strap. Winterized, waterproof boots or running shoes covered with a gaiter are the preferred footwear. Gaiters are a covering of material worn by cross country skiers and snow shoers to keep snow and moisture from getting inside their shoes/boots. They come in pairs and attach to the shoe/boot and span up to below the knee. Some snow shoers prefer to use poles; others go at it just with the shoes. Snow shoeing can be done on groomed trails, but adventure really begins off trail. Off trail snow shoeing in deep snow can be demanding, so adjust the time you are out there to accommodate for the heightened intensity so as not to overdo it. If you want to cover a long distance, the groomed trails might be a better pick.

Risk: Falling in snow shoes is always a possibility but because of the low speed and snowy landing it is usually harmless. If you want a quiet walk in the snow, then snow shoes are the way to go.

Equipment: The equipment consists of snow shoes, poles, and gaiters. You can rent everything but the gaiters. If you want to buy snow shoes, decide whether you will be predominantly walking or running. The designs for each vary slightly. Some snow shoes are easier to get in and out of than others; some are longer than others. Renting before buying is best. It is also helpful to talk to people who have snow shoed about the differences between the styles and brands. Mail order catalogs are helpful, convenient resources for answering your questions and for buying, especially if your choice of retail stores is limited.

Aerobic Activities Indoors

Indoor exercise is reliable, convenient, limits your exposure to outside risks, and can be more social if you so choose. Indoor exercise can be done at home, at a gym/club, or in a class. If you prefer indoor exercise and frequent a gym/club, you can expand your exercise options by having a backup activity to do at home. There are new indoor inventions coming to market all the time. The best indoor exercise is the one that works for you. Experiment with several before you hone in on one or two and be receptive to trying the new pieces of

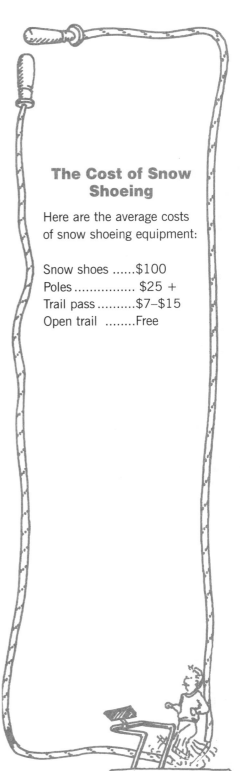

The Cost of Snow Shoeing

Here are the average costs of snow shoeing equipment:

Snow shoes $100
Poles .... $25 +
Trail pass ....$7–$15
Open trail ....Free

equipment that show up in your gym. The stationary bicycle might feel good when you work on your feet for 8 hours a day. But when you are promoted to the office job and spend more time on your glutes, the stair climber might sound pretty good.

Posture, technique, and cheating: When your elementary school teacher told you that "cheating only hurts you," it was the truth. When you exercise, proper posture and technique are essential to maximizing your effort and avoiding injury. Many exercisers respect the importance of posture and mechanics about outside sports but give little thought to it when exercising indoors on equipment. Consider this; it matters.

Most commercial equipment in health clubs has the instructions on the equipment. If after reading them you are still unclear about how to use it, ask the staff for instruction. Someone should be happy to help you. If you are going to buy a piece of used equipment, make sure you get a demonstration (and a warranty if buying from a retail store) on how to properly use it as well as an instructions manual.

Here are some tips for using aerobic exercise equipment:

1. Learn how to use it *before* you use it.
2. Use manual mode for complete control of the intensity (speed, elevation, and resistance).
3. Pay attention to your intensity level. Use distractions (music, reading, talking, thinking) to pass the time, not to distract you so that you overdo it.
4. Stay hydrated and drink during exercise.
5. Use a fan to keep from getting uncomfortably heated.
6. If you wear headphones and like to sing, remember that others can hear you.

Following is a review of indoor exercise equipment that has proven to be enduring, safe, effective, and, yes, somewhat fun (see Chapter 6).

Treadmill

Once you get used to the feeling of the ground moving beneath your feet, you can truly appreciate walking and running on a treadmill. The treadmill is obedient and will keep the speed/pace and elevation steady. Intensity is determined by the speed and elevation settings. You can either control the settings yourself through the *manual* mode or experiment with the preprogrammed workouts. Many home models will

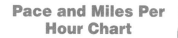

Pace and Miles Per Hour Chart

To figure your pace, divide the number 60 by your speed in miles per hour: Example: Treadmill speed = 3.5 mph.

60 divided by 3.5 = 17 minute mile.

6 mph = 10 minute mile
5 mph = 12 minute mile
4 mph = 15 minute mile
3 mph = 20 minute mile
2 mph = 30 minute mile

allow you to program your own workouts and keep them in memory as a preprogrammed workout.

Here's another bonus about using a treadmill: You can choose to run or to walk. If you are a runner who wants to walk on the treadmill but have difficulty elevating your heart rate, walk your fingers over to the elevation control and press "up." Your heart rate will go up quickly in response to even slight elevation changes such as 1 to 2 percent. Do not focus so much on heart rate that you forget about your muscles, which may not be used to elevation. Elevate gradually and give your muscles time to adjust. The muscles used while walking at high elevation are different from those used when running. If the elevation doesn't agree with your hips, knees, or ankles but you still want to elevate your heart rate while walking, wear a back pack and put some light weight in it. You can use a telephone book or weight plates but use low weight such as 1 to 5 pounds. Just that seemingly small amount will elevate your heart rate. It will also give you an appreciation for what it would feel like if you weighed that much more and had to carry it around with you all the time.

The treadmill makes for an efficient workout because it eliminates the distractions that outdoor exercise can pose (traffic, road debris, etc.) and allows you to maintain intensity. A good treadmill has a shock-absorbing pad built into the platform that makes the force absorbed by the body gentler than what it absorbs from concrete or asphalt pavement outdoors. A treadmill workout allows you to focus upon form. You should avoid holding the handrails continuously during exercise; use them mostly to steady or regain your balance.

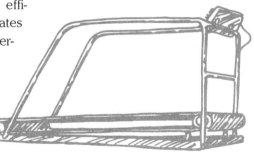

Treadmill

To start: Begin each treadmill session by walking slowly. Tread easy until you are oriented to the motion. Warm up for 5 minutes, then gradually increase the speed and elevation to your desired levels. Most have display settings—for your speed, elevation, the distance covered, and approximate calories burned—that will entertain you while treading.

Safety First!

Before using a treadmill, learn how to control it:

1. Know where the STOP button is located or the emergency pull cord.
2. Practice grabbing the handrail and straddling both feet so that they rest upon the nonmoving side panels. Then stop the machine or turn the intensity down.
3. Do not look directly down at your feet. A reflection off a mirror is okay and can help to maintain balance.
4. Stay focused and avoid turning your body, even if your kids are calling you.
5. A moving treadmill can be dangerous to curious children, pets, and so on. Keep them away and secure the operating key out of reach when not in use.
6. Position the back of the treadmill away from a wall so that you do not go splat against it.

You can use the information to challenge yourself by comparing your progress. Pace is another motivating unit of measure. It conveys your speed relative to the distance traveled. In the United States, pace refers to the number of minutes it takes to travel 1 mile. A 12-minute pace means it took you 12 minutes to cover 1 mile. In other countries, pace is the number of minutes it took to travel 1 kilometer. Pace is used for many activities—walking, running, or riding your bike. When it comes to pace, the lower the number, the faster the pace—and a sure sign that you are getting fitter.

Stationary Bicycle

If you like bicycling without the worries of the road, then stationary bicycling is for you. And if being mindless during exercise is your desire, you can best "slip away" more safely on a stationary bike than on other indoor aerobic equipment. There are computerized and non-computerized bikes and upright and recumbent bikes. *Upright bikes* position you as you would be on a traditional bike. *Recumbent bikes* position you in a semireclined position, which means the pedals and your feet are out in front of you. They were designed to support the lower back. If you suffer from "fanny fatigue" on an upright, you might want to try a recumbent. Neither style is better, so select that which is more comfortable for you.

Different bike, same concepts: Even though stationary bikes may seem like pseudo-bikes, you still apply the bicycling concept of spinning to them. *Spinning* is when you pedal in quick circular revolutions at a tension that allows you to push the crank (what the pedals are attached to) without straining. *Cadence* refers to the pedaling rhythm and, in bicycling, is accounted for by how many *revolutions per minute (rpms)* you pedal. Many bikes are equipped with a control panel that will display your cadence in rpms. With a cadence range in mind and a heart rate monitor, you can familiarize yourself with what levels are aerobic and comfortable. The biggest cycling error comes from pedaling too high a resistance (high gear or setting). Exercise should challenge your body, but it is not supposed to hurt. Your goal is to spin with an intensity that elevates your heart rate but does not make you strain. The second error associated with bicycling is improper seat position. On any bike, you want to have a slight bend of the knee, about 15 to 20 degrees, when your leg is in the down position of the

Are You Straining on the Stationary Bike?

Do you feel tension in your knees, hips, or groin?

Are you wishing you had two more legs to help you pedal?

Are you pushing so hard with your legs that you wobble from side to side on the seat?

Are you gripping the handlebars with the force of a rock climber?

If you answer yes to any of the above, you could be straining.

pedal stroke. Another general way to set the seat height is to stand behind the bicycle facing the rear of the seat. Your pubic bone should be even with the top of the seat. If the bike is mounted on a stand, then stand on top of the support feet and then align the pubic bone. You should not wobble from side to side on the seat. If you are still unsure of where the seat height should be, use the two suggestions above, then get on the bike and pedal for a minute or two with your eyes closed. This will help you focus your attention on how it feels.

Variable resistance: The most important feature you want on any stationary bike is the ability to change the leg resistance. There are some stationary bikes being sold that use a fan or flywheel to create the resistance but offer no gearing or other way to change the resistance. Spinning at a comfortable cadence is difficult to do on these bikes, and it means you are stuck with the factory-determined range of resistance. One such bike is popular because it produces a cool fanning effect for the rider. The fanning effect is a great feature, but because it has no option for varying the resistance, it is not optimum. This style can produce injury, ineffective levels of intensity, or both.

Spin cycle bikes: A spin bike is an indoor stationary bike that delivers the feel of an outdoor bike because of its stability, pedal action, and variable resistance. Spin classes are instructor-led group bicycling sessions that feature varying levels of intensity, music, and guided-imagery. Although the popularity of these bikes comes from the class setting, you can ride them as you would any stationary bike when class is out of session. They have brought a new enthusiasm to indoor bicycling like never before. The pedal action is smooth and circular like that of a fine outdoor bike. The seat is narrow like a road bike but a bit more forgiving. It also has adjustable settings for height and fore and aft positioning. A flywheel generates the resistance, and the bike's shifter allows you to vary the resistance. The shifter makes a slight click when the resistance is changed. The pedal is two sided; it allows you to use conventional exercise shoes on one side and cleated bicycle shoes on the other. Spin cycles do not have all the electronic feedback of other styles, so if you miss the spin class and want to combat boredom, bring along your headset. Aside from not having an electronic feedback panel, when you compare the cycle-feel of this bike to other stationary bikes, it is the closest to the real thing.

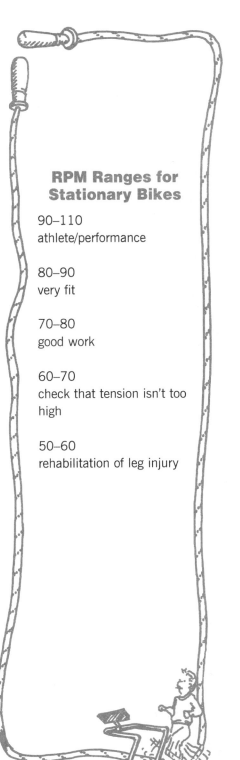

RPM Ranges for Stationary Bikes

90–110
athlete/performance

80–90
very fit

70–80
good work

60–70
check that tension isn't too high

50–60
rehabilitation of leg injury

Stair Climbing Machines

You may have heard of the Harvard Step Test, the test in which students' heart rates were monitored while stepping repetitively onto a 12-inch platform. The stair climber, stair stepper, or stepper can be thought of as the grandchild of the classic testing tool. (Running the bleachers and stadium steps can be thought of as the second generation of the step test.) This machine was made popular by StairMaster and continues to be the leader in the industry. When used properly, it will get you aerobic and build leg strength and endurance. In addition to getting the average person fit, it is a terrific cross-training exercise and will more than sufficiently prepare skiers, runners, and hikers for their primary sport. It is gentle upon the skeletal system, and many love it for its ability to challenge them aerobically while giving their bones and joints a rest.

Skill: In terms of actual movement, the stair climbing machines are the no-brainers of aerobic exercise equipment. You stand; you step. Well, there is a little more to it than that, but for the most part, it's pretty simple. However, the biggest "skill" that seems difficult for many is maintaining correct posture during the exercise. More than on any

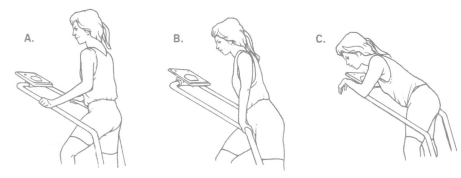

Stair Climbing Machine Posture

A. Proper stair climbing posture. Back is erect, arms are bent yet relaxed, hands and wrists in overhand position and used only to balance, feet are fully on the pads not hanging off the ends, leg extends down to an almost touch-the-bottom range of motion.

B. Improper, compensating, and potentially dangerous stair climbing posture. Leaning one's body weight onto wrists in an upturned position makes wrists and shoulders vulnerable to injury and is not recommended.

C. Improper stair climbing posture. Leaning over the machine can cause backache, lower leg soreness and undermines the work load by shifting weight away from the leg area.

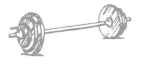
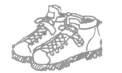
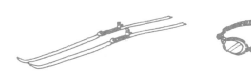

Stair Climbing Properly
(and 6 things people do to sabotage it)

1. Stand erect and lean *slightly* forward at the hips.
   Common error: There is severe over-leaning, or hunching, over the machine. This transfers weight off the pedals and onto the front railing, which negates the intensity level of the exercise.

2. Place your entire foot on the pedal.
   Common error: Exercisers stand with the balls of their feet on the edge of the pedal with their heels hanging off the ends. This can strain the calf muscles and even the knees.

3. Use your hands for balance only, not for gripping.
   Common error: The ego turns up the resistance to a higher level, but the legs respond, "Hey, this is too much. Move off." The exerciser either grabs the rails forcefully or leans to compensate. Either way the extra resistance is negated, the posture sacrificed, and the exerciser may experience sore hands, sore lower back, or both.

4. Hands and wrists should be in an overhand position. Elbows should be bent at a 45- to 90-degree angle in front or to the side of your body.
   Common error: The wrists face up or out rather than down, hyperextending the elbows and wrists. Don't do it!

5. Step with even full, deep steps but do not let the step touch bottom.
   Common error: The exerciser takes short, quick bouncy steps, which means more compensating.

6. Let the legs do the stepping.
   Common error: To compensate for lack of leg strength, the exerciser leans and sways deeply from side to side. This is neither race walking nor tryouts for the Florida A & M marching band. The hips should not swivel to and fro. The motion comes from the legs and hips moving up and down evenly.

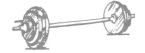

Pity This Posture

For 2 years a woman religiously read her newspaper while using the stair climbing machine and complained that she was not getting any fitter. She assumed her F-I-T was adequate enough to produce improvements—frequency, five times per week; intensity, level 5; time, 30 minutes. Upon watching her, it became obvious that her posture, leaning forward and gripping the side rails, was incorrect, which counteracted the intensity level of the exercise. Stair climbing machines use the person's body weight to appropriate the intensity level. Her weight transference from legs to arms negated much of the intensity level. Once she started using the correct posture she was truly using her legs and reaching a higher aerobic level.

other piece of equipment people either innocently or carelessly cheat themselves from the benefit of stair climbing by negating the intensity level of exercise. They adopt compensating postures that are primarily caused by lack of strength, which is exactly what they need and why they should perform the exercise properly!

Equipment: Most health clubs have a stair climber. Home varieties are available, but if you are accustomed to the smooth action of the commercial varieties, you might be better off buying a used commercial variety. One brand is so bouncy that it feels like a priming activity for upright bungee jumping rather than for stair climbing.

NordicTrack and Other Ski Machines

Designed to simulate cross-country skiing, this machine used properly is highly effective in building aerobic conditioning, muscular strength, and endurance. For years NordicTrack was *the* ski machine and entire category. Other variations are now available, but for the purest action and most thorough workout, none compare to the original. The dual action movement of the upper and lower body challenges your ability to balance and coordinate two different movements. It takes more than what is needed to walk and chew gum but less than what is needed to walk on ice.

Leg action: The skier stands with one leg on each of the two skis that glide over a front and rear set of rollers (one for each ski). The feet slip into small cuplike stirrups. The hip pad is attached to a vertical post and is the pivotal spot for establishing balance. The pad is positioned below the navel and is flush with your hipbones. You want to maintain an erect, though not stiff, posture while leaning with your hips into the hip pad. Leaning too far forward will cause your legs to fly out behind and you to fall forward, and leaning backward will cause your skis to fly forward and you backward. You use your abdominal and back muscles to maintain the position during the skiing action.

Heel and foot: At the back of the leg stride, lift your heel (pivot onto the ball of your foot) but keep your toes in the stirrup. This allows for the continuous gliding motion.

Arm action: The arm action comes from a pull cord with left and right handles attached to a flywheel. The flywheel can be adjusted to increase or decrease arm tension by turning the knob right and left, respectively (see sidebar). Some machines are designed without the upper flywheel. Instead they have a moving set of side poles. The pole version is not as demanding nor does it require the coordination of the independent flywheel, but it still has you working your upper body.

When pulling backward, squeeze the top of the shoulder and back of the arm muscles (deltoid and triceps). Extend and keep the elbow fairly straight but relaxed. An error novices make is bending the elbows on the pulling motion. This not only puts stress on the elbow joint, but it also throws off your balance. On the flywheel version, the forward stroke is passive and mostly just a return to the starting position.

Head: Keep your head up and face forward. Do NOT look down at your feet; that is the quickest way to invite a slew of undesirable outcomes.

Putting it all together: Think "diagonal stride." The leg action alternates left and right and resembles a front and back scissors kick. The arm action also alternates left and right and is independent and opposite from the leg action. When your left leg moves forward, your left arm pulls back. The term *diagonal stride* is also used to describe classic cross-country skiing. The challenge of using a ski machine is coordinating the arm and leg action at a pace and force that are comfortable. A good rule of ski machine skiing is to let the legs lead and the arms follow. That means you let the legs dominate the pace and resistance and then adjust for the arms.

Beginners should start with the leg action first and get comfortable with it. For some this could mean minutes; for others it could mean days. You will still get an aerobic workout, plus the strengthening benefits for the legs and hips. You also use the muscles of the back and abdomen simply by maintaining the upright position. When you are ready to add the arm action, be prepared to watch your heart rate jump quickly. Even though the arms have smaller muscle groups than

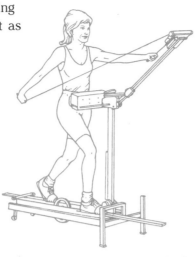

NordicTrack® Ski Exerciser
A ski exerciser is an efficient exercise machine that exercises upper and lower body muscle groups.

Ski Machine Tips

- **Upper Body Tip:** Keep your elbows straight. If you have ever water skied, you know what happens when you bend your elbows and begin to pull in on the rope. Your skis move forward, and you go splash in a hurry. On ski machines, there is no splash, but keeping your elbows straight will help to keep you balanced on your feet.

- **Lower Body Tip:** If your feet feel as though they are sliding out of the foot cup, then lift the foot ever so slightly and move it forward into the foot cup on the forward leg stroke.

- **Balancing Tip:** When possible, use a ski machine in front of a mirror. Watching your legs and feet can help you stabilize yourself on the skis. It is also a good reminder to keep your posture erect and your head up and forward.

1

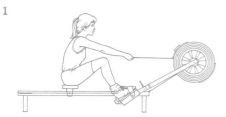

2

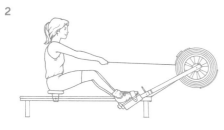

3

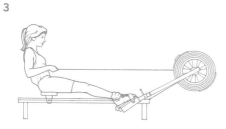

4

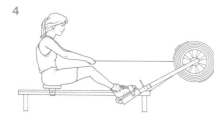

5

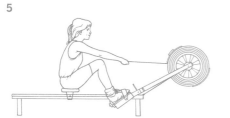

the legs, the arm movement elevates the heart rate quickly because of their proximity to the heart. This machine is not for everyone. It may take some time but be patient and give it a try; the benefits are many.

Indoor Rowing Machine

Row row row your boat, gently . . . the Concept II indoor rowing machine was designed by two competitive rowing brothers who wanted an indoor rowing option. This and other good rowers have a cable, handle, flywheel, and fan. The stroke is a two-part stroke—the drive and the recovery, which are blended together to make for a smooth and continuous action. Other companies have made miniature versions that do an average job of simulating the motion, but the one you'll find in most gyms and health clubs is the Concept II.

Instruction: Follow these steps for good rowing technique:

1. The drive: Reach forward with your knees bent, arms extended, and body leaning toward the flywheel. The drive is begun with your legs and back doing all the work. Note that the arms are straight and the shoulders relaxed.
2. Halfway through the drive, the legs and back are still doing all the work. The arms are still straight with the shoulders still relaxed.
3. At the finish of the drive, the arms and shoulders pull the handle into the abdomen. The legs are straight, and the body is leaning back slightly. Note that the height of the handle is neither at the chest nor in the lap.
4. Recovery: The first motion of the recovery is to extend the arms and swing the body forward at the hips. This puts the handle in front of the knees to avoid interference between the knees and hands as the seat moves forward.
5. The body is drawn forward with the legs to the starting position for the next stroke. The rower is now ready to begin the next drive. Remember that the motion is continuous and that your body never comes to a complete stop until you are finished.

Elliptical Trainer

An elliptical trainer is a large electronic machine with two foot pads/pedals that look as though Goliath's feet could fit on them. There are two poles on each side that move in conjunction with the leg motion and work the upper body. The motion is oval-like (ellipse) and feels like a combination of classic cross-country skiing, stair climbing, and walking. The machine works on a similar principle as the other indoor equipment (treadmill, stair climber)—you have to keep up with the pace of the machine. It gives you a good workout, as well as feedback from the electronics console.

Elliptical Trainer
Elliptical trainers provide an effective cardiovascular workout, work all the major muscle groups in the legs, and do so with low impact upon your joints. They can be programmed to move in forward or backward motions. The backward motion emphasizes the gluteal muscles (buttocks).

Arm Ergometer

This is a best-kept-secret piece of equipment. If you have a lower body disability or temporary injury that keeps you from using your legs, an arm ergometer will give you a workout. The arm ergometer rests on a tabletop and looks like the crank arm and pedals of a bicycle. You use your arms to pedal. It is an excellent upper body and cardiovascular tool used by many wheelchair athletes for training, as well as a common rehabilitative tool seen in physical therapy offices. Ask your health club if they have or would consider having one.

Jumping Rope

Sometimes basic equipment is refreshing because it is so simple and hassle free. You probably played with one as a kid or

Indoor Rowing Tips

1. All movement is with your legs and buttocks, not your back.

2. Never extend your knees all the way. At the point of fullest extension, your knees should be slightly bent.

3. The faster and harder you pull, the greater the resistance.

4. Think "continuous motion." Do not stop or pause at either the extended or bent positions.

have seen boxers train with them for agility, footwork, and aerobic conditioning. They make great travel companions because of the intense workout in a short amount of time and the minimal space they take up in your travel bag. If done slowly, it can be a warm-up activity, and when jumped at a faster pace, if desired, it can be used for interval heart rate training. Wear your heart rate monitor to see just how intense it can be.

Skill: The natural tendency is to jump on the balls of your feet, but this can lead to calf stress and cramping if done for long periods. Try intervals, alternating the faster pace by landing on the balls of your feet with a slower pace by landing on the balls and heels of your feet. The challenge of jumping rope comes from jumping properly, with the knees slightly bent, while staying low to the ground, such that your feet are only slightly off the ground.

Intensity: To add to the intensity of the exercise, use a quarter- to half-pound "heavy" rope; stay clear of ropes with weighted handles (they can stress your wrists without building the strength you desire). To spare your hands, you can either wear gloves over wooden handles or use the foam and soft rubber handles.

Equipment: To determine the correct rope length, stand on the center of the rope with both feet and pull the handles up toward your armpits. A good length is where the handles are close to your armpits. Do not jump in bare feet; rather wear supportive running or workout shoes. Your feet are the landing pads for this moderately impactful activity, and you will feel better for having a good pair of shock absorbers on your feet.

Cost: Jump ropes can be found at most sporting goods stores; the price range is from $5 to $35. It is actually difficult to find one made from rope anymore. Most are made from molded plastic and other very durable materials.

Medicine Ball

Here's a form of "medicine" you do not have to swallow. You do not have to plug it in, program it, adjust it, or maintain it. You need only include it in your fitness program to build strength, endurance, flexibility, and a good sweat.

It began with the Greek physician Hippocrates in the fifth century and then received notoriety with President Herbert Hoover in 1928. Since President Hoover, basketball teams, including the world champion Chicago Bulls, have used medicine balls as a regular part of their training. They are once again gaining popularity.

Originally, they were made from sewn animal skins stuffed with sand. Today they are made from recycled materials, sand, and ground-up stones and bolts encased in leather or synthetic rubber. They weigh anywhere from 2 pounds to 35 pounds and can be as small as a softball, bigger than a basketball, and also in between. They cost between $15 and $150.

So how can this heavy ball make you fit? By tossing, throwing, and catching the round weight every which way. It builds muscles of the chest, stomach, back, arms, shoulder, legs, and hips. Medicine ball exercises are fun and seem more like play, yet you can get aerobic and build strength and flexibility. Having a partner is helpful, but you can use them alone too. You can exercise with them outdoors or indoors, but when indoors, make sure you have a clear space near you. One caution is to start with the lightweight balls; even they provide plenty of resistance. (See the Appendix for instructional books and for the Web site where you can order medicine balls.)

Aerobics—High/Low Impact

Aerobic routines are dance-style movements that get you moving and shaking and your heart a-poundin'. In low-impact aerobics, you move horizontally (up and back, side to side) a lot but without absorbing much jarring and pounding. You usually have at least one foot on the ground, which rules out the high-impact activities like jumping and hopping. In high-impact aerobics, you experience more vertical movements, hopping, and jumping, which naturally have a stronger impact on you when you land. Weight-bearing exercise is good for you, so you should not be too quick to assume that the "impact" part of high and low impact is a good or bad thing. It depends upon your fitness goals. There are also combination high/low classes. If those are

Rule of Screws and Mechanical Pieces

"Righty tighty, left loosey"—when you want to tighten something or secure it, think "righty tighty," meaning if you turn it to the right it will get tight; and to unscrew or loosen something, you turn it to the left. You can also think in terms of clockwise and counterclockwise, but that is not as poetic nor as memorable as "righty tighty, lefty loosey."

not available, try alternating between the two-class styles. Classes vary by styles of movement, intensity of exercise, and types of music. Most instructors are well intended, but you should watch out for those who use the class as a good excuse to get paid for a workout. You want an instructor who is interested in you and your ability to follow along in the class. Having a certified instructor can weed out a lot of bad experiences. Verbal projection and instructional skills are two qualities you want in a good instructor. If you do not care for the instructor's choice of music, ask if that is the normal type of music in the class and, if need be, find another class.

Skill: If you have rhythm, coordination, and the ability to follow or remember dance-style movements, you will catch on quickly and have a great aerobic workout. However, if this is your first-ever dance class experience or if you opted for tennis and skipped dance at summer camp, you could be in for a tough time.

Intensity: Monitoring your heart rate in an aerobics class keeps you aligned with your fitness goals. However, manually monitoring your heart rate in class when the music is loud is difficult and prone to inaccuracy. In the time that you stop and search for your pulse, your heart rate has already dropped significantly from what it was during exercise. Unless you are trying to determine your recovery heart rate, what you have is an inaccurate reading for an exercising heart rate. The best way to monitor your heart rate in an aerobics class is to wear your heart rate monitor and check your intensity level while you are moving. Some classes may not challenge you enough; others might push you too hard. In either case, it is good to know your aerobic level of exercise.

Step Aerobics

A step is the complete movement of one leg. Step aerobics is another activity that was made popular from its class offering, but it can be conveniently performed at home. The classes are fun if you like loud music and group energy. Step aerobics is a dance-style step routine set to music that you perform using a rectangular, circular, or square platform. You step onto, off of, and up

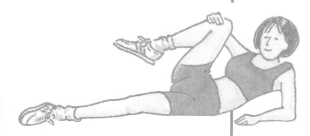

on the step with varying degrees of intensity. The pace of the exercise/music and height of the step determine intensity. The height is adjusted using plastic molded fittings intelligently named risers.

Skill required: Step aerobics will pleasantly challenge you if you have rhythm, coordination, and good movement memory, but it will frustrate you if you do not. Unless you have a secret passion to be a choreographer, you will want to buy a few good step aerobics videotapes that will lead you through your workout at home. Step does an excellent job of toning your legs and buttocks muscles and pushing you aerobically. However, if you suffer from back, knee, or ankle ailments, you should either consider another form of exercise or give it a go by stepping with a low-platform height at a slow pace until you build strength.

Equipment: All you need is a step platform, riser(s), and videotapes, or you can attend a class.

Cardio Kickboxing

It is still too early to tell whether this is a fad exercise but classes of it have popped up all over. As the name implies, it is a cardiovascular workout that utilizes martial arts type movements, including forceful kicks and punches. If you take a class or use a video in the presence of others, make sure everyone knows their right from their left and front from back, otherwise someone could get ko'ed! It is very rigorous and has been criticized for the number of injuries it produces. Defenders claim that injuries are mostly the result of exercisers advancing too quickly from the low-intensity to high-intensity sessions. In either case, ask to observe a class before signing up for a series of sessions.

Minitrampoline

If you like to dance, jump, or run, try doing so on this small, portable, bouncy, inexpensive apparatus. Minitrampolines are the miniature circular version of the larger ones seen at summer camps, gymnastics training centers, and even in some household backyards. Most minitramps have a small nylon sheet held by springs to a frame. It is not as sturdy as the larger version; to

Risers

Sold as a single unit, a riser is a molded plastic unit that fits underneath a step platform to increase the step height. A riser is 2 inches tall so you can easily and incrementally adjust the platform height. For some unknown reason (design flaw, opportunity to sell more?) the riser is not long enough to elevate and support the entire length and width of the step platform. It means that if you want to increase the height, you have to use risers in increments of 2 in order to keep it level.

• • •

Rule of Step

When you step up, your knee should be even with or lower than your hip.

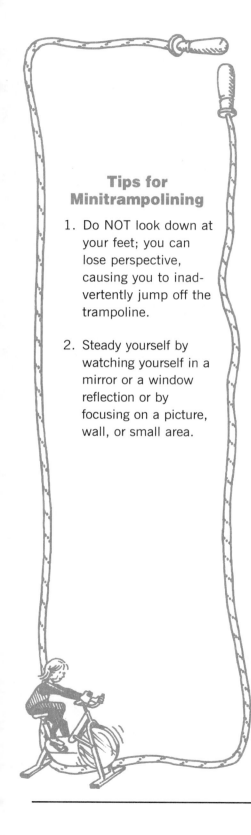

avoid tipping over, you need to distribute your body weight equidistant from the center.

The minitrampoline is fun and will give you an effective cardiovascular workout with little to no impact on your skeletal system. Unfit persons can dance, jog in place, or do intervals of each. Very overfat persons should stay low to the nylon base. Fit persons can get aerobic by running in place, remembering to swing the arms. To raise the heart rate even more, exaggerate the leg motion by kicking back behind you. For extremely fit individuals, a fun workout involves running in place on the minitrampoline for 5 minutes and alternating with jumping rope for 2 minutes and then repeating the sequence for a total time of 20 to 30 minutes.

The minitramp is light and portable enough that you can easily carry it inside or out. When using the minitramp indoors, make sure you have at least 3 to 5 feet clearance over your head at the point of your maximum jump height. For maximum pleasure, listen to rhythmic, uplifting music and either dance, jump, or jog in place. After five or six of your favorite songs, you will have been aerobic and will bask in the afterglow of a fun exercise session. You may well be humming a few tunes too!

Equipment and clothing: Most sporting goods stores have minitramps, and oftentimes you can score a very cheap one at a garage sale. It stores easily by leaning it up in a closet or against a wall. Do not minitramp in socks; they will cause you to slip and slide easily. Wear walking or running shoes and your heart rate monitor for feedback so that you can be sure that your pace is aerobic. Music from a radio, cassette tape, or CD player will enhance the session. Women should wear supportive jog bras; depending upon how rigorously you dance, run, or jump, you may feel qualified to be the next wear-tester for a jog bra company.

Cost: New minitrampolines cost $25; garage sale minitramps go for as low as $5.

Tips for Minitrampolining

1. Do NOT look down at your feet; you can lose perspective, causing you to inadvertently jump off the trampoline.

2. Steady yourself by watching yourself in a mirror or a window reflection or by focusing on a picture, wall, or small area.

Exercise for the Mind: Physically Fit and Mentally Refreshed

Many people do not stick with their exercise programs because they do not enjoy the actual time during exercise. They cite boredom as a factor in not enjoying exercise. Would you like to *enjoy* your exercise time rather than tolerate it? If you experience boredom or find yourself wishing away the minutes, try these remedies. These valuable mind activities are really mental refreshments that can take you to new places in your mind and your exercise. They will help you exercise with greater enjoyment and appreciation and will also boost your mood and elevate your spirit. In addition to feeling physically charged from exercise, you will feel mentally and emotionally refreshed. Give these an honest try. You have nothing to lose and everything to gain. Listed among the ten ideas for enjoying your exercise time are a variety of ways to either enjoy your time or to use it as a productive life-enhancing medium. Read through all of them. There is nothing as invigorating as a new idea.

Ten Ideas for Enjoying Your Exercise Time

What and how we choose to think affects the direction and outcome of our lives. People have used positive mental imaging, such as visualizing healthy cells eating up bad cells, to heal their illnesses. More and more we are seeing the impact of the mind/body connection and the idea that what we focus our conscious attention on permeates into the subconscious mind and teaches us how to heal ourselves and how to make ourselves happy.

So what does all this have to do with enjoying your exercise time? The continuous rhythmic and repetitive nature of aerobic exercise is a formidable platform for consciously focusing on the ideas you want to see happen in your life. When engaging in solo aerobic exercise (walking, jogging, ski machine, stair climber), use the time to focus on ideas you would like to make realities. Ask yourself, "What do I want?" Do you need or want to be more creative in

Tae Bo and Kleenex?

Tae Bo is the signature cardio kickboxing brainchild of Billy Blanks, a former martial arts champion. Blanks packaged his exercise sessions as invigorating spiritual-physical experiences and offers them by class sessions in southern California (LA) and by videotape. The marketing of Tae Bo has been so effective that many use the name Tae Bo when they want to describe the activity of cardio kickboxing. One could say that Tae Bo is to cardio kickboxing what Kleenex is to facial tissue.

your work, to be more kind to others, or to achieve a specific goal? Whatever it is, attach a positive verbal and visual image to it and rehearse it during your aerobic exercise session. You will come out of your sessions energized and be on your way to mentally achieving that which you affirmed for yourself.

1. **Affirmations for exercise or "moving meditations"**
   a. The ABCs of affirmation. Starting with the letter *A*, think or say a word or idea that describes something positive that *you are* or *aspire to be*. Connect the powerful words *I am* to it. Proceed one letter at a time, repeating the entire sequence each time you add a new letter/thought. See if you can make it through the entire alphabet. For example: *A*, Alive—Say: I am alive. A-L-I-V-E. I am alive; *B*, Blessed. Say: I am blessed. B-L-E-S-S-E-D. I am blessed. Then repeat, I am alive, I am blessed. Then *C*, Creative. Say: I am creative. C-R-E-A-T-I-V-E. I am creative. Then repeat, I am alive, I am blessed, I am creative.

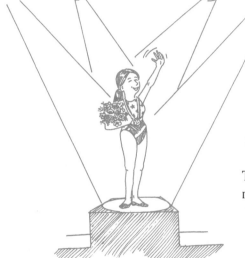

Keep adding the next letter and repeat the entire sequence. This is terrific mental exercise too. If you practice this during a 30-minute aerobic exercise session, you will be amazed at how "time flies when you are having fun!" And you will come away from it with some positive constructive thoughts and feel mentally refreshed.

   b. Variation on above: Focus on one letter and come with as many words with that one letter as you can.

2. **Powerful affirmation.** Is there something you want to bring about in your life? If so, put the idea in place and then recite: *I can; I will; I am able to.* Repeat the words and picture the image; say it and see yourself achieving it. Imagine the steps you will take to achieve it. Attaching this affirmation to the idea gives it power and possibility.

3. **Body blessing/appreciation, and thanks.** As you exercise, think about your body parts and their functions and give thanks for them. If some of them need extra attention, take your mind's energy to them and lovingly bless them. Remember to focus

on what they do for you. If an area needs improvement, think positively about it, bless the function it serves, and see it improving. *Nurture*-ment is nourishment and more effective than belittlement.

For example, I give thanks to my brain; it allows me to think. I give thanks to my eyes; they allow me to see, to experience color and image. I give thanks to my lungs; they allow me to breathe, which allows me to live. I give thanks to my heart, arm, knee, hip, and so on.

4. Laugh out loud. Ever notice how good you feel after a genuine, hearty laugh? Laughter creates a relaxing physiological response (lowers blood pressure, lowers stress). In *Anatomy of an Illness*, Norman Cousins wrote how he healed himself of a serious illness through laughter. Try these laughing exercises. They are fun, they feel good, and they are good for you. If you are afraid you will look or sound silly, maybe that is precisely what you need. Keep your sense of humor and do not take yourself too seriously. Remember, you want to feel better! Give these a try.

a. Laugh by design. This is a tried and true exercise. If you are alone, you might prefer a more private setting (at home indoors or outdoors on your bike). It is fun and it feels great. Try laughing in threes (ah-ha-ha, ah-ha-ha, ah-ha-ha) continuously for 1 minute, exhaling deeply as you do. Listen to your laughs. Watching or hearing laughter can induce laughter, even when it is your own. It sounds so funny that you start to genuinely laugh.

b. Recreate the moment. Think of some funny event that has happened in your life that made you laugh. Get back into that moment, recreate it, and allow yourself to laugh in it again. What was the most recent thing you have laughed at or about?

c. Recall. Revisit a funny event that you saw on television or a movie. Remember when Lucy and Ethel were working at a furious pace at the chocolate factory? That has to bring a smile to your face.

5. Serious stuff. Visualize yourself and your goal. Mentally rehearse your goal. See yourself graduating school, running in the marathon, receiving news of a clean bill of health, and so forth.

Home Exercise Versus Club/Gyms

Any of the gym/health club or class activities can be done at home as long as you have the specific equipment and space. Any of the home activities can be done at the gym as long as your gym has the equipment. If there is a piece of equipment you would like to have at your health club, talk to the director. Chances are that if you like it, others will too.

6. Loving focus. Concentrate upon a loved one, a favorite place, an enjoyable experience, a poem, or a song. Think of loving, caring things to do for yourself and others.

7. Create entertaining distractions. Get an audio headset and listen to books on tape (the library has them too) or to music. For indoor activities, you have more options, such as renting a movie (multiday rental) or watching a video, the television, or a sporting event.

8. Create social opportunities. Exercise with a partner— human, canine, or other.

9. Nothing . . . Do nothing. Relax your mind.

10. Your breath. Focus on your breath; see it filling your body with new life.

These ten ideas for enjoying your exercise time can make the difference between getting through your exercise or leaving you wanting more. Don't knock them until you have tried them. They work.

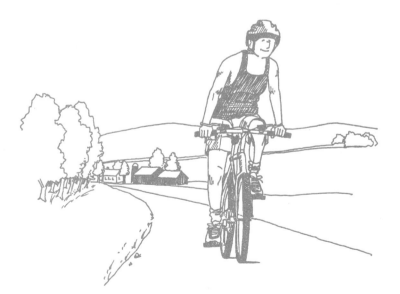

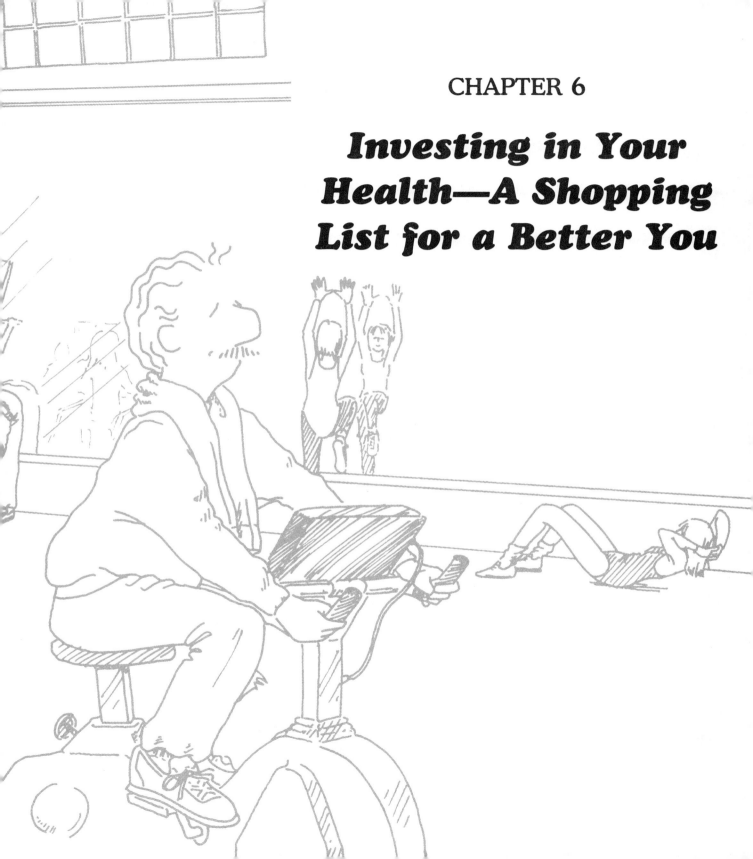

CHAPTER 6

Investing in Your Health—A Shopping List for a Better You

Movement as Medicine

Whenever a health challenge pops up, most people do not hesitate to spend money to see their doctor or to buy medicine. While those are prudent and necessary expenses, they are "after the fact" treatments. The next time you buy anything related to your fitness, remind yourself that you are investing in your health, "before the fact," and are taking a preventive action that is a real investment in your wellness and preventive health.

From the Beginning

Buying appropriate and comfortable equipment *from the beginning* gives you the best chance for staying with it. The "right stuff" increases the probability of you enjoying the activity or being comfortable, which translates into sticking with it. How many times have you told yourself, "Once I prove to myself that I'll stick with it, I'll buy . . . " If your introductory /initial experiences are unpleasant and uncomfortable, you are not likely to continue. Give yourself a fair chance to be comfortable and enjoy the activities. Start in the beginning, or you may sabotage your well-intended efforts.

Buying comfortable, appropriate equipment from the beginning also makes good financial sense. It saves you money because you will not need to upgrade later to the "better" equipment (that you originally wanted).

Items such as new running/walking shoes, a decent stationary bicycle, a sturdy treadmill, or other equipment in good condition can make all the difference in the world. Get whatever you need to be relatively comfortable. If you do not feel good or are uncomfortable during your activity, you will not stick with it. Forget the old motto "no pain, no gain." It will only undermine your success.

As you invest in your fitness comfort, allow yourself to feel good about it. Remember, you are investing in something that is going to improve the quality and, probably, the quantity of your life in more ways than you can imagine.

Selecting and Purchasing Equipment

Selecting and purchasing equipment is more convenient now than ever before. But do not let convenience distract you from doing your

You Can't Take It with You

Spending money on fitness and fun is a lot healthier and productive than spending it on junk food, alcohol, drugs, and doctors' appointments. You work hard for your money. Grant yourself permission to spend it on that which you enjoy and makes you feel good.

research prior to your purchase. Read about the equipment you are considering buying, through manufacturer's brochures, fitness magazines, and Web sites (see Appendix for information). Talk to other people who do the activity and use the same type of equipment (the exact same, if possible) and ask what they like and do not like about it. Make a list of your priorities (space, noise, expense, convenience, etc.), match them to your research, and see whether or not there is a good fit. A good motto for purchasing fitness equipment and apparel is this: Whenever possible, *try it out or try it on.* If that is not possible, make sure you can return it for a credit and/or refund. Most reputable companies offer money back guarantees if you are not satisfied.

Once you have narrowed down your priorities and decided what is right for you, the shopping will be much easier. Through Web sites, mail order catalogs, exercise specialty retail stores, mass merchandise, and outlet stores, you can hunt for the features that are important to you and make an educated and appropriate purchase.

Once you have become familiar with how your equipment works and how it eventually wears down, you can shop your local newspaper's want ads and garage sales for used equipment, as long as you know what to look for. Remember that the sale is final, with no guarantees.

See the Appendix for listings of manufacturers and distributors of exercise and related equipment and apparel.

Tip: Buying Used Equipment

Before you commit to buying a piece of used equipment, ask the seller if the owner's manual is available. A seller is more motivated to find it before the sale than after your money is in hand. If it is not available, contact the manufacturer to see whether they have another copy available.

Aerobic Equipment
Heart Rate Monitor

This is one of the best pieces of exercise equipment you can buy and use anywhere! You can use it with any activity: indoor or outdoor, wet or dry, sport, machine, and so on. The heart rate monitor will help you make sure you are exercising at an intensity level that is productive. Heart rate monitors are currently a three-part device, although strapless monitors are in the making. The battery strap is flat and somewhat flexible plastic, and an elastic, adjustable, two-ended strap fits into the battery strap and keeps it on your torso. These two connected

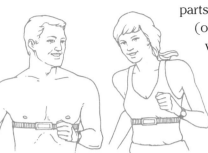

parts are worn just below the breast area (on men, beneath the nipples; on women, beneath the bottom of the bra line). The third part is the actual monitor, which looks like a wristwatch and can be worn as one. It can also be attached to a nearby apparatus for easier viewing, such as on the handlebar of a bicycle, on the rail handle on a ski machine, or wrapped around the rail/handle of the stair climbing machine (remember to remove it when you finish!).

Heart Rate Monitor: Battery and Sensor Strap, Elastic Strap, and Wrist Monitor
The heart rate monitor takes the guesswork out of how hard you are exercising. It is an effective and motivational tool that displays your level of exercise intensity.

Types and Manufacturers: Types and manufacturers include Acumen, Cardiosport, HeartZones Polar, and Sensor Dynamics. The price range is $49 to $300.

Considerations: Comfort is important; check specifically the width, thickness, and weight of the strap and battery strap. Most exercisers will not even notice it is there, but on very lean bodies, it can be more noticeable. The strap should be snug to the body so that you can barely fit one finger between the strap and your body, but not so tight that it leaves an imprint.

How it works: The reading is accomplished by communication between the sensors (not the battery) on the front of the belt and the monitor. To engage the heart rate monitor, moisten the inside of the sensors that are in contact with the skin. Usually the battery is in the middle of the belt, and the sensors are on both sides of the battery. Moistening can be accomplished by licking or running the sensor under water. Next, attach the adjustable strap and sensor belt to the body and hold the monitor (watch) in front of the sensors. The heart rate will display in a few moments.

Functions: Visibility and readability are most important, you have to be able to see number(s) displayed, and on some models they are tiny. With a single read (displays only heart rate), the numbers are usually the biggest; they only display one set of numerals. Obviously, the more information (heart rate, elapsed time, time of day) displayed, the

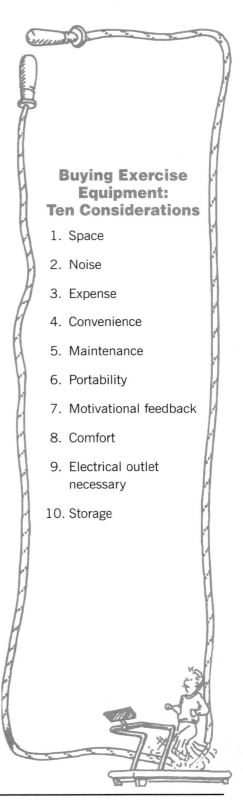

smaller the numbers, due to the shared space. For the average exer-ciser, the single read is adequate, although some of the other compo-nents may eliminate your need for a heart rate monitor and a sport watch. Other displays are stop watch/chronograph, alarm, lighted back-ground for dark viewing, and beeper and flashing numbers for high- and low-target heart zone settings. If you exercise alone, you will not need this next function, but if you work out around others who wear monitors or machines equipped with them, you will want a watch equipped with cross talk elimination. It keeps your monitor from reading the heart rate of someone exercising near you.

For those really into heart rate monitoring, there is a computer downloadable function that will track and store your workouts. And for women, there is a style that addresses the comfort issue by offering the heart rate monitor built into a jog bra.

Mount: If you plan to use your heart rate monitor on a bicycle or want to attach it to your home, office, or gym exercise equipment, order a handlebar mount or make your own. It is a simple piece that wraps around the apparatus handle, which allows the monitor to then be wrapped around the mount. Without the mount, most handles are too narrow, and the monitor/watch will not stay in place.

Warranty and battery: A typical warranty period is for 1 year. The battery can last up to 3 years on a single read and less on those that beep and flash a lot. Beeps, flashes, and lighted backgrounds use more battery power. To extend battery life, you can turn off the beeps and flashes when you do not want to use them. When the time comes to change the battery, some models are easier to change batteries on than others; some want you to send them back to the manufacturer in order to keep the warranty alive.

Stationary Bicycles

Considerations: Consider comfort in the saddle/seat and overall body position, adjustable settings for intensity, seat height fore and aft, and handle bars. Also consider noise, portability, and maintenance. Motivational feedback from a speedometer (speed), tachometer (rpms), odometer (distance), resistance settings, programmable workouts, and a built-in heart rate monitor are helpful. Beware of bikes that do not allow you to adjust the tension to levels low enough so that you can spin at rpms comfortable for your knees, and heart rate.

Buying Exercise Equipment: Ten Considerations

1. Space
2. Noise
3. Expense
4. Convenience
5. Maintenance
6. Portability
7. Motivational feedback
8. Comfort
9. Electrical outlet necessary
10. Storage

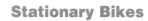

Stationary Bikes

Types and manufacturers: The following list should prove helpful:

- For nonelectrical/computerized uprights, consider BodyGuard, Monark, Schwinn, and Tunturi. The price range is $250 to $500.
- For computerized uprights, consider Cateye, LifeCycle, Precor, Schwinn, and Tectrix. The price range is $500 to $3000.
- For nonelectrical/computerized recumbents, see Schwinn and Precor. The price range is $500 to $1200.
- For computerized recumbents, see LifeFitness, Precor, and Schwinn. The price range is $500 to $2000.
- For spin bikes, see Reebok and Schwinn. Their price range is $530 to $900.
- For transforming your bike to a stationary, use trainers and rollers. Check out catalogs from Bike Nashbar and Performance. The price range is $100 to $170.

Treadmill Running and Walking

Considerations: Commercial treadmills can accommodate persons of most body weights; home models are typically built to withstand body weights not greater than 250 pounds. If you plan to run or eventually run on the treadmill, a minimum horsepower of 1.5 to 2.0 is recommended. If you plan to only walk, you can get away with fewer horseys. Ask if the machine has elevation change capability. Elevation capability gives you more variety in the types of workouts you can do or may grow into doing.

Noise is difficult to detect on the showroom floor but listen for it anyway. Compare the surroundings to those where you may put your machine. If it seems a bit noisy in the showroom and you plan to put it in a small room with little insulation, expect that it will be even louder at home. How much space does it take up? Take measurements to make sure you have enough room for the treadmill you are considering, and for safety purposes, avoid positioning the treadmill so the back of the deck is close to a wall. One small misstep and you could be thrown into an unplanned chiropractic adjustment, as well as in need for some home remodeling. Which leads to the next essential feature.

Safety features: You absolutely want an *emergency pull/stop mechanism*. In the event that you would unexpectedly fall (or move more than a few feet from the treadmill), a light emergency cord connected to the treadmill control panel would disengage and instantly stop the motor. Some prefer to wear it clipped onto their clothing; others prefer for it to rest on top of the treadmill within reach. Either is an effective and valuable safety feature. A *railing* is a safety factor and also a personal preference for many people. Front rails are best; side rails are steadying but, for some, can get in the way during exercise. This is another reason to get on the treadmill and feel the differences between the models.

Deck, speed, and other features: Deck flexibility will make a difference in how your bones and joints feel in response to the impact. There is no standard word to describe how flexible the deck is, but you need to inquire if the treadmills you are considering have such a system. Good treadmills have some type of flexible deck system. You also want a smooth belt action, which means that the machine can pull its own weight (and yours) without hesitation or knocking. What are the maximum speed and maximum elevation the machine can deliver? If you consistently run a blazing 6-minute mile, some treadmills cannot run as fast as you, and you would not want to buy them. The more components you want to see displayed on the console, the higher the price. But do not let that discourage you. Envision yourself walking/running for years to come, and think about how much enjoyment and motivation you will derive from knowing how you did in those seemingly trivial areas. The components panel may display your distance, speed, calories burned, elevation, programmable workouts, and heart rate monitor. Lastly, note which creature comforts, if any, are important to you, such as cup and magazine holders. Make a list of questions and bring it with you when shopping so that all your concerns are addressed before buying.

Do not waste your money on nonelectrical or human-powered treadmills. They have a limited capacity for generating any degree of exercise happiness and satisfaction. The movement of the belt is stiff, sluggish, and uneven and it doesn't feel like something you'd want to stay on for more than one minute. The mental and physical energy spent trying to make it feel better can be better spent doing something more pleasurable and/or easier to do.

Manufacturers: Manufacturers include BodyGuard, Precor, Quinton, Trotter, StarTrek, and Pacemaster.

Price range: The price range is from $800 to $3000 plus.

Rower

Considerations: The top of the category are those rowers that utilize a flywheel, fan, cable, and handle, and have a smooth gliding seat. The shortcut versions have arm handles that you could choose to think of as oars and a seat that rides along a short track. Chances are good that you will not stick with this one. The glide is not smooth, and the tension is inconsistent, which means you will not be comfortable. That means you will not stay on it long enough to get enthused about your exercise.

Manufacturers: Manufacturers include Concept II and Precor.

Ski Machine

Considerations: NordicTrack is all you really need to know. You can buy them in NordicTrack retail stores, at their Web site, through their 800 number, or through the classified ads of your newspaper. The

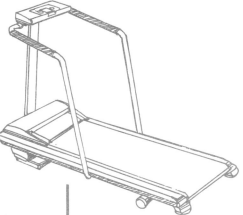

Treadmill
The versatility (walking and running), ease of use, convenience, safety, and reliability of a treadmill make it a top choice for in-home exercise equipment. Features to consider before buying include: the user's body weight, horsepower, length of deck and user's length of stride, side or front rails, noise output, space, emergency pull cord to stop, display panel with motivational information (speed, distance, calories burned, heart rate monitor), manual and programmable workouts, speed and elevation capability, warranty, maintenance, flexible deck, and cup/water bottle holder.

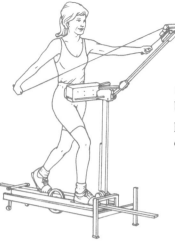

NordicTrack® Ski Exerciser
The NordicTrack ski exerciser is a durable, reliable, and somewhat portable workhorse piece of aerobic equipment.

company was bought out in the late 1990s, and the skier line was reduced to one model, the Classic Pro. This machine is so well built that it rarely, if ever, breaks or needs to be replaced.

Conjecture is that slow sales were due in part to the superior craftsmanship; loyal customers loved their machines, but because they were built to last, they never had reason to buy another one. Of course, competition became much fiercer too, but it is one solid performance piece of exercise equipment. Regardless, the machine is still a great buy.

Cost: It sells new for $600 and used for between $250 and $400.

Considerations: The arm and leg settings are independent of each other, which is a thoughtful design. You can work just the legs if you prefer (it is suggested that you get comfortable with the legs before you add the arm action), or you can tighten up the leg tension so that the skis will not move and just work the arms. As for maintenance, the rollers that the skis run on top of need to have a drop or two of oil applied once or twice a year. Wipe off sweat after each use. Pretty simple.

The electronics compartment gives speed, distance, calories burned, and heart rate. And if you prefer to use your own heart rate monitor, it can attach to the console. The Nordic Track is portable and folds up for storage. It is not ideal to have to do that with every use, but it can be done if necessary.

Climbing Machines
Stair Climber

Considerations: If you are used to the commercial gym stair climber, you might consider purchasing a used one (refurbished, of course) from either the health club or from an exercise equipment company. The commercial variety typically uses chains and/or cables, which is what gives them a smooth pedal action. Less expensive steppers utilize air pressure or hydraulic pistons, and they may feel less smooth and even a bit bouncy because of it. Extras you may want are the plastic cup and magazine holder.

Manufacturers: Manufacturers include HydraFitness, LifeStep, Precor, StairMaster, and Tetrix.

Climbing/Stepping Machine: Versa Climber

Imagine climbing up a mountain using your arms and legs but in the safety of a nonaltitude, indoor environment. In 1981 Heart Rate, Inc., introduced the first climbing/stepping machines. The Versa Climber and Climbmaster machines effectively and simultaneously build cardiovascular fitness, muscular strength, and endurance. The design ensures good posture and mechanics, which is often sacrificed by users of single action stair climbing machines. Commercial models are available in many gyms, and home models are available.

Cost: Home model starts at $1430.

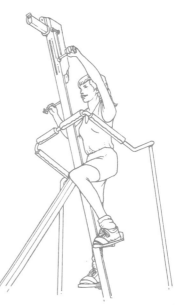

Versa Climber Climbing/Stepping Machine
Climbing machines are versatile because they can function as either a stair climbing machine or as a dual-action (arm and leg) climbing machine. Climbers use all of the major muscle groups of the upper and lower body during this aerobic exercise.

Exercise Clothing

Each of the products in this section will prove to be good investments if you use them. Getting started is the first step, so use whatever tools you have available to make that happen. After you have been successful over time, you can always re-evaluate your needs.

Shoes

Shoes support the foundation of your body weight, so you definitely want the right shoe to accommodate the specific activity. Some simple ailments of the ankles, hips, and knees are easily avoided with the purchase of the appropriate shoe. For fitness activities whose foot movements are largely up and down and compression related, such as standing or pedaling, an average running shoe will provide excellent support. For activities whose movements are predominantly lateral, such as aerobics or racquet sports, either a sport-specific shoe (a tennis shoe for tennis) or a cross-trainer shoe is appropriate. Most people at some point will buy a running shoe for either running, walking, or casual walking. To be better prepared, review this section before buying your next pair of shoes. The more you know, the better the chances that you will buy the right pair of shoes for your needs, without overspending. We all like that!

The Anatomy of a Running Shoe

When you've tried on running shoes, how many times have you used phrases such as "this doo-hickey" or "this cushy piece" to describe a part of the shoe that feels a certain way on your foot? With a little basic running shoe knowledge, you can become a more informed buyer and satisfied user. This anatomy session can help you get the shoe that's right for you.

Toebox: The toebox is the toe section of the shoe. It should be roomy enough to comfortably fit your toes. There should be approximately half an inch between your longest toe and the end of the shoe and half an inch between the top of your highest toe and the top of the toebox.

Laces: You should lace your running shoes with cotton laces that are not too long or slippery. If too long, cut them down and use lace locks.

Upper: The upper refers to the material that encloses the foot. Breathable fabrics such as mesh keep feet from overheating but are cooler in the winter time. Be sure the upper fits properly; it helps the shoe stabilize the foot.

Tongue: The tongue should be thick enough to protect the top of the foot from pressure of the laces but not so long that it rubs against your foot just above the ankle.

Heel notch: The heel notch is the slight depression cut into the shoe's heel collar to reduce Achilles tendon irritation and provide a more secure heel fit.

If the Shoe Fits . . .

- Wear running shoes for running, jogging, combination jogging/walking, stationary bicycling, stair climbing, and weight training.

- Wear sport-specific shoes or cross-trainer shoes for aerobics, step aerobics, racquet sports, and dance.

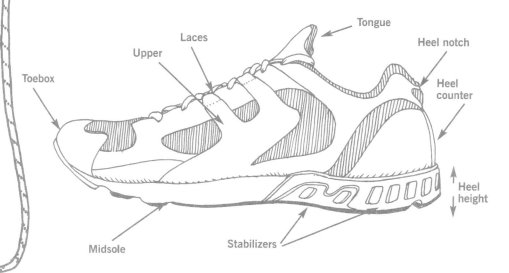

Heel counter: This is the rounded place where your heel fits snugly yet comfortably. Too loose a fit can cause blisters on your heels. If you need extra stability (your feet wobble a lot), look for a stiff heel counter or an external heel counter or ring that wraps around the outside of the heel.

Heel height: Look for heel heights that match your cushioning needs. If you are a big person, chances are you are more of a heel-striker and want more midsole foam under the heel, so you need a greater heel height. Faster runners tend to strike more in the midfoot and need a lower heel.

Split heel: On the bottom of the shoe, look for a two-part heel structure that separates the outer and inner sides and contributes to a smoother heel-to-toe transition.

Stabilizing Technology: These are devices that reduce over-pronation. These are usually in the shoe's midsole on the arch side of the shoe. Some shoes have firmer densities of midsole foam to combat overpronation.

Midsole: You want one of two midsole foams, polyurethane or EVA. Polyurethane is denser, heavier, and more durable than EVA. EVA has a softer, cushier feel. Generally, big persons do well with polyurethane midsoles. EVA is more common because of its lightness and more cushioned feel.

Outsole: This is the stuff that covers the bottom of the shoe. You want one of two kinds, carbon rubber or blown rubber, or a combination of the two. Carbon rubber is more durable but heavier and stiffer than blown rubber. Some shoes have carbon rubber in the high-wear areas of the rearfoot and the cushier blown rubber in the forefoot, for a softer feel.

Costs: Running shoes are priced from $30 to $140.

Adapted from *Runner's World*, September, 1999. For running shoe companies and contact information, see the Appendix.

Dressing for the Part: Selecting Exercise Clothing

You want to stick with your exercise program, but you don't want your exercise clothing to be sticking to you. The wrong kind of clothing can cause imprints, chafes, and blisters. Some people mock fashion for exercise (they must be nonexercisers!), but authentic exercise clothing

Lace Locks

These tiny devices are used by runners and triathletes to save the time (and to compensate for the absence of fine motor skill dexterity) it takes to tie one's shoelaces during a race. Within each lace lock is a small hole with a spring, which, when compressed with the fingers, creates an opening through which to thread the laces. Once the laces are fed through the hole, the spring is released and the laces are locked into place. Laces secured with lace locks do not come untied and they allow for easy and quick shoelace adjustment. Once you use lace locks you'll wish you could use them on your dress shoes too. There is one caution. Since tying one's shoes is a valuable lifetime skill, young children shouldn't use them in place of learning how to tie their shoes.

The Arch Test

Before drying your feet, step out of the shower onto a dark towel so that you leave a footprint. A full-foot image indicates a low arch; a curvy incomplete foot image indicates a high arch; in between indicates a medium arch. Use this information when shoe shopping and match the shoe to your arch style.

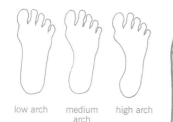

low arch   medium   high arch
            arch

The Post-Shower Arch Test
Immediately after your shower, step onto a dark towel so you leave a footprint. A full foot image (image 1) indicates a low arch, a curvy incomplete foot image (image 3) indicates a high arch, and in between (image 2) indicates a medium arch. This information can be used to match an appropriate shoe to your arch style.

is designed for function and to perpetuate the stick-to-it-ness of your program, as you will learn here.

Does the thought of riding a stationary bike in tight-fitting blue jeans send a chill up your spine? Or how do you like it when your shorts or shirt have chafed your skin? How confident do you feel when you wear worn-out, torn, and faded garments? Do such garments make you feel more outgoing and friendly, or do they make you want to avoid contact with others? Wearing comfortable, functional, colorful clothing during exercise can greatly enhance your comfort and enjoyment. If you want to elevate your exercise mood, wear exercise clothing that feels good and that you feel good about.

Support Materials

Undergarments provide support to very important parts of your anatomy. Make sure that they have the right amount of elasticity, strength, and support to do their job, but not so much that they constrict or chafe. The use of a non-petroleum lubricant such as BodyGlide can prevent or ease chafing and skin irritations.

Athletic Supporters, Jock Straps, Compression Shorts

Personal preference will dictate the use of these invaluable protective and supportive devices for boys and men. For contact activities (martial arts) and even some nonintentional contact sports (soccer), athletic cups and supporters may be preferred. Two garment styles that have taken the place of the more traditional supporters are running shorts with built-in liners and compression shorts. They reduce movement and vibration, which leads to greater comfort.

Sport Bras

Unlike the male support materials that have been around a long time, sport bras were first introduced in the late 1970s but didn't become as widely accepted (worn without a shirt over them) until the 1980s, as the running boom hit. One of the originals, named "Jog bra," has become for many people the categorical description. Now more universally known as the sport bra, the impact of this supportive garment on women's health and independence has been revolutionary. It liberated big-breasted women, who were previously inactive; today, large-breasted women have numerous options for exercising in comfort.

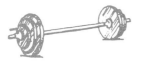
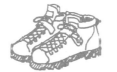
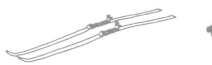

Sleepy or Slipping Feet? Try These!

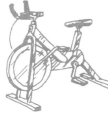

One very bright exercising professional complained that his feet would go to sleep only during exercise and that his shoes were not tied too tightly. For weeks this went on, until finally he tried a new lacing system. If you have sleepy feet or feet that slip out of the heel cup, try these lacing techniques.

- **Narrow foot** If your foot slides around in your shoe and tightening your laces doesn't fix the problem, try the lacing pattern here. Notice the "lace lock" near the forefoot.

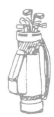

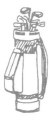

- **Shoe Lacing 101** How you lace your shoes can make a world of comfortable difference. Does your heel slip in your shoes? Does the top of your foot get irritated or fall asleep? If so, these lacing remedies just might help you.
- **Heel slippage** If your heel moves side to side or up and down, try the "lace lock." It will bring the heel of the shoe closer to your heel, alleviating the slipping.
- **High instep** If the top of your foot falls asleep or gets irritated, you may have a high instep. A high instep causes your foot to take up an excessive amount of space in your shoe. If so, follow the lacing pattern here. It should give you the extra space to alleviate the pressure.

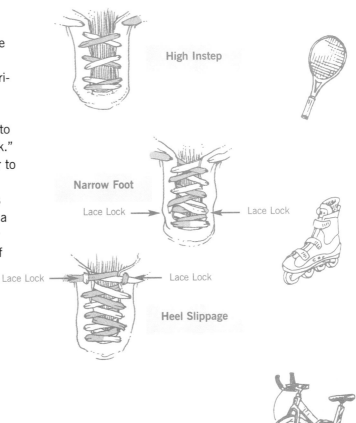

High Instep

Narrow Foot

Lace Lock → ← Lace Lock

Lace Lock → ← Lace Lock

Heel Slippage

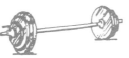

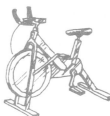

Types: There are three types of sport bras: compression, encapsulation, and combination. Compression style uses fabric pressure to squeeze or press the breasts inward toward the chest, which limits movement. This style is favored by small- to medium-breasted women. The encapsulation style limits movement by surrounding and supporting the breasts with reinforced seams or wire and is a favorite of large-breasted women. The combination compression-encapsulation sport bra utilizes both principles.

Options: There are many options for sport bras, and women are all the healthier and happier for them. Comfort should ultimately dictate a woman's choice. The options include underwire, wireless, rear clasp, front clasp, no clasp, front zipper, cross-over-the-head, cross-in-the-back, cross-in-the-front, halter style, nursing compatible, prosthetic compatible, heart rate monitor encapsulable, high impact, and low impact. Fabrics include Lycra, Coolmax, Supplex, polyester/Lycra, Drylete, cotton, spandex, and mesh.

Best sources: If your local sporting goods or running stores do not have what you need, two women's apparel catalogs with great selections of sport bras are Title Nine Sports and Athleta (see the Appendix for contact information). At last count, Title Nine had more than twenty sport bras offered in their catalog, and Athleta had fifteen. Brands or manufacturers include Adidas, Champion, Hind, Moving Comfort, Nike, and Reebok.

Cost: Sport bras cost from $18 to $40.

Exercise Clothing "Partnerships"

Exercise and 100% cotton garments have outgrown each other as optimum partners. Why? Because 100% cotton items become wet and stay wet, which can cause chafing, odor, and chills. New fabrics are used in every form of exercise clothing on the market, including shirts, tops, singlets, vests, jackets, arm warmers, hats, ear muffs, headbands, sport bras, shorts, tights, leg warmers, sweats, compression shorts, socks, swim suits, and wet suits. Wearing 100% cotton exercise clothing is the equivalent of using rotary dial telephones. You can still use them, but your options are severely limited. Old fabrics are not as efficient, productive, or comfortable as the newer fabrics.

The blended, engineered fabrics to look for in your exercise garments are Coolmax, Drylete, Lycra, polypropylene, polyester, spandex,

Supplex, cotton blends, wool, and wool blends. These are the champions of removing moisture from the body. This action quickens evaporation of perspiration, which is what keeps you dry, temperature regulated, and comfortable. This moisture-wicking action also makes you less "nose-able," that is, less noticeable in an odoriferous way! The moisture-releasing properties make laundering these garments better and easier because of their quick-drying capability. This can be a big plus when you only have a few athletic garments, are traveling, or need to wash and wear them again the very next day. So select these fabrics for your exercise clothes and experience the many pleasant comforts and conveniences.

Socks

Some people tend to take socks for granted, perhaps because of the "out of sight, out of mind" theory. But it only takes one blister to bring your feet to your attention. The fit of your socks can make a tremendous difference in your exercise comfort. Your socks should not constrict your skin or make a deep imprint upon it, especially at the ankles or calves. Socks are meant to support, reduce friction, regulate foot temperature, and promote comfort and circulation, not constrict it. Socks should not bunch up inside your shoes or slide off your feet, and you should be able to move your feet and wiggle your toes comfortably.

Again, 100% cotton, once recommended, is no longer the winner. Socks made from Coolmax, Supplex, Kevlar, acrylic, Merino wool, wool blends, combed cotton, nylon, or cotton blends help keep moisture, blistering, and bunching to a minimum, which leads to overall greater comfort. A high-performance sock label reads like the chemistry panel for a scientific experiment, but these are highly functional, comfortable socks designed for long-term wear and endurance athletics.

Cross Dressing?

Most exercise clothing is adaptable and agreeable to numerous activities. Just as you can cross train, you can cross dress. You can wear running tights for bicycling, cross-country skiing, and in-line skating. You can wear running shoes for the climbing/stepping machine, NordicTrack, and stationary bicycling. Glad that's clarified!

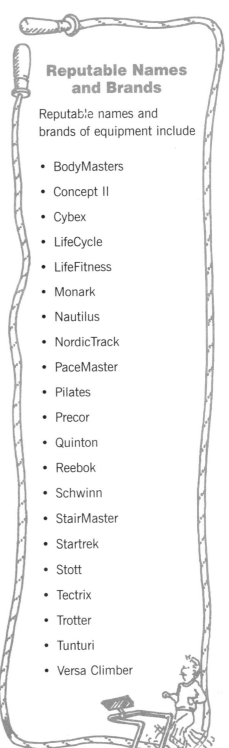

Reputable Names and Brands

Reputable names and brands of equipment include

- BodyMasters
- Concept II
- Cybex
- LifeCycle
- LifeFitness
- Monark
- Nautilus
- NordicTrack
- PaceMaster
- Pilates
- Precor
- Quinton
- Reebok
- Schwinn
- StairMaster
- Startrek
- Stott
- Tectrix
- Trotter
- Tunturi
- Versa Climber

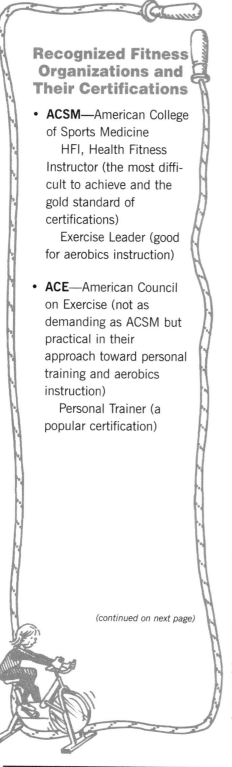

Recognized Fitness Organizations and Their Certifications

- **ACSM**—American College of Sports Medicine
  HFI, Health Fitness Instructor (the most difficult to achieve and the gold standard of certifications)
  Exercise Leader (good for aerobics instruction)

- **ACE**—American Council on Exercise (not as demanding as ACSM but practical in their approach toward personal training and aerobics instruction)
  Personal Trainer (a popular certification)

(continued on next page)

Tops

Exercise tops come in all of the fabrics above and in many styles, including long-sleeved, turtleneck, mock T-neck, short-sleeved, sleeveless, muscle t, tank, and short crop. Feel free to enjoy making a fashion statement, but first and foremost, find the style that is comfortable and does not interfere with your activity. Prices vary.

Bottoms

Also available in many fabric styles, exercise clothes for your bottom half include compression shorts, cycling shorts, running shorts (loose fit), tights, loose fit sweats, and tri-shorts. With some fun experimenting, you will find the styles and fabrics that work best for you. Prices vary.

For a complete listing of clothing manufacturers and suppliers, see the Appendix at the end of the book.

Health Clubs, Gyms, and Classes

Many people enjoy the camaraderie, support, and enthusiasm of exercising around others. The club and class environment gets you mentally prepared even before you begin. And even if you do not want to be conversational, the visual impact of being around others exercising is validating, and the collective energy is contagious.

Classes

These exercise formats work well for many because they provide a definite and specific commitment of day and time. They are not only terrific for exercising but also fun, and they provide socialization. Group settings for exercise are like "exercise parties," social celebrations of your good health. Classes are available at many places including community centers, universities, high schools, religious centers, and private businesses that offer classes. Remember, if you enjoy what you do, you are more likely to continue doing it. The benefits of signing up for classes (versus joining a health club) are that classes are offered by skill levels and given for a definite period of weeks. If cost is an issue, you have more flexibility with a class. You can sign up and pay for only the time of year that you are available to participate, versus paying a continuous/monthly club fee when you know you will be gone for 2 weeks in the winter and 4 weeks in the summer. Ask to attend or observe a class with the designated instructor before you sign up to make sure you haven't subjected yourself to the nightmare-loudmouth you had for a drill sergeant.

Health Clubs/Gyms

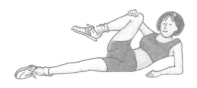

Location, location, location: This isn't buying a house or opening a retail business, but the same law of success applies. If the health club is more than 10 minutes from your home or office, chances are you will not go.

Big or small? It depends what you want from the club. Larger clubs offer more of everything including equipment, variety of classes, a bigger locker room with more showers, people, and so on. Small clubs can feel less intimidating to beginners and more personal.

Costs: While many gyms and health clubs are friendly and helpful and are exciting to join, the experience of joining a gym with an "attitude" can be about as pleasant as buying a car from an obnoxious dealer. Remember that you are the potential customer, the lifeblood of any business. If you are getting hard-sell pressure tactics, tell them you want to think about it and walk out. Even when they throw limited time offers as bait, you can always walk back in and offer that under *that* condition you will join. Memberships usually include an initiation or membership fee plus a monthly fee. Many offer discounts on these fees once or twice a year, during slow times such as May or November. Many clubs offer fitness evaluation sessions that will rebate or reduce some of the fees. They are usually worthwhile and good benchmarks for you to establish your fitness levels before you begin.

Monthly fees: To fairly evaluate these fees, divide them by the number of times per month you anticipate using them to get an estimated cost per session value. This puts the fees into a better perspective without overwhelming you with a total cost. Understand the total value you receive for the investment. For example, if you join a club and it costs $60 per month, figure that to be $2 a day for your health and fitness. Or, if you go four times per week, that comes out to $5 per session with amenities; five times per week is $4 per session plus amenities. Is it a place you like going to? Do they have the equipment you like to use? Do you like the instructors/trainers/other participants? Is it clean? Is

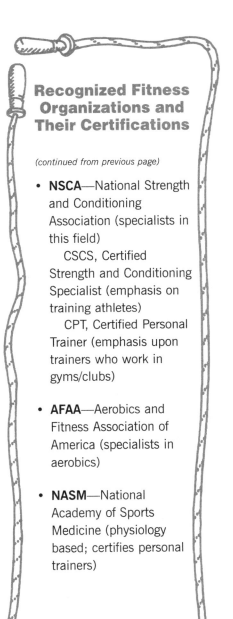

Recognized Fitness Organizations and Their Certifications

(continued from previous page)

- **NSCA**—National Strength and Conditioning Association (specialists in this field)
  CSCS, Certified Strength and Conditioning Specialist (emphasis on training athletes)
  CPT, Certified Personal Trainer (emphasis upon trainers who work in gyms/clubs)

- **AFAA**—Aerobics and Fitness Association of America (specialists in aerobics)

- **NASM**—National Academy of Sports Medicine (physiology based; certifies personal trainers)

Exercise Gym and Health Club Etiquette

1. Do you wear head-phones and listen to music or radio talk shows while exercising? If so, remember that others near you can hear your singing or the comments you are making in response to the radio talk show host.

2. The stair-climbing machine and stationary bicycle are not telephone booths. Take your cell phone to a private area (like where the telephones are located). No one wants to hear your conversation.

3. If someone is using the weight machine that you want, ask if you can work in (take turns or alternate each set). However, if you have to readjust the seat and add or subtract weights each

(continued on next page)

the equipment well maintained? Do you have shower facilities? Do they provide towels? These components all cost money, and if they are all part of what keeps you going, then it is worth it. Once you consider all the components, the cost-to-value ratio can be a healthy one.

Time, day, and closures: Some clubs close on Sundays; some are open 24 hours a day, 7 days a week. Make sure your schedule matches the hours of operation. Ask for their policy on "leave of absence." Some wisely offer temporary leaves without monthly fees or reinstatement fees. Does your potential club close in the summer for 2 weeks for maintenance and refurbishing? If so, do you pay during that time, and do they have an alternative place for you to exercise?

Equipment and classes: This is the entrée and what you came for. Do they have the classes and equipment you want? Does it look like a lot of equipment, or is it sparsely outfitted? Are the brands of equipment reputable?

The members: Surround yourself with those who will motivate you, whatever that means to you. You do not want to be judgmental or alienate yourself from joining just because you think everyone but you looks like the cover photo for a fitness magazine. On the other hand, do you want to go to a gym where no one looks like they have made any progress? New friends can come in all sizes, shapes, and designs. Keep an open, friendly attitude, and you can have a surprisingly positive experience.

Staff: In the beginning you may need more assistance, until you know what you are doing. Observe the staff to see whether they appear competent, caring, and friendly. Are the instructors certified and knowledgeable?

Maintenance: When you walk in first thing, does the place smell bad? If so, there is your first clue that cleanliness is not valued or practiced as much as it is needed. Do you ever see staff cleaning the equipment, the floors, sinks, showers, mirrors, and locker rooms? Can you see through the water of the jacuzzi? Can you breathe clean or odorless air in the sauna and steam rooms? Are the bathrooms well stocked with supplies? These are a large part of what you pay for in your fees, and management should deliver the clean goods.

Other features: You may not need any of these other features, but if you do, make sure you inquire as to whether they are offered. Does the club offer day care, towel service, laundry service, privately owned lockers, a snack bar, massage therapy, social gatherings, nutritional services, and televisions near the aerobic equipment?

Personal Fitness Trainers

Personal fitness trainers can be helpful in teaching you how and what to do, specifically in your exercise sessions. It is in your best interest to learn the how and why of what you are doing as well as to enjoy their company during your sessions. Then you can work toward becoming less dependent upon them for the long term. But trainers can be invaluable in showing you proper technique and helping you avoid valuable losses of time due to injury and/or frustration "spinning your wheels" doing something improperly. Trainers also can provide valuable motivation and help break you into exercise as a habit and commitment.

Expectations: Your trainer can help you with as much or as little as you commit to in your program. If you have the cardiovascular fitness component of your exercise program well under control, your trainer can help you with strength training or flexibility. Be specific about what you want, and if you are unsure about what you want, ask the trainer for a recommendation. Your trainer should make sure through close observation that you perform your activities with proper form and mechanics and at the proper levels for you and give you corrective and supportive feedback regularly. Your trainer should also help you to update your progress and continue to overload you as warranted for building and maintaining your fitness.

Certifications: The science of exercise and sport has matured tremendously in the past 20 years, and it is much easier these days to find someone knowledgeable to guide you. Trainers with bachelor's degrees in exercise science, exercise physiology, health and human performance, physical education, and the like are highly valued. Those with current master's degrees in the field are probably of the highest caliber that you will encounter. But even for trainers with a degree, certifications are important; most require continuing education in order to recertify every few years. Trainers with college degrees and current certifications are optimum, but do not discount the value of a trainer who has no college degree and holds only a current certification from a reputable organization. As with any educated professional, their competence has as much to

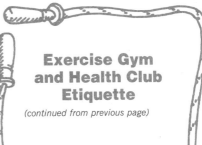

Exercise Gym and Health Club Etiquette

(continued from previous page)

time, you are better off waiting until the person is finished.

4. If someone appears eager to use the machine you are using, either tell them how much longer you anticipate using it or invite them to work in with you.

5. Use your towel (or disinfectant spray and towel, if provided) to clean up the equipment, seats, or benches you used.

6. Remove heavy weight plates from barbells when you are finished so that others can use the barbells.

7. Remember that most people are on a tight time schedule, so don't just hang out on the equipment if you are not using it.

Locker Room Etiquette

1. If it is rush hour and others are waiting in line for the shower, be considerate and make it short.

2. Spray your cologne, perfume, deodorant, or hair spray out of range of others.

3. Share the dressing area and mirror. Don't "stake your claim" and then go away for more than a couple of minutes.

4. Remove trash, cups, hangers, and other items from the locker.

5. Be courteous. It's a common locker room, not your personal dressing room.

do with the personal integrity, interest, experience, and enthusiasm of the person as it does with the credential achieved. There are many certifying bodies, with differing emphases. Select the one that fits your needs. You wouldn't want an expert aerobics teacher instructing you on weight training unless s/he holds a certification in that field too. Trainers should possess a good knowledge of anatomy, physiology, the principles of exercise, and overload and, like any professional, have a personal interest in you and your goals. Some trainers offer the choice of coming to your location, and some will have you go to theirs.

Business related: Some trainers charge by the hour, others by the session. Fees can range from $25 an hour to $150 an hour, depending on the market. Ask if your trainer has a business license and liability insurance. These are good signs that they are legitimate business owners, committed to their customers.

Fitness Consultants

This new breed of fitness professional is testament to the growth and need for expanding fitness services. Fitness consultants are independent fitness experts who offer a variety of fitness-related services, from program design, classes for senior, prenatal or postnatal or other population specific groups, nutritional counseling, sport-specific training programs, exercise testing, public speaking, corporate consulting, writing, and anything else related to fitness. They may hold the same or higher degrees and certifications as trainers. Consultants emphasize education, instruction, motivation, and independence. If you want someone to evaluate, educate, instruct, and motivate you, but not necessarily accompany you on your workouts, engaging the services of a fitness consultant could be money better spent than the services offered by a personal trainer.

Cost: Consultants usually cost more than trainers, but there are fewer sessions. The fee is $60 to $200 an hour, depending on market.

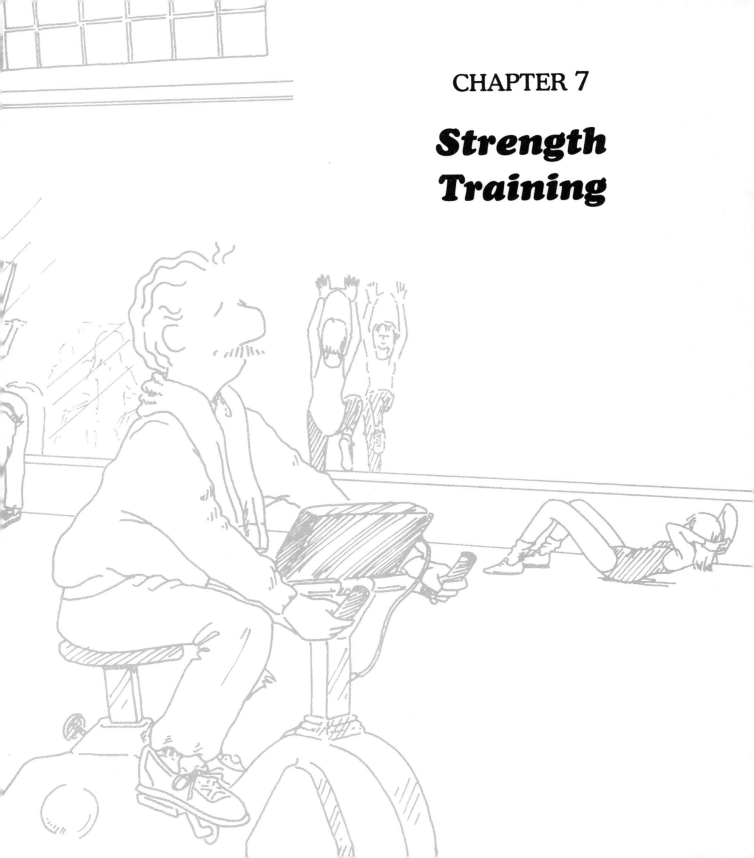

CHAPTER 7

Strength Training

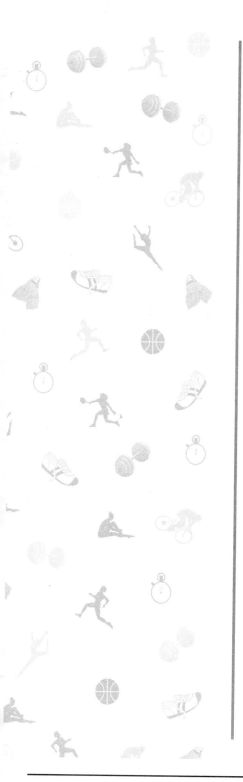

We all want muscles; without muscles we have no strength, little function, and cannot live an independent life. Muscles are *body tools* that help us perform work. It has also been proven that the work we perform to maintain and improve our muscles has other positive effects on our health.

Strength training benefits everyone, including children, women, men, older adults, and athletes. It is effective in developing and maintaining muscular strength and endurance; developing muscle mass; stimulating bone density (which helps prevent osteoporosis); reducing body fat; preventing and treating low back pain, diabetes, obesity, and orthopedic injuries; and reducing falls in elderly persons.

Increased muscular strength allows you to perform the basic and functional movements of life, such as picking up your small children or pets, carrying your groceries and luggage, taking out the recycling and trash, or moving from a lying position to a raised position without back pain. With increased strength, you can participate with greater ease in seemingly simple activities, such as standing and walking the sidelines all day at your child's soccer tournament, hiking and experiencing new sights, riding your bike farther than usual, or pushing your wheelchair-bound friend outside for a real outing of 1 hour rather than 10 minutes. Increased strength gives you the ability to improve other areas of your health, such as aerobic fitness. And lastly, strength training is empowering because it enables you *to do* what before you could not do, to do it with ease and without negative consequences.

Injuries associated with strength training come from training improperly or from doing too much. We will cover strength training *fun*damentals (yes, it can be fun) to make sure you know how to properly include this valuable fitness component into your life.

Bulk Is in the Eye of the Beholder

Do you fear that by strength training you will become big and bulky? Many men and women who have an inflated, unnatural muscular appearance do so with the help of an unhealthy additive, anabolic steroids.

Unless you decide to spend hours and hours lifting very heavy weights, you will not get bulky. First of all, women do not have enough natural testosterone to produce major size. And secondly, men will build bulk only if they spend many hours each week lifting extremely heavy weights. But as you will learn, there are many other ways to lift weights that will not produce such an effect.

What is bulk anyway? Bulk is merely something with great volume, something that takes up a lot of space. Fat is bulky and muscle can be bulky. But fat lacks definition, and it can be all over the place.

Strength training develops the shape of your muscles. Shape has a definite outline; shape is not "all over the place." The word *definition* refers to the shapeliness of one's muscles. Strength training may cause you to become shapely, but you should not confuse shape with bulk. You will learn in this chapter how to tailor your weight training to your goals. Bulk may be in the eye of the beholder, but—don't kid yourself—muscle is healthier, better looking, functional, and takes up less space than fat.

Overload Principle: The way we stimulate muscle growth is by applying the Overload Principle (Chapter 4), pushing the body (in this case, your muscles) a bit beyond what it is accustomed to. To strengthen muscles, overload is accomplished by offering them resistance, or an opposing force. Think of it as "taking them out of their comfort zone." The opposing force comes from gravity and weight. In this chapter, you will learn how to use different types of resistance (as the opposing force) to build strength (the terms *resistance training* and *strength training* are used interchangeably and simply mean the process used to produce strength; the term *weight training* refers to using weight(s) for resistance that produces gains in strength).

Anatomy Review

You may not be interested about the intricacies of your automobile, but you probably know where the parts that need more frequent attention are located, such as the gas tank, the oil stick, the tires and air valves, the wiper fluid well, the coolant well, and so on. If you plan to exercise and want to do so most effectively, being familiar with the names and specific functions of your muscles will serve you well. You don't have to memorize them, but understanding where they are located, what they do, how big or small they are, and what they look like will give you the knowledge to work out with your brain and not just brawn.

Steroids

Anabolic steroids were produced in the 1930s as a supplement for malnourished and undernourished persons. Steroids helped individuals to gain weight and muscle size until the time when proper nutrition could be established. Other people, for whom the steroids were not intended, began experimenting with steroids and were enthused by the quick weight and strength gains that could be achieved.

The problem with steroid use is the serious and damaging side effects it has on the body. Steroids cause aggressive behavioral abnormalities, damage to the liver and kidneys, and impair bodily functions. There is also suspicion that they can cause some types of cancer.

Here's a list of body parts and related muscles:

- **Shoulders**

    Deltoids are the muscles that run over the tops of your arms. They are responsible for moving your upper arm in many directions.

    The *rotator cuff* is a group of four muscles underneath your shoulder. They are used for throwing and catching, carrying or reaching.

- **Back**

    Trapezius is the elongated diamond-shaped muscle that runs into your neck across your shoulders and down to the center of your back. It is used for most back functions as well as lifting your arms out sideways to wave to someone.

    The *Latissimus dorsi* is the largest of your back muscles, which goes from below your shoulders to your lower back. It is used for pulling. Developed "lats" balance against rounded shoulders.

    Rhomboids are small, rhomboid shaped (like rectangles) muscles underneath the trapezius at the center of your back. They are used to keep your shoulder blades together, which helps your posture.

    Erector spinae run the length of your spine, but you want to emphasize strengthening the lower segment of the back. These enable you to straighten your spine, to go from reclining or bending, to standing or straightening.

- **Chest**

    Pectoralis are the main muscles of your chest. And yes, even if you have breasts, you have pectoralis muscles underneath, vying for your attention. Activities that require you to push with your arms happen because of your "pecs." They help to push a wheelchair, shopping cart, or lawn mower.

- **Upper Arm**

    Biceps are the two most famous muscles at the front of your arm. Anytime you bend your elbow, you engage your biceps (e.g., when carrying small children or pets and lifting groceries).

    Triceps are the three-headed muscles opposite of your biceps, on the back of the upper arm. They straighten your elbow and help out your "pecs" when you push something.

Abs Versus "Stomach Muscles"

Whoever first called abdominals the stomach muscles must have missed anatomy 101 class. Abdominals are muscles that run from below your chest down past your navel. Your stomach is the receptacle and organ that digests your food. Your abdominals have nothing to do with digestion.

- **Forearm**

  There are many forearm muscles with too many names to mention here; think of them as your wrist muscles. Developing these helps prevent or alleviate symptoms of carpal tunnel syndrome and tennis elbow.

- **Abdominals**

  This set of four muscles allows you to bend at your waist, twist, and keep your torso stable. The abdominals (abs) and back muscles are neighbors, and when strong, they support your posture and back.

  Rectus abdominis are the long running muscles that start under your chest and end below your umbilicus (navel, belly button).

  Internal and external obliques run obliquely or diagonally down the sides of your rectus abdominus. These enable you to twist or bend at your side.

  Transversus abdominis are the deepest of the four abdominal muscles. The transversus abdominis comes along for the ride when you exercise the other ab muscles. It is most active when you sneeze, cough, or exhale deeply.

- **Buttocks and Hips**

  Gluteus maximus, medius, and minimus are the largest muscles on your body. They are involved in nearly everything you do with your lower body, including walking, running, stepping, jumping, and getting up.

- **Legs**

  Quadriceps are the group of four muscles on the front of your thigh. These allow you to straighten your leg at the knee.

  Hamstrings are the group of three muscles on the back of your thigh. These allow you to bend your leg at the knee.

  Gastrocnemius and soleus are better known as your calf muscles. The gastroc is the rounded muscle at the back of your lower leg, and the soleus is just underneath. Women who wear high-heeled shoes may have some calf development (and chronic soreness) because the constant angled position causes these muscles to contract or tighten.

  Tibialis anterior (shins) are on the front of your lower leg and go from just below your knee cap to the top of your

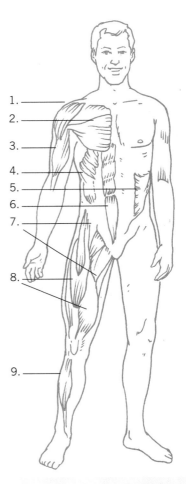

Our Muscles: Front View

1. Deltoid
2. Pectorals
3. Biceps
4. External Obliques
5. Internal Obliques
6. Rectus Abdominis
7. Adductors
8. Quadriceps
9. Tibialis Anterior

ankles. These muscles allow you to extend or point your toes. They work in opposition to the calf muscles, so you want to keep them balanced.

Types of Resistance Training

You probably have heard of the three primary forms of resistance training: dynamic, isometric or static, and isokinetic (equal force throughout motion). We are going to focus on the dynamic form, the more common and effective type used to build strength in healthy persons.

Dynamic exercises involve shortening and lengthening movements of the muscle against a constant or variable resistance. Free weights (weights that are free from machinery, such as dumbbells and barbells), weight machines, and calisthenics exercises are the most commonly used in dynamic exercises. For now, we are going to focus upon the concepts of strength training as applied to free weights and machines.

EXTREMES OF STRENGTH TRAINING

Goal: Muscular Strength and Size	Goal: Muscular Endurance
High (load) Resistance	Low Resistance
Low Repetitions	High Repetitions

Muscular strength refers to the ability to do or perform work. In addition to being able to perform heavy work the muscles become more defined in their size and shape. *Muscular endurance* refers to the ability to do or perform work over time. These two outcomes are opposites along the total spectrum of strength training.

The table above shows the two extreme objectives of strength training and how you would achieve each one. If you were to train with the exclusive purpose of developing muscular strength and size (as do some body builders) you would lift high loads/weight for a low number of repetitions. But if muscular size and strength were not your goal and instead it was to develop muscular endurance (as do some distance runners) you would lift low weight/resistance for a high number of repetitions. To achieve a general level of fitness, most individuals need to train somewhere in between the two extremes.

Our Muscles: Back View

1. Trapezius
2. Deltoid
3. Rhomboids
4. Triceps
5. Erector Spinae
6. Latissimus Dorsi
7. Forearm
8. Gluteus Medius
9. Gluteus Maximus
10. Hamstrings
11. Gastronemius
12. Soleus

You can tailor your strength training program for the result you want by adjusting the load, reps, and sets you perform. To build maximal muscular strength and size, you lift a heavy load, one that is close to the maximum amount you can lift for that exercise. To build muscular endurance, you lift a low to moderate amount of weight. And this is where the reps and sets enter the picture. Your weight training goals will determine the load and numbers of reps and sets you perform.

How Much Weight to Lift?— Two Schools of Thought

One of the biggest unknowns for beginners is how much weight to lift. You certainly don't want to hurt yourself or to cause an injury, but neither do you want to feel you are wasting your time. The amount of weight to lift will vary with the exercise and the muscle or muscle group being exercised. For small muscles and muscle groups, you want to lift less weight than what you will lift for large muscles and muscle groups (see the anatomy review for large versus small muscles).

There are two schools of thought used to determine how much weight you will lift: the *practical approach* and the *maximum repetition approach*. If you are a beginner or not very fit, the practical approach is for you. If you have some level of fitness, strength, and even some weight training experience, you could use the maximal repetition approach. Here is a brief summary of each.

Practical Approach

For those getting started or who have little strength or experience with weight training, start by lifting a very low amount of weight, one that you can pick up and exercise with easily and with proper form. Use that weight for a session or two and notice how you feel the day after; if you feel very little or no aftereffects, then increase the amount of weight to the next increment. Do so until you arrive at the amount of weight that is manageable and so that the last repetition really challenges you. This is the safest approach, especially if you are coming from a sedentary or unfit background.

Maximum Repetition Approach

The other school of thought for determining how much weight to lift is the maximum repetition approach. Although theoretically sound, if

Shin Splints

The term *shin splints* is used to describe sore tibialis anterior muscles. *Shin splints*, although painful, are usually a temporary condition. They can be a result of "waking up" the muscles; when you begin exercising, they are not yet used to the activity, and so they just get sore. Shins are vulnerable to different angles or surfaces, for example, when running or walking on a harder or softer surface than usual, changing shoes, or walking or running on a road or path with a slight camber (the rounded portion of the road). When you do make changes in those areas, light stretching immediately after the activity can help reduce soreness. Treat shin splints with ice massage, stretching, light massage, and, when necessary, rest.

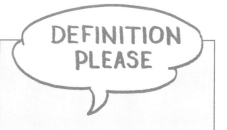

DEFINITION PLEASE

Simple Lingo

The language for basic strength training is pretty simple yet significant.

The *load* is the resistance; it is the amount of weight lifted in pounds or kilograms.

A *rep* (short for *repetition)* involves one complete movement of an exercise, including the start, the middle, and the finish.

A *set* is a series or group of repetitions.

For maximum strength and advanced size, lift very heavy weight: 6 to 8 reps, 5 to 6 sets.

For muscular endurance, lift light to moderate weight: 15 to 20 reps, 3 sets.

For general fitness and strength and endurance, lift moderate weight: 8 to 12 reps, 1 to 3 sets.

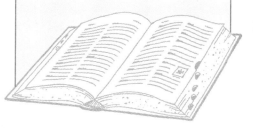

you are not fit or have little muscular strength, it can derail you before you even get started.

The term *maximum repetition* refers to the maximum amount of weight you can properly lift for one repetition and is used as the benchmark for determining how much weight you will lift during your exercise session. The use of maximum repetition in strength training can be compared to the use of maximum heart rate in aerobic exercise (see Chapter 4). You rarely, if ever, exercise at your maximum levels. They are simply used as points of reference to help you establish specific levels for exercise that will overload you. This approach takes more time and commitment than the practical approach, but it is effective.

Determining your maximum repetition. To determine your maximum repetition, you perform each exercise and find the heaviest weight that you can properly and completely lift one time. For example, to determine maximum repetition for the biceps curl, you would pick up the 5-pound weight and properly perform the exercise one time. If 5 pounds seemed very easy, then try the 8- or 10-pound weight. If you can *properly* perform one biceps curl without much effort, then try the 12- or 15-pound weight. At some point, you will perform the exercise with a weight that will either be too difficult for you to perform completely or properly. When that is the case, return to the heaviest weight that you could properly and completely perform for one repetition. That is your maximum repetition, written 1 RM (1 repetition maximum). You would then perform the same maximum repetition for each exercise.

Once you have established your 1 RM for each exercise, review your goals (maximal strength, muscular endurance, or general fitness, which is a combination of both). Then apply the percentages of effort for the goals you desire. This enables you to determine how much weight to lift for each exercise.

Let's assume that your goal is general fitness. Having established your 1 RM for each exercise, multiply the percentage of effort for general fitness, which is 60 percent, times the 1 RM. That number will be your starting weight for each exercise. To determine the numbers of sets and reps, once again apply the guidelines for general fitness, which are 8 to 12 reps for 1 to 3 sets. Do not start out with the maximum number of reps or sets. Instead work up to them.

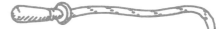

Strength Training and Women

Some women are hesitant to participate in strength training exercises because they fear they will get big muscles, something they consider unfeminine. Some men are afraid the women in their lives will lose their femininity. These men and women need to consider several facts.

- Muscles and their development are part of the human body and necessary for daily independent function.
- Strength training is a healthy exercise practice that helps keep males and females physically functional and independent.
- Women do not naturally have the hormone levels that men have that produce bulky muscle formation. Some women body builders use artificial methods to build bulky muscles; without them, they could not build bulk.
- Strength training reduces body fat. Muscle is a workhorse; fat is a storehouse. Your body wants more workhorses and fewer storehouses.
- If muscle is unfeminine and fat is feminine, tell that to the increasing numbers of active, vital, productive feminine women (actors, politicians, businesswomen, homemakers, students) who have taken up and enjoy the benefits of strength training (including former Gov. Anne Richards of Texas).

Modes for Strength Training

You can strength train with barbells, dumbbells, weight machines, bands and tubes, your body weight, Pilates-based exercise, medicine balls, and with buddy sticks and cords. Each has its own set of pros and cons regarding location, convenience, space, time/expediency, equipment required, cost, skill required, and whether or not a spotter is required.

Free Weights

These weights are unattached to chains or cables and are not part of a machine. Free weights are bars with weights attached at the ends. The shorter and stubbier-looking free weights are called dumbbells, and the longer bars are known as barbells. The beauty of free weights is that because they are not attached to anything, you can conveniently use free weights at your home, your office, or your gym. You can do

Frequently Asked Question

"While lifting, how do I know if I am lifting the right amount of weight and using the right numbers of reps and sets?"

Answer: Regardless of whether you lift 1 set of 12 reps or 3 sets of 15 reps, **the last repetition should be very challenging,** such that you can still perform it properly and completely but are glad it is your last one.

• • •

How Much Weight to Lift

For maximum strength and size, lift 80 to 85 percent of your 1 RM.

For general fitness, lift 60 to 80 percent of your 1 RM.

For muscular endurance, lift 60 percent of your 1 RM.

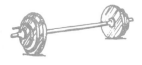
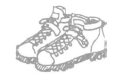
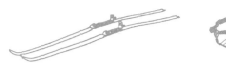

The Practical Approach

For those getting started or with little strength:
Day 1: Perform the following exercises:

Biceps curl—3-pound weight   (small muscle on front of the arm)
Triceps curl—2-pound weight   (small muscle on back of the arm)
Shoulder press—3-pound weight   (small muscle on top of shoulder)
Bent over row—5-pound weight   (larger muscle group, upper to middle of back)

If the day after performing these exercises (Day 2) you feel nothing different in your muscles (light soreness, etc.), then you should proceed to the next highest amount of weight as follows:

Day 3: Perform the following exercises:
Biceps curl—4- or 5-pound weight
    Increase in small increments of 1, 2 or 3 pounds.
  Triceps curl—3- or 4-pound weight
Shoulder press—4- or 5-pound weight
Bent over row—6-, 7-, or 8-pound weight

If the day after this session you feel some light soreness, then you should continue with these weights and adjust the numbers of reps and sets as desired.

The Maximum Repetition Approach

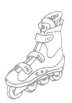

For those resuming a program or with moderate strength:

EXERCISE	MAX REPETITION (1 RM)	X % FOR GOAL	= WEIGHT TO LIFT
Biceps curl	20 pounds	x 60%	= 12 pounds
Triceps curl	10 pounds	x 60%	= 6 pounds
Shoulder press	20 pounds	x 60%	= 12 pounds
Bent over row	30 pounds	x 60%	= 18 pounds

*For this example, we are using the low end for general fitness, 60 percent of 1 RM.

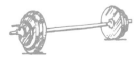
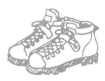
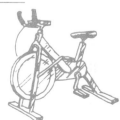

numerous exercises with a single barbell and a few weight plates; once you learn the basic exercises, you are set. The exercises are not difficult to learn. There is some skill involved in learning the exercises, but nothing as complicated as learning to tie your shoes or a necktie.

With a barbell exercise, you use two hands to perform the exercises. The length of the barbell and the ability to position weight plates at the ends gives you a mechanical advantage of spreading out the weight. Therefore, you are able to lift heavier weight than with dumbbells. Plus, using barbells also develops your coordination and balance.

The Olympic style barbells found at gyms and health clubs weigh 45 pounds without any weights or collars attached. Barbells sold for home use vary and will weigh less, so you should inquire about how much they weigh. If you intend to push yourself to lift very heavy weight, then you will need a spotter to assist you. With free weights, your muscles exercise in movements that are close to those you perform in everyday life. Although a free weight exercise may be named for a single muscle, they most often call upon other muscles to help out. So you essentially get more bang for your buck. And many people believe they get quicker results from free weights than from machines. A time consideration is that with free weights you have to add or remove weight plates in between exercises. This will add a little time to your session.

Dumbbells

Using dumbbells is a very convenient, very effective mode of weight training. Dumbbells are easy to use and take up little space; they are small enough that you can keep them at your home or office. Dumbbells are the most universal and prevalent weight training equipment around, so you will definitely see them at the gym. You are likely to see dumbbells in many hotels, which is great for when you travel and want to work out. You can do a lot with dumbbells in a short time. This is partly because you do not have to adjust them and because you rarely have to wait for someone else to finish using them, as you often do with machines. There is some skill involved in learning the exercises but, again, nothing as complicated as learning to tie your shoes. With dumbbells you provide your own balance, support, and coordination. You do not get this from machines; in fact, it is easy to sacrifice posture, mechanics, and range of motion on machines.

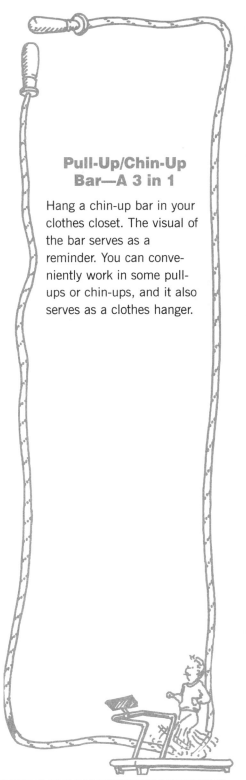

Pull-Up/Chin-Up Bar—A 3 in 1

Hang a chin-up bar in your clothes closet. The visual of the bar serves as a reminder. You can conveniently work in some pull-ups or chin-ups, and it also serves as a clothes hanger.

For some exercises you will use only one dumbbell at a time; for some you will use a set of dumbbells. A set means you have two individual dumbbells in the designated weight denomination. Because you do not lift the same amount of weight for every exercise, you will need a few different pairs. Dumbbells are inexpensive; depending upon where you live, you can expect to pay between $.50 and $1.00 per pound (which, if you think about it, is cheaper than a breast of chicken!). If you use dumbbells, you will want to buy a bench that adjusts for different incline positions.

Strength Training Machines (Cybex, Nautilus, etc.)

If you want to use machines, you will more than likely need to join a gym/health club or buy a home gym setup. Most commercial machines have instructions on them, showing proper positioning and movement of the exercise. But in the beginning, you are best to have a trainer check that you are positioned correctly. Performing an exercise in an incorrect position can stress your joints painfully and unnecessarily. Although there is not as much skill required as with other exercises, it is still important that you perform the exercises correctly. One rule that is true for any type of weight training is that you do not want to let the weights come crashing down to the stack or to the ground. That is a symptom of lifting too much weight.

One drawback to using machines in a gym or club setting is that oftentimes you have to wait for others to finish using them. Whenever you use machines in a gym/club, always check and change the weight/load for your need. Machines are designed to isolate specific muscles, so if you are trying to rehabilitate a previously injured area or target a weakness, they are very effective.

Dynamic Exercises

These are exercises that move your muscles through a range of motion and utilize gravity or body weight for resistance. They are very convenient, require some skill, do not cost much at all, and will develop balance and coordination in the process of strengthening your muscles.

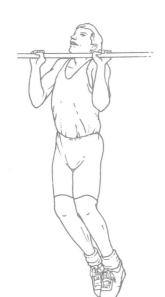

Pull-Ups

On a sturdy, horizontal bar, hang from the bar using an overhand grip (palms facing away from you), and with arms and elbows straight. Pull your body up toward the bar until your chin is just above the bar. Then lower your body slowly to the starting/hanging position. Exhale when you pull your body up; inhale when you lower it.

Variation: If you can't do a complete pull-up, use a lower bar and grasp the bar with bent elbows while you are standing on the ground.

Bands and Tubes

At first they sound like hocus pocus magic trick paraphernalia. But in reality stretch bands and tubes are very simple, inexpensive, compact devices that are effective for strength training especially while traveling or for rehabilitative exercises and initial strength gains. They are made of rubber, which explains how they allow for the exercise movement, yet provide resistance. Bands and tubes vary in thickness but generally speaking the thicker and shorter, the greater the resistance. The biggest difference between the two is that a band is a flat latex rubber strip (3 feet) that wraps around your hand(s) and a tube is a stretch cord with handles about the length of a jump rope.

You will need to learn how to use these stretch-resistance devices for each exercise, but once you do, you've got it. In most of the exercises you use your hands or feet to secure at least one end (sometimes the middle) of the band/tube while you use the other hand or foot to perform the resistance exercise. Band and tube distributors such as DynaBand, Spri, StretchCordz, and Collage Video Specialties can provide you with resources for purchasing the bands and tubes and learning the exercises. You can exercise nearly all the major muscle groups with bands and tubes and, as with free weight exercises, apply the general fitness guidelines (8–12 reps, 1–3 sets) for determining the numbers of reps and sets. If you are an "exacting type" who likes to know the exact load you are lifting, then bands and tubes may not appeal to you. With bands or tubes, it is difficult to measure and reproduce the identical workload from session to session. It is also difficult to translate what the numbers of sets and reps for dumbbell exercises would be in band or tube exercises. Bands and tubes break down over time from regular use and from exposure to severe heat or cold. Check them for signs of wear and tear and replace them when necessary. You do not want one of them tearing or breaking while you are in the middle of an exercise. When using bands and tubes, control the resistance for the entire range of motion, from start to finish. If you wrap bands around your hands, make sure you do not cut off your circulation. And when stepping on them, make sure they are secure enough to stay put and not surprise you with a snap and a pop. Check with the exercise equipment company who sells bands and tubes for video instruction and band and tube exercise routines. (See the Appendix at the back of this book for resources.)

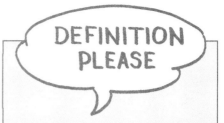

DEFINITION PLEASE

Spotter: A spotter is someone who offers assistance to the person lifting weight in the event that the lifter has trouble lifting the weight. The spotter does not assist in actually lifting the weight unless the person begins to fail at the rep.

Collars: These are the pieces that are used on each end of the weight plates to secure them onto the barbell. Collars come in a few different styles. Some are lightweight chrome and look like circular clothespins. You squeeze them to slide them onto the barbell until they are next to the weight plates, securing them into place. The older collar style is heavier and uses a screw-pin that when made tight secures the weight in place. This style can come loose on its own, so it is best to always tighten the collar before lifting the barbell. Remember: "Righty tighty, lefty loosey!"

Your Body Weight

The least expensive medium for exercise resistance is your body weight. If you were stuck someplace and had no other equipment, you could stay fit by performing push-ups, abdominal curls, leg lifts, and other calisthenics. And even if you're not stuck someplace, push-ups and the others are excellent exercises to keep your strength up. One fun way to include pull-ups and chin-ups in your life is to install a chin-up bar in your closet. As mentioned previously, the visual reminder will prompt you to do them, and the bar can also be used for hanging or drying clothes on hangers.

Push-Up Military Style

Start in the up position. Your hands and feet are shoulder width apart. Your contact points with the ground are your palms (face down) and your feet (on your toes). Keeping your body in a horizontal line, lower your entire body until your nose is inches from the ground or your upper arms are parallel to the floor (elbows may bow out). Next, push your body up to the starting extended arm position. That is one repetition.

Military-Style Push-Up

Push-Up Modified Style or Bent Knee

The lower body contact point/position is the only variation from the military push-up. However, it makes this exercise possible for those who lack the strength to perform the military style.

Instead of the toes being in contact with the floor, bend the knees and, keeping the body in the horizontal line, proceed with lowering and pushing up. Some find it helpful or comfortable to cross their feet behind them.

Bent-Knee Push-Up

Isometric Exercises

Also called static exercises, isometrics involve holding muscle contractions for seconds at a time. They became popular in the 1960s because of their convenience.

Isometric exercises are best suited for rehabilitative, orthopedic purposes, especially for limbs that have been isolated and immobilized. But isometrics are not recommended for people with high blood pressure and coronary conditions because of the increase in intrathoracic (chest area) pressure. Isometrics are not as useful for fitness purposes because they do not strengthen the muscle throughout its entire range of motion.

Pilates-Based Strength Training

Born in 1880, Joseph Pilates' early life began as a frail child but soon he became a boy on a fitness mission. He became a gymnast, a boxer, and a circus performer. He also studied yoga, karate, and other eastern movement disciplines. During World War I Joseph Pilates was imprisoned in an English internment camp. There he combined his prior studies and interests to develop a style and series of exercises that kept him mentally and physically fit. Mr. Pilates' creativity literally sprung forth as evidenced by his use of springs, frames, and mattresses of prison beds and chairs as he designed his own exercise equipment. Other prisoners and guards noticed his relatively superior health (considering the prison environment), and before long he was teaching others his body core (abdomen and back) based exercises.

Years following the internment camp, he arrived in New York City with boxing friend Max Schmelling. There he became acquainted with many prominent dancers of the time and his exercises made their way into dance training/environments.

Dancers used Pilates' style exercises and equipment to build strength and to maintain and improve flexibility. They still do today and without amassing (here comes that word again) bulk! Pilates' popularity is growing as evidenced by the greater availability of Pilates® equipment, floor exercise classes, and instructional videos currently offered for the general public.

The exercises are performed on Pilates® machines, which are the refined versions of the original ones made by Pilates himself. A common first impression of a Pilates® apparatus such as "The Reformer" conjures up feelings of fear and intimidation. With the springs, straps, and movable parts, it appears as likely to be a torturous experience as it is therapeutic. Fortunately it is the latter. Pilates® floor exercises are also performed as one would perform calisthenic exercises, on a mat. The exercises are performed slowly and gently, yet with effort. The only drawback is that if you plan to do the exercises on your own, you need a dancer's abstract ability to learn the proper technique. They work your muscles, your memory, and require patience to learn them.

Weight Bench

To work out all parts of the body, you will want to use a weight bench. Weight benches are padded and can be either a single flat bench or one that inclines and declines. Some weight benches look like very narrow seats, but you would not and should not use them for anything other than your weight exercises. Benches cost between $40 and $150.

• • •

Machine Etiquette

Always carry a towel and wipe up after yourself. Better yet, use the spray bottle and cleanup towel provided by many gyms.

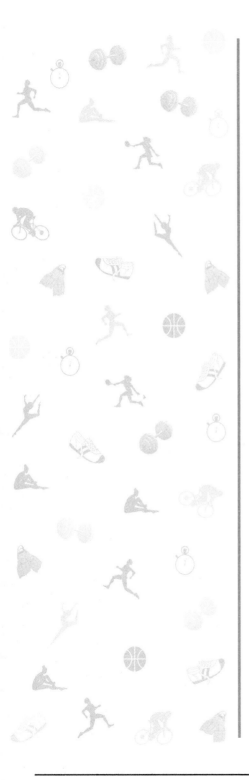

Pilates instruction is available in therapeutic and rehabilitative settings as well as in exercise class settings. There are Pilates videos that lead you through in-home exercise sessions. Pilates® certified instructors are making their way into the mainstream fitness community. And as an example of how passionate some are about the concept, there is a long-time, on-going legal challenge concerning the use and marketing of the Pilates name and trademark. Makes you wonder what Joseph Pilates would think about it all. In any event, his core strengthening exercises are well worth trying. See Appendix for Pilates® certified resources and instructors in your area.

Essentials of Strength Training

These guidelines can be applied to any of the strength training modes we've just covered.

1. Safety first. Always wear close-toed shoes and clothing that provides movement but does not hang. You do not want the end of the dumbbell to get caught in your ove-sized T-shirt and cause you to drop it on your foot. Check for clear space around you. If you want to meet the person behind you, there are better ways to go about it than punching him or her with a dumbbell during a triceps exercise. Warm up your muscles first so that they are ready to go. If you plan to strength train and do aerobic exercise on the same day, strength train after aerobic exercise. If you have an aerobic rest day, then do a light jog or stepping (even in place) or some arm circles for 5 minutes.

2. Breathe—*ex*hale with *ex*ertion. NEVER hold your breath when strength training, though it may be tempting to do so. Holding your breath during strength training increases chest pressure, which is close to the heart and brain and not a good idea.

A simple word cue for remembering to breathe is *ex*hale (blow out) with *ex*ertion. Breathe in when you return the weight to the starting position. ***Ex*hale = *Ex*ertion.** And if all else fails and you get confused remembering when to breathe, just breathe while you are lifting and you will be fine. If your face turns colors, that is a clue that you are holding your breath.

3. Posture, mechanics, and the mirror. Weight training exercises will accentuate whatever you are doing, right or wrong. It is effective at targeting the muscle and surrounding tissues; when/if you perform the exercises improperly, you will pay the price for it in discomfort. Next to learning how to perform the exercises properly and not lifting beyond your capabilities, the best insurance you have for avoiding discomfort and injury is to use mirrors to check that you continue to perform the exercises with good posture and the correct mechanics. Mirrors are the best feedback for checking your posture and mechanics.

If you want to enjoy the outdoors while using dumbbells, stand in front of a window and use its reflection as your feedback. It is very easy to forget what the proper posture and mechanics feel like, especially when you are just beginning. Novices mistakenly attribute the mirrors in the weight room to vanity. Even though some may use them for admiring themselves or others, mirrors are there to make sure that you are doing the right moves.

4. Posture and stance. Stabilize your body weight and keep an erect back, not arching. For most of the standing exercises, your feet should be shoulder-width apart. Think of a cord coming out of the top of your head pulling your entire spine erect. Rarely will an upright exercise call for your feet to be close together or touching each other. That is a sure way to lose balance. You don't want to be stiff, but you should strive to keep the erect posture throughout the entire exercise. Start with lighter weight than you anticipate being able to lift, and if form or posture suffers, lighten the load.

5. Objective intelligence. Decide the reps and sets you will perform before you start and stick to your plan. This keeps you from overdoing it. (Refer to the earlier section of this chapter for deciding how much weight to lift.)

6. Perform both phases of the exercise. In dynamic exercises, there are two phases of the exercise, the concentric and the eccentric. Those are technical terms for shortening and lengthening. Both phases work the muscles. When you bend your elbow to perform a biceps curl, you can see the muscle balling up or shortening; that is the concentric phase. When you slowly release the weight to the starting position, you are lengthening the muscle; that is the eccentric phase. During the exercise, you want to exhibit control during both

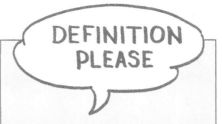

DEFINITION PLEASE

The **concentric** phase is the first phase of the exercise; it shortens the muscle. The **eccentric** phase, the equally important "return to position" phase of the exercise, lengthens the muscle. Strength gains occur in both phases.

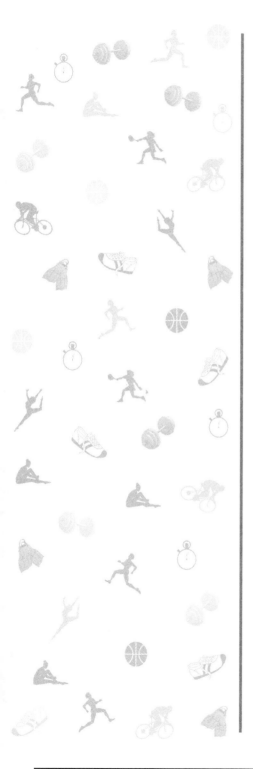

phases of the exercise, smoothly and slowly. Take approximately 2 seconds to complete each phase of the exercise. A common error is to work hard while performing the concentric, shortening phase of the exercise and then relaxing and letting gravity return the weight to the starting position. This is a waste of a strength-gaining opportunity, and it sets you up for injury by not balancing the strength gain.

7. Squeeze! When lifting weights, squeeze the muscles being called upon rather than passively allowing gravity to do the work for you. This actively recruits the muscle fibers, and your muscles will work more efficiently and respond more favorably.

8. Muscle balancing. Just as you want to perform both phases of the exercise, you want to work the muscles that anatomically oppose each other (but actually work together to keep you strong). For example, if you exercise the front of the legs (quads), you should exercise the back of the legs (hamstrings) to decrease the chances of muscular imbalances. Have you ever watched track athletes grabbing the back of their upper legs following their event? Many athletes with muscular imbalances in their legs injure their hamstrings during short explosive running events because the opposing leg muscles, the quadriceps, are stronger.

9. Which muscles? The answer is, just the ones you want to keep relying on.

But let's add a bit of common sense to this issue. *Ideally*, you want to exercise all of your muscle groups, with a few exercises per group. The groups you want to include are back, chest, shoulders, triceps, biceps, abdominals, gluteals, hamstrings, quadriceps, and calves. But if that list overwhelms you and you find it impossible to fit all the groups into your life right now, then select one or two areas to get started; as you become familiar and comfortable with them, you can add others to your routine. One way to decide which to start with is to give the most attention to the least exercised area. If you are performing other regular exercises (aerobic) that use one or more of the major muscle groups, you could start your weight training program by working the areas that do not get as much attention. For example, if you are a cyclist and you use your legs a lot but rarely use your upper body for exercise, begin your program by adding the upper body exercises (shoulders, back, chest, and arms) first, since they get less attention than your lower body. A little bit of weight training is better than no weight training, and

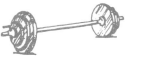
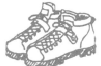
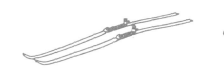

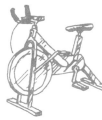
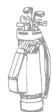

Example of a Split Routine for Upper and Lower Body

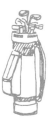

SUNDAY	MONDAY	TUESDAY	WED	THURSDAY	FRI	SAT
back	glutes	back	glutes	back	glutes	REST
chest	quads	chest	quads	chest	quads	REST
shoulders	hamstrings	shoulders	hams	shoulders	hams	REST
triceps	calves	triceps	calves	triceps	calves	REST
biceps	abdominals	biceps	abs	biceps	abs	REST

In this split routine, you are splitting and alternating the upper body and the lower body. Upper body muscle groups include the back, chest, shoulders, and arms (triceps and biceps). Lower body muscle groups include the gluteals, legs (quadriceps and hamstrings and calves), and abdominals (actually, the abdominals can be worked in on either day since they are upper and lower).

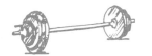
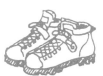
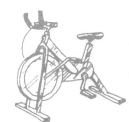

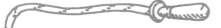

Adjustable Ankle Weights

Adjustable ankle weights are perfect for seniors who may lack leg strength, for those rehabilitating a knee injury, or for anyone who wants to lift very light weight. They wrap around your ankle and are secured by a velcro strip at the end. You change the workload by either adding or removing cylinder-shaped weights from the weight pockets. This clever device makes leg exercises possible without machines. You can perform the leg extension exercise in a chair and the leg curl exercise on your stomach. The price range is $20 to $50.

if you ease into it, you may be more successful. Once you see the results, you will be motivated to work in all the muscle group exercises.

10. Order of exercises. As a general rule, you should exercise larger muscles before smaller muscles. Smaller muscles help the larger muscles perform their work; if they are too exhausted from being worked out, the larger muscles will not be able to work as hard. (See the anatomy review illustration to find out which muscles are large and which are small.)

11. Rest period. Never weight train the same muscle group on 2 successive days. If you worked out your arms on Monday, do not work the arms again until Wednesday. This rest period is the time when muscle fibers repair and come back even stronger. If you want to strength train 6 days a week, then split up your routine so that rest and recovery can occur.

12. What if I am sore? Do I work out or wait for it to go away? You should feel something in your muscles after you work out; typically, you will notice it most the morning after you exercised. Muscle soreness is actually a good sign (but acute pain is not; keep reading to learn how to distinguish between soreness and pain). Muscle soreness is a sign that those areas are the ones that will be improving. Rather than being upset that you are sore, be glad that what you did is working and know that you can expect those areas to become stronger in the weeks ahead.

So, should you exercise with sore muscles after your rest day or not? The answer is yes. You want to get those sore muscles moving; when you do, you stimulate blood flow to the muscles, which facilitates recovery and growth. Think of the activity as massaging the muscle. But use your head. That does not mean that you work out sore muscles as hard as you can. Ease up on them a bit, and you will notice how even after a few minutes of exercise your sore muscles actually feel better. Muscle soreness is also a healthy reminder to do some stretching and flexibility exercises (see Chapter 8).

13. How often? What is a split routine? You can weight train each muscle up to two or three times a week. One way to keep your total workout time from getting too long is to split up the body parts to exercise. The simplest is to split up the body between upper and lower muscles. For example, on 3 alternating days, you would exercise your back, chest, shoulders, triceps, and biceps. Then on the other 3 alternating days, you would exercise your gluteals (buttocks), quadriceps, hamstrings, calves, and abdominals. There are other advanced split routines to use, and if you are interested, ask a trainer to advise you. This 6-day-a-week program is merely an example and not meant to overwhelm you. You could do the same program by exercising each part once or twice a week.

14. Set your ego aside. Some days you may not feel as fresh or able to lift as much. Listen to your body rather than your ego and adjust your workout accordingly. In the gym, there will always be someone stronger and someone weaker than you. Focus upon your own progress and work within your current parameters.

15. Soreness versus pain. There is a difference between soreness and pain. Soreness or tightness following a weight training session (usually when you wake up the next day) can indicate a challenging and appropriate workload. Pain, however, is a sharp, acute feeling and indicates that you may have lifted improperly or with too much intensity (load, reps, or sets). Exhibit patience. Be conservative when strength training. It is easier to exhibit patience and take a little longer to reach your goal than it is to have to stop completely while waiting for your body to heal.

16. When and how to increase? For simplicity's sake, let's assume you are strength training for fitness. You are performing most of your exercises at 75 percent of your 1RM, 12 reps, 3 sets. You have been feeling stronger and have noticed in the past few sessions that the exercises are becoming VERY easy. You also notice that the morning after lifting you do not feel "low level soreness" or "like I did something"—as you experienced previously. These are signs that you may be ready to add to your strength training "overload." So which do you increase, the weight, the reps, the sets, all of them, or some of them? Help! Here is a "stair-step-slide" approach to increasing your "overload" that is prudent and effective.

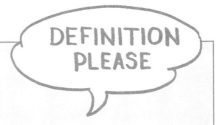

DEFINITION PLEASE

"Ready" to increase overload or "mastering" your current load means that you performed the exercise with ease and that during the rest day in between, you did not feel any tightness or soreness (or pain, of course). You are "ready" to increase the work intensity.

After building up to and "mastering" 3 sets of 12 reps, slide back down to 3 sets of 8 reps and increase load (weight). Once you have progressed to 3 sets of 8 repetitions, then move up to 3 sets of 10 rep-

Alternating

A benefit of using dumbbells is the ability to isolate and specifically address each side of the body. One side may lack coordination; the other may lack flexibility or strength. By working one side at a time, you can focus and devote the proper attention to each side. Alternating makes for an efficient, concentrated use of time. The nonworking side is resting while the other side is working. This applies for some but not all dumbbell exercises.

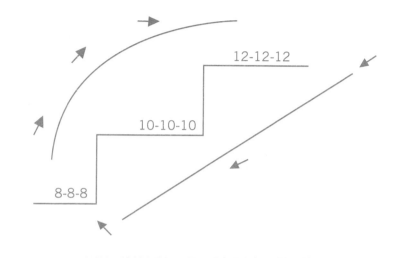

Example of the "Stair-Step-Slide" Approach

etitions. If you experience improvement "symptoms" again, then progress next to 3 sets of 12 repetitions. Once you have mastered 3 sets of 12 repetitions, return to the 3 sets of 8 repetitions but increase the weight (load) slightly (from 1 pound to 2, or from 5 to 8 or from 8 to 10). Repeat the sequence as needed. A word of caution: When you return to weight training after having missed a few sessions, you may need to "step down" and decrease some aspect of the intensity (either load, reps, or sets). The ego's need to "pick up right where I left off" can result in unnecessary and preventable injury.

17. Pay attention and heed the warning signs. Do you feel pain or strain? STOP immediately. Stretch lightly; ice the area if injured. Stretch following your workout to decrease soreness, promote flexibility, and prevent injury.

Let's Do It!

Now that you are excited to start weight training, let's give you a short workout that could get you started the most expediently. To keep it simple, we will use dumbbells. You already know now to determine how much weight to lift and how many sets and reps you want to perform. For those of you who do not yet have the strength to use dumbbells, you can do these without using weights to begin. The movement and exercise will be taxing enough. Following are some excellent basic exercises for upper and lower body. If you are pressed for time but still want to get in a healthy dose of strength training, these five great upper dumbbell exercises can be performed in 15 minutes or less (that is, 3 sets of 12 reps).

Five Upper Body Dumbbell Exercises

These exercises are not offered as a total or complete workout; rather, they are just a few to get you started. For simplicity's sake, let's assume you have only a set of dumbbells and your weight bench has not arrived yet. (For a complete workout, see the Appendix for resources on weight training exercise instruction.)

Use a mirror or window to check for proper body position and mechanics throughout the exercises. You will perform these five exercises in either the standing or bent-over positions and will use the overhand or underhand grip. Once your bench arrives, you can use it for the bent-over exercises if you prefer. However, supporting your own body weight develops balance and coordination.

First, here are the positions and grips:

1. Standing position. Face the mirror. Stand with your feet shoulder-width apart, knees slightly bent (not locked), head and shoulders as level as possible (not slanted), and your back erect.

2. Bent-over position. Stand sideways with the working arm/side toward the mirror. Stand with your feet shoulder-width apart in a diagonal stride. That means one leg (the one opposite the working arm) is ahead of the other, creating a diagonal line effect. Bend at the waist and bend the forward knee. Strive to flatten out your

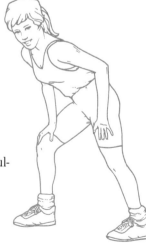

Bent-Over Position

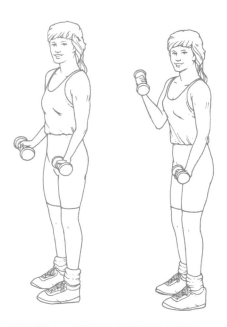

Biceps Curl (start and finish)

back as best you can. Rest/support the nonworking arm on the same-side thigh.

3. Overhand grip. Grab the dumbbell with a fist so that your palm is facing down and knuckles are up.

4. Underhand grip. Grab the dumbbell with a fist so that your palm is facing up and knuckles are down.

And here are the exercises (for each of these upper body exercises, use only one dumbbell at a time):

1. The biceps curl works the two-headed (bi-ceps) muscle on the front of the upper arm.

Standing position—Your arms hang at your sides. Grasp the dumbbell with an underhand grip. Keep your elbow "attached" to the side of your body so that it does not flounder or chicken wing out to the side (visualize a dowel running through your elbow that keeps it attached to the side of your body). Curl one arm/dumbbell toward your chest as far as it will come (this is the concentric/shortening phase). Next, control the weight as you let it down (this is the eccentric/lengthening phase). That is one repetition.

2. The triceps kickback works the three-headed (tri) muscle on the back of the upper arm.

Bent-over position—Grasp the dumbbell with an overhand grip so that your palm is facing your body. The movement comes from the elbow joint (the shoulder does *not* rotate). Extend the working arm (squeeze the triceps/back of upper arm) back straight behind you, but do not hyperextend. While controlling the weight, bend the elbow and return to the starting position. That is one repetition. As the name suggests, you are "kicking back" the dumbbell—but do so gently, not explosively.

3. The front raise works the front of your shoulder (deltoid) muscle as well as the side of your neck.

Standing position—Grasp the dumbbell with an overhand grip. The arm (with the weight) hangs in front of your body with the palm side resting on the

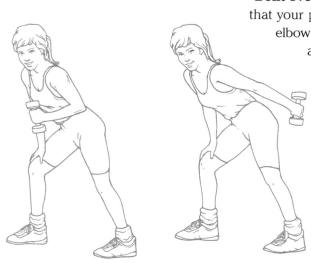

Triceps Kickback (start and finish)

center of your same-side thigh. With a straight arm, extend it by squeezing and raising the shoulder up and toward the midline of your body (your nose and mouth are at the midline), creating a slightly diagonal line, until the arm is parallel to the floor or between your nose and mouth, but not higher. Control the weight as you return it to the thigh. That is one repetition.

4. The shoulder press works the top and center of your deltoid as well as your upper back and triceps. You will also feel this on the side of your neck.

Standing position—Grasp the dumbbell with an overhand grip, at shoulder height. Bend your elbow and position your palm to face away from the body. Raise the working arm up until the arm is fully extended just slightly in front of your head (NOT directly behind or over your head). Control weight as you return (recoil the elbow) your arm to the starting position. That is one repetition.

5. The bent-over rows work your lats (back) as well as biceps and shoulders.

Bent-over position—*Imagine rowing a rowboat bent-over with one arm, or pulling the starter cord on a lawn mower.* Grasp the dumbbell with an overhand grip, with your palm facing your body. Raise the working arm toward the level of your armpit. Feel and squeeze your back muscles as you perform this exercise so that you do not overemphasize the biceps action. Allow your elbow to bow out

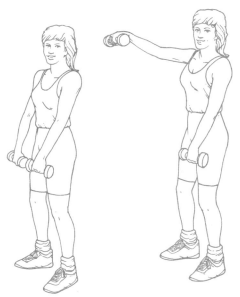

Front Raise (start and finish)

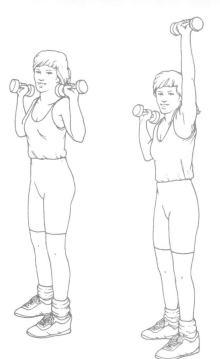

Shoulder Press (start and finish)

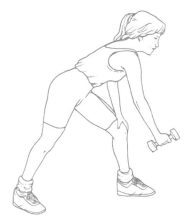

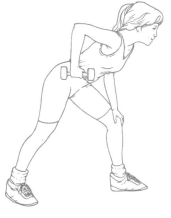

Bent-Over Row (start and finish)

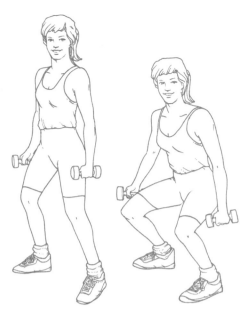

Squats (start and finish)

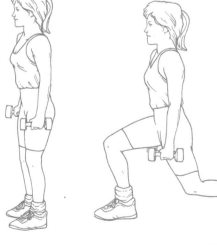

Lunge (start and finish)

a bit, but do not break your wrist. Control the weight as you return to the starting position. That is one repetition.

Four Lower Body Exercises

For the first two of these lower body exercises, use two dumbbells at a time.

1. Squats work the legs and hip (gluteal, quadricep, and hamstring muscles). You may be wondering, "How can holding a dumbbell in each hand work my legs?" The dumbbells only add resistance to the exercise. Your arms do not move. Your knees bend to create leg movement. If you have hip, knee, or lower back conditions, do not perform the exercise as deeply.

Standing position—Holding a dumbbell securely, let your arms hang. Your hands rest on each side of your thighs. The motion is as if you were going to sit down and raise up out of a chair. The *lowest* you should squat is where your thighs are parallel to the floor. Your knees should not extend over the plane of your toes. Keep your back erect and do not allow it to arch. If your knees hurt, then squat down only to the point where you feel no pain. When you return to the starting position, that is one repetition.

2. Lunges work the gluteals, quadriceps, hamstrings, and calves.

Standing position—Holding a dumbbell securely in each hand, let your arms hang. Your hands rest on each side of your thighs. Keep your back straight. As you lift the lead leg and step forward about one stride's length, you want to gently land on that heel and roll onto the entire foot. When your foot is flat against the floor, bend both knees until your lead thigh is parallel to the floor and the other thigh is perpendicular to the other thigh. The heel of the rear leg will and should lift off the floor (this stretches the back of the leg). To complete the exercise, press off the ball of the lead foot and return to the standing position. That is one repetition.

What follows are two of the best leg exercises you can do. The use of a machine is preferred. However, they can be performed using light weight with adjustable ankle weights. With or without a machine, the leg action is the same.

3. Leg Extensions. Sit with your back and buttocks against a supportive chair. Squeeze the top of your thigh as you straighten your leg until your knee is straight. Hold for the position for just a second and then control the weight (don't let gravity make it come down) as you return it to the starting position. That is one repetition.

4. Leg Curls. Lie on a bench (if you can't lie on a bench, use the floor) on your stomach with your arms at your sides and your legs extended. Turn your head to one side. Bend your knee so that you are curling your leg toward your buttocks. To maximize flexibility, bring your heels as close to your buttocks as possible, squeezing the backs of your thigh as you curl your leg. Control the weight as you return it to the starting position. Use your abdominal muscles to keep your hip bones flush against the floor/bench. That is one repetition.

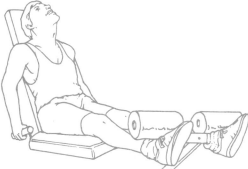

Leg Extension

Leg Curl

Two Exercises for Strong Abdominal and Back Muscles

As mentioned earlier, you want to have strong abdominal and back muscles to reduce the possibility of low back injuries. The following exercises are effective in building those areas and do not utilize weights. The posterior pelvic tilt (PPT) is prescribed by many physical therapists for patients with back ailments and is considered the cornerstone for building abdominal strength. Start with PPT and graduate to the basic abdominal crunch. Watching someone perform PPT, you would have no idea how challenging it really is. But after doing it, you will have an appreciation for how it will build your abdominal and back strength. The basic abdominal crunch is the next advanced level of abdominal conditioning and is *not* to be confused with the old-time sit-up exercise, which is strongly discouraged.

1. The posterior pelvic tilt (PPT). This exercise can be performed on a mat, on carpet, or on a soft floor.
Position: Lie on your back, with your knees bent, your heels resting on the floor, and your toes pointed up. Arms are at your sides.

The Exercise—PPT part 1: Just for a moment, take one of your hands to feel the slightly curved space between your lower back and the floor. This is the natural curve of your back. Now return your hand to the side of your body. Next, visualize your navel (belly button) and use it to pull your abdominal muscles toward the floor, flattening out the curve of your low back. This will cause your pelvis (hip area) to tilt slightly up and forward in the process. Keep your buttocks on the floor. There should be no space between your back and the floor, and you should feel your abdominal muscles tightening, going to work. Hold this position with your abdominal muscles for several seconds, then relax and repeat. Repetitions: 10. Sets: 1 to 3. Frequency: 1 time/day. Unlike weight training exercises, these can be performed every day.

PPT part 2 (more advanced PPT): From the basic PPT position, slowly and gently slide your heels forward and away from your body so that your legs begin to straighten. Continue to use your abdominal muscles to keep your back against the floor. Do not lift your heels and keep them on the ground as you do so. Allow your heels to slide slowly to the most forward position, where your back can still maintain contact with the floor. When you reach the point at which you can no longer maintain back-to-floor contact, stop sliding the heels forward and slowly slide them to the starting position. The out-and-back is one repetition. You will know you have made gains when you are able to reach the fully straightened position while maintaining the back-to-floor contact.

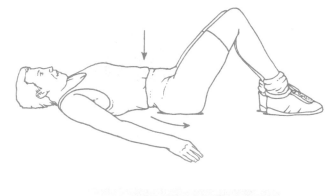

Posterior Pelvic Tilt

How many, how often? Repetitions: 10. Sets: 1 to 3. Frequency: 1 time/day. Unlike weight training exercises, these can be performed every day.

2. Basic Abdominal Crunch. If we had a contest for "the best butchered exercise," it would be a close tie between the stair climbing machine exercise and the basic abdominal crunch. Read these instructions carefully and pay attention to your form.

Position: Lie on your back with your knees bent and your feet flat on the floor shoulder-width apart. **What to do if your feet come up. It may help (but is not necessary) to secure your feet under the edge of a table or bed to keep them from moving.** Place your hands at the back of your head with your thumbs pointing down behind your ears. Do not interlock your fingers. If you have a small head, your hands may overlap. Keep your chin up just slightly so that it does not dig into your chest. Spread your elbows out to the sides.

Motion: Curl up from your spine, pulling with your trunk to the point at which your shoulder blades are off the floor. Pause, and then slowly control your trunk as you bring it back to the starting position. That is one repetition.

Frequency—Sets/Reps: Although the abdominal muscles are small and recover quickly, they too need a rest. Alternate the days that you perform ab exercises. Apply the same reps and sets format to abdominal exercises that you do to your others. If you perform 3 sets of 15 reps and you feel that you are not challenged, add the more advanced variations to your abdominal workout.

Variations on the Crunch:

1. For beginners—**cross-arm crunch**: Fold your arms across your chest. You have now eliminated lifting the weight of your arms, so the exercise is easier than the basic ab crunch.

2. More advanced—**alternate crunch:** To work the oblique muscles, twist and alternate crunches to three successive positions: left, center, and right. From the starting position, the movement would be curl up to the center, go down, curl up to the left, go down, curl up to the

Isokinetic Resistance Training

Isokinetic resistance training exercises can be performed with partners but are most effectively performed on speed-controlled equipment. They involve moving the muscle against a resistance that matches the force produced by the muscle throughout the entire range of motion. The exercises and the equipment are not commonly seen in gyms or clubs. Mostly they are seen in athletic and rehabilitative environments/settings.

Advice about Curls and Crunches

In performing abdominal exercises, it is unnecessary and undesirable to raise the trunk more than 30 degrees off the ground. To stay within that parameter, curl your spine so that you lift your shoulder blades off the floor and no more.

• • •

Why Not Sit-ups?

The old sit-up ("full" sit-up) stresses the lower back and only uses the abdominal muscles for a small part of the exercise. Partial curls or crunches should be substituted for a full sit-up. It makes greater use of the abdominal muscles and decreases stress to the back muscles.

center, go down, curl up to the right, go down, and repeat the sequence.

3. More advanced: **crunch with weight:** Put a light weight plate (5 pounds) on your abdomen and perform the exercise. A weight plate is a flat weight that slides onto a barbell.

4. Very advanced—**crunch with feet/legs up:** Keeping your knees bent, lift your legs up and off the floor and cross your ankles. Perform the exercise.

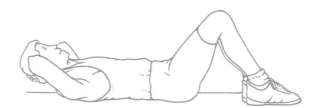

Abdominal Crunch

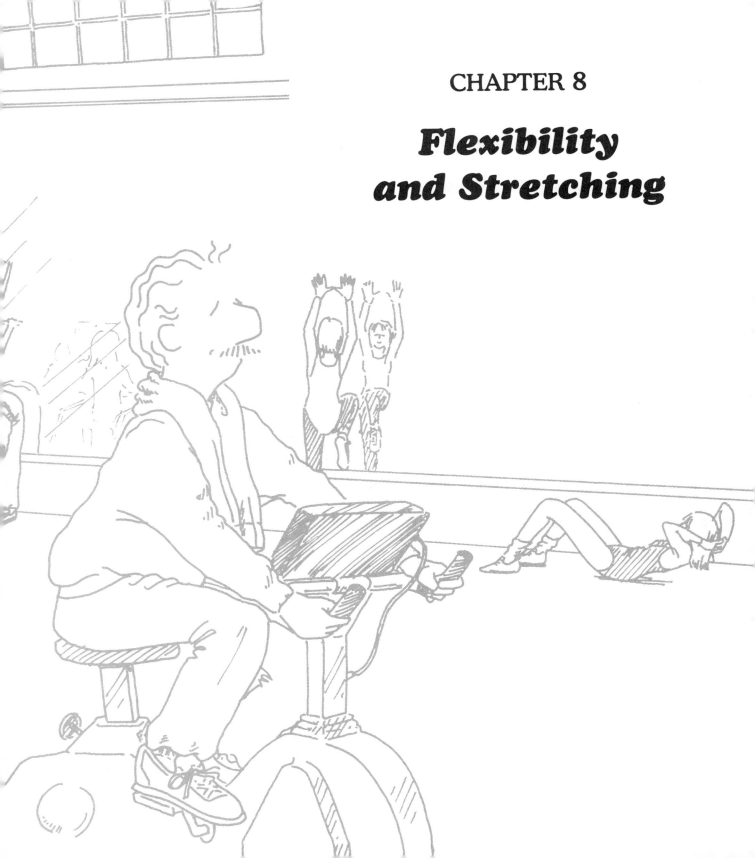

CHAPTER 8

Flexibility and Stretching

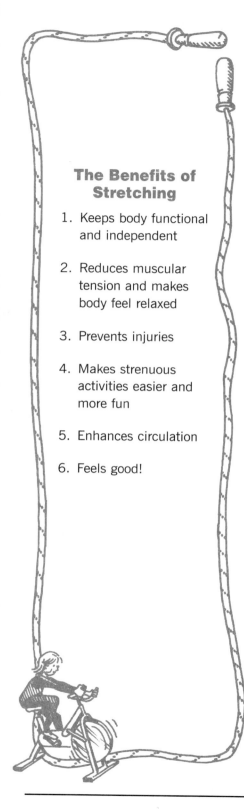

The Benefits of Stretching

1. Keeps body functional and independent

2. Reduces muscular tension and makes body feel relaxed

3. Prevents injuries

4. Makes strenuous activities easier and more fun

5. Enhances circulation

6. Feels good!

Sleeping is very underrated. So is stretching.
—SUZY BECKER, *ALL I NEED TO KNOW I LEARNED FROM MY CAT.*

When you awaken from sleep, do you *stretch* and yawn? After sitting for long periods of time and especially after being confined to a small space (been on an airplane lately?), do you find yourself wanting to move around, to *stretch*? Have you noticed how other mammals, particularly cats and dogs, stretch and shake after sleeping or lying? These examples remind us that we instinctively stretch to be flexible and that it feels good.

Flexibility is the ability to move a joint (where your bones meet) throughout its full range of motion without discomfort or pain. Flexibility keeps you independent and functional. It makes bodily movements more efficient, decreases the chances of muscular injuries, decreases soreness following activity, and helps prevent and reduce low back pain (the number one reason for absenteeism from work).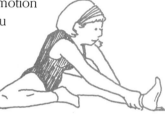

As a child you probably had a tremendous degree of flexibility. And sometime after adulthood you probably reached a general decline in flexibility. It is unknown whether this reduced flexibility is an aging-related phenomenon or whether it is related to becoming more sedentary. One thing is for sure: flexibility can be improved by regular stretching and physical activity. It is another effective tool you can use to keep yourself feeling good and reducing the potential for injury or stiffness. Stretching does not require that you spend a lot of money, and you need only yourself to do it (unless you want a stretching partner, sometimes a towel). And lastly but importantly, stretching is relaxing and *not* competitive.

When and where to stretch? Stretch anytime and anywhere, at home, at work, in the car, while standing, while waiting (airplane bathroom), after exercise, before exercise, as exercise, when you feel stiff, when you feel limber, while watching TV, while working on the computer, while talking on the telephone, and anytime you can!

The temperature factor. When was the last time you tried to bend or twist an item that came out of the freezer? Were you successful right away, or did you have to wait for it to thaw a bit? Just like the item that needed to be thawed before it could be manipulated, the body stretches best in a warm environment, either external or internal, and after it has been warmed up. If you are going to perform a series of dedicated stretches, you might choose to walk, jog, or step (in place if necessary) as a means of elevating the temperature of your muscles and to assist them in optimum stretching.

Warming up versus stretching. Warm up *before* you stretch. Although both are beneficial, warming up and stretching are different. Warming up is what you do before engaging in an activity and, as its name indicates, is about raising the body temperature. Once warmed up, your muscles, tendons, and ligaments become more flexible and better able to perform the intense exercise that will follow.

Warm-up: same but slower. Sometimes, the best warm-up is a slower, less intense version of the activity itself. For example, if you were preparing to run several miles, a slow jog for 5 minutes would be an effective warm-up. You would be warming up the same muscles that would be involved in the more demanding activity, running in this case. In contrast, if you were to forego a warm-up and went right into specific and isolated stretches before running, you would not be as flexible, and your stretching would not be as productive. You would also be doubling your risk for injury by stretching cold tissues and from bypassing your warm-up. Stretching cold muscles and tissues is a sure way to injure yourself and should be avoided. Warm up first; stretch later.

Types of Stretching

There are three types of stretching: proprioceptive neuromuscular facilitation (PNF), static, and ballistic.

1. PNF. Don't let the name scare you; this is a very effective way to stretch. Think of PNF as a two-step process, a contract-relax technique. First you tire out the muscle, then you stretch it. By tiring out the muscle, you eliminate some of the natural resistance or "fight" that the muscle initially puts up; thus, it is better able to stretch. PNF stretching requires a partner, a wall, or a towel to provide resistance.

To perform a PNF stretch, first squeeze the muscle against an immovable resistance (person or

PNF Stretching

wall) without moving it for 5 to 6 seconds. (This is called an isometric contraction.) Then relax the same muscle and have your partner (if you are solo use a towel) slowly move and stretch the muscle to a new point of limitation, holding it for 15 to 20 seconds. PNF stretches are most commonly used for stretching the hamstring (back of the thigh) muscles but can be performed on many others.

2. Ballistic stretching involves quick jerky or bouncy movements. Sports teams, especially contact-type sports, use ballistic stretching as part of their conditioning. However, it is recommended that they be performed after warm-up and all other stretching, whether it is static or PNF stretching. For general fitness purposes, ballistic stretching is not recommended (as the other forms of stretching are) because of the potential for injury.

3. Static stretching involves slow movements; it is safer than ballistic stretching and produces less soreness. A partner is not required.

Stretching Facts

Here are five steps to a good stretching technique:

1. Focus. The correct way to stretch is by focusing your attention on the muscles being stretched and to slowly and gently elongate (or stretch) the selected muscle. When you stretch properly and regularly, movement will become easier for you.

2. Breathe—never hold your breath when stretching! Breathing should be slow and rhythmic. A stretch that interrupts your natural breathing indicates that you are out of your comfort zone and should ease up to the point at which your normal/natural breathing is returned.

3. Move gently. Move into the stretch gently, lightly, and slowly, until you feel slight or mild tension. Exhale and relax "into the stretch." The slight tension should pass as you hold the position. If it does not, then ease off slightly and find some milder tension that is more comfortable to maintain.

4. Hold for 10 to 30 seconds. In the beginning, it is helpful to count. As you make stretching a regular part of your fitness, you will soon be able to "feel" the stretch and abandon the counting. Stretch; do not bounce.

5. Gently, slowly come out of the stretch. Do not bounce out of a stretch. Give the tissue a few moments to readjust.

Use PAIN as your indicator and STOP!

Begin the stretch→ slight discomfort→ discomfort→ PAIN
(begin)   (continue)   (continue or ease up) (stop!)

Stretch reflex. The *stretch reflex* is what keeps the muscle(s) from being injured. When muscle fibers are stretched too far, the nerve reflex responds by sending a signal to the muscles to contract or stop the movement. This keeps the muscles from being injured. When you stretch, pay attention to your muscles. During a stretch, the muscle group should loosen. You know whether you are stretching properly when the longer you hold the stretch, the less you feel it. If the muscle begins to tighten (after the initial loosening), relax the stretch. The stretch reflex is sending you a preventive message.

Holding a stretch as far as you can or bouncing up or down strains the muscles and activates the stretch reflex. More is *not* always better! These actions cause pain and microscopic tearing of muscle fibers, which causes scar tissue to form, leading to loss of elasticity, which leads to tightness and soreness. So the bottom line is that you should avoid it.

Where you feel the stretch. It is possible that when you perform a stretch for a specific area, you may actually feel the stretch in a different area. For example, when you are performing a stretch for the calf, you may feel it mostly in your lower ankle or Achilles area. It does not necessarily mean you are doing the stretch incorrectly. It means that your lower ankle area is tighter than your calf, so that is the place where you feel it most. Stick with the stretch; you will eventually feel it at the primary stretch spot.

What areas do you want to be stretching? Stretch most everything that moves, including your neck, shoulders, face, upper back, arms, lower back, trunk/torso, hips/gluteals, hamstrings, quadriceps, groin, ankle, and Achilles tendon.

How to Stretch

In stretching, there are two words to focus on, *slowly* and *gently*.

1. Focus.

2. Breathe/exhale.

3. Move in slowly and gently.

4. Hold for 10 to 30 seconds.

5. Come out slowly and gently.

6. Stretch both sides. Some stretches isolate one side of the body.

The F-I-T Principles of Stretching

Frequency—Stretch at least 3 times per week and preferably daily.

Intensity—"No pain, period!" Discontinue the stretch if discomfort turns to pain.

Time—Hold each stretch for 10 to 30 seconds.

• • •

Stretch Tip

Stretch by how you feel, not by how far you can go. Stretching is a process, not a destination and it doesn't help to hurt.

What are the few best stretches? It can be overwhelming to try to decide which stretches to include in your general fitness program. What follows are a few excellent stretches for areas of the body where most people need improved flexibility. (If you have a specific area that is not addressed in these stretches, see the Appendix for resources that will likely have what you are looking for.)

Inclusive and flexible—an attitude. One great characteristic of stretching is that you can secretly and quietly work many stretches into your day. Some can be performed in bed when you first awaken or when you go to sleep, while getting dressed, in the shower or while toweling dry, in a chair, or in your car during your commute.

Seemingly simple motions like reaching, pushing, and pulling are stretching opportunities in disguise. When you adopt an inclusive and opportunistic attitude for stretching, you can easily and conveniently improve your flexibility. Ask yourself, "How and where can I include stretching in the normal part of my day?" Just by asking the question, you will start noticing the many opportunities to improve your flexibility. Here are some stretches and appropriate opportunities for including them in your life every day.

Stretching Exercises
Hamstring (Back of the Thigh) Stretch

Tight hamstrings are a contributing factor to low back pain. Start from a standing position with your feet shoulder-width apart pointed straight ahead. Slowly bend over at the waist, keeping your knees slightly bent. Allow your hands to drop in front of you toward your feet and relax your neck. Give a big exhale (saying "ahhh" really helps). Bend to the point where you feel the stretch in the back of your legs and hold for 10 to 15 seconds. The goal is to feel the stretch. When you regularly do this stretch daily, you will notice how much more flexible you are. With time you will progress from reaching your thighs, to your knees, to your ankles, to your toes, and maybe even to the floor.

Opportunities for Hamstring Stretching
1. Stretch while dressing. Unless you live in a nudist colony, you have to get dressed anyway, so here is a convenient way to work in a hamstring stretch. Dressing presents many opportunities for

stretching, such as when you first put on your shoes, socks, and pantyhose and then again when you remove your shoes, socks, and pantyhose at the end of the day. Twice a day (and more if you work out midday and change clothes again) you have the opportunity to improve your lower back and hamstring flexibility.

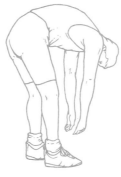
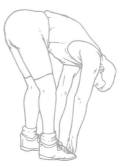
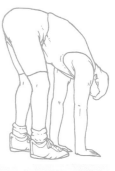

Hamstring Stretch
When stretching the hamstrings, bend to the point where you feel the stretch and hold for 10–15 seconds. Daily practice will improve your flexibility.

2. Pick it up. Years ago, the television journalist Andy Rooney of *60 Minutes* did a story about how few if any people would pick up a penny if it was on the ground. Although the story was about the devaluation of the penny, it is a great reminder that we have many "pick it up" opportunities for stretching. When you see something such as a penny or a winning lottery ticket on the ground, do the hamstring stretch to pick it up. Or for twice the reward, beautify your environment and stretch in the process by picking up trash off the ground or items that have fallen to the floor. See and seize the opportunities.

Stretches for Lower Body: Lower Back, Hips, and Gluteals
Squat

If you sit or stand a lot, you will love this stretch. *Avoid this stretch if you have knee problems or are pregnant.* Rumor has it that squatting was once used to induce labor and delivery. Another side benefit of the squat is that it can induce peristalsis, which is the fancy name for the wavelike contractions of the intestine. The squat stretches many areas including your shins, knees, back, ankles, Achilles tendons, and groin.

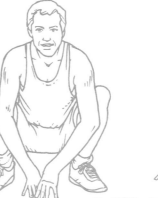

Squat Stretch
Squat down with your feet flat, toes pointed just slightly out, and heels spread about a foot apart. Shoulders and elbows should line up inside the knees. Knees should be directly above the big toes in this position. Hold for 30 seconds. The squat stretches the back, ankles, Achilles tendons, and groin as well as the front of the lower leg.

For balance or support, squat with your back toward a wall.

The squat stretch: Start from a standing position with your feet more than shoulder-width apart and your toes slightly pointed out. Slowly bend your knees as you squat down, keeping your feet flat. Keep your knees outside of your shoulders but directly above your big toes. Your arms hang in front of you, and your hands rest on the floor at the midline of your body. Remember to let out a big exhale and feel

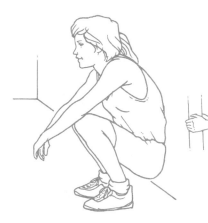

Squat Stretch
For balance or support, squat while holding onto a pole or other heavy, immovable item.

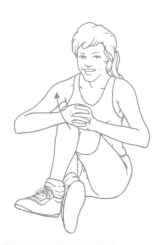

Spinal Twist Stretch
Sit with your right leg extended on floor. Bend your left leg, cross your left foot over the right leg, and rest it to the side of your right knee. Next, bend the right elbow and rest it on the outside of your upper left thigh, just above the knee. The elbow is used to exert the controlled pressure that creates the stretch.

the tension run out of your body. Coming out of the squat, stand up using your quadriceps (front of the thigh) and keep a straight back as you rise.

Variation: Grab a pole, bed frame, or other level item that allows you to balance and stretch further.

Leg Crossover from a Sitting Position

One of the best, but not the only, times to incorporate these stretches into your day are following your aerobic exercise session. Most aerobic activities involve the legs and buttocks muscles, and performing stretches immediately following will keep your muscles from getting tight. The leg crossover from a sitting position and spinal twist, a variation, are easy stretches to work into your day because they can be performed in an office chair.

The exercise: Sitting on the floor with your legs extended, bend one leg at your knee and cross it over the extended leg. Pull or hug your knee across your body toward your opposite shoulder (left knee to right shoulder; right knee to left shoulder) until you feel your hips and buttocks stretching.

Do not make the common error of leaning forward, bringing your shoulder to your knee. Bring the knee to the shoulder. The goal is to stretch the hip/gluteal area.

Variation—**Spinal twist:** This variation will stretch more of your upper back, spine, and rib muscles, which will increase your flexibility when you turn to look behind you, as when driving your car in reverse.

Position: It's the same as the leg crossover from a sitting position, except instead of hugging your knee to your opposite shoulder, use the elbow opposite of the bent knee to press the leg across your body. The other hand rests behind you. Slowly turn your head and rotate your upper body as you look over your shoulder in the direction of the hand behind you. This is called spinal twist for a good reason.

Leg crossover from a lying position. In addition to doing this stretch immediately following your aerobic exercise, you can conveniently do it in bed when you awaken or before going to sleep. Just don't kick your pet or companion next to you.

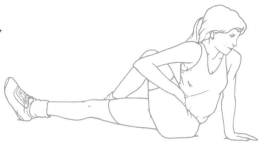

The exercise: Lie on your back with your arms and legs fully extended so that you look like a *T*. Do not cross your legs or ankles. Here comes the crossover part of the stretch: Bend and bring one knee up toward your hip and then rotate your hip so that your knee crosses over your other leg. *Keep your shoulder blades on the floor; otherwise you will lose the stretch entirely.* Use your opposite hand (of the leg that is bent) to pull the bent knee over the body and intensify the stretch. While keeping your head resting on the floor, turn it toward the arm that is still lying flat on the floor.

Leg Crossover Stretch, Sitting Position
Pull or hug your knee across your body toward your opposite shoulder until you feel your hips and buttocks stretching.

Variation for your spine: Extend your leg and slowly "walk" your foot down toward the other foot, feeling the stretch progress down your spine. Then "walk" your foot up toward the level of your arm and feel the stretch progress up the spine.

Variation for gluteals: From the crossover position, reach under your leg and behind your knee. Slowly pull the knee toward the opposite shoulder until you feel the stretch in your gluteals. As in the basic crossover stretch, keep both shoulders flat on the floor.

Finishing the stretch. To come out of the crossover stretches, roll slowly onto your back, then gently untuck your legs so that you are back at the starting position. You will feel it in your spine, and it should feel good.

Fetal Position Stretch

This is an oldie but goodie. Do you remember way back when?

1. Lie in the fetal position—on your side, knees drawn up toward your chest, with your head resting on your hands. That's it.
2. To intensify the stretch, use the "up side" arm to bring the "up side" leg higher toward the chest.
3. To come out of the fetal position stretch, simply roll onto all fours and prop yourself up.

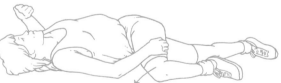

Leg Crossover from a Lying Position
It is essential that you keep your shoulder blades on the floor during this stretch. Apply controlled pressure to intensify the stretch by using the opposite hand to pull the bent knee toward the floor.

Achilles Tendon, Gastrocnemius, and Soleus (Calf Area)

Stand facing the edge of a stair or curb. Place the ball of your foot on the edge of a stair or curb so that your heel hangs down. Keep your leg and ankle straight as they stretch. Balance yourself by holding onto the wall or handrail.

Quadriceps (Front of Thigh), Knee, IT Band (Iliotibial)

Many knee problems are a result of weak and /or tight quadriceps muscles (front of the thigh) and supporting tissues (the iliotibial band runs along the outside of the leg). This exercise will stretch them all.

The stretch: From a standing position, bend one knee so that the foot comes up behind toward your buttocks. Grab the foot with the *opposite* arm (left foot, right arm; right foot, left arm), which keeps your knee bent at a natural and comfortable angle. Gently pull your heel up and toward your buttocks. To intensify the stretch, point the bent knee straight down.

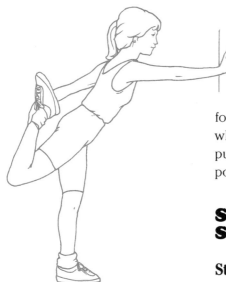

Quadriceps Stretch
Stand facing a wall. Bend your right knee so the foot comes up behind toward your buttocks. Grab the right foot with the left hand and gently pull your heel up and toward your buttocks. Use your free hand (in this case the right) to balance against the wall.

Variation: To simultaneously practice your balancing abilities, remove your hand from the wall and steady yourself on the one leg.

Stretches for the Upper Body: Chest, Back, Shoulders, and Arms

Opportunity for Stretching: After Bathing—Towel Stretches

Grab the towel with an end in each hand and extend your arms in front holding the towel horizontally. Pull with just enough pressure to keep the towel straight. Raise the straightened towel over your head; exhale. Then bring the towel down behind your back. To increase the stretch, move your hands closer together, keeping your arms and the towel straight. If you cannot bring the towel behind your head, move your hands farther apart.

Chest stretch: Hold the towel behind you even with your shoulder blades.

Side stretch: Still grasping the towel so that it is straight, bend at your waist over to one side of your body, exhaling as you bend. Remember to stretch both sides.

Other Upper Body Stretches

The bow down stretch, or the "I lost my contact lens" stretch. Kneeling on the floor, bend your knees so that they are under your abdomen (belly). Extend your arms in front of you and either grab the end of the mat or rug or gently press your palms into the ground and pull back.

The in the car or on the train shoulder stretch. Use your abdominal muscles to lean into the seat back (like a sitting PPT exercise) and horizontally extend your arms around the back of your seat or extend your arms so that one arm is behind the other seat (assuming you are in the front of a two-seated vehicle).

Now you have some ideas for implementing stretching into things you do daily, like bathing and dressing. And you have a few good stretches to include immediately following your aerobic exercise. Some other effective methods of stretching involve the practices of yoga, yoga-related exercises, and Pilates or Pilates-derived exercises.

Conclusion

It is easy to take our flexibility for granted, that is, until you experience a stiff neck or shoulder, low back pain, or tight hamstrings. Flexibility is one of the major components of a complete fitness program. Now you have a better idea of how to include it in yours. The best ways to keep and improve flexibility are by stretching and lengthening the muscles you use most often and by strengthening and lengthening the muscles opposite those performing movement. See how often you can include stretching in your day and how much better you feel when you do.

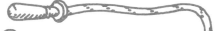

Yoga

Yoga is a Sanskrit word that means unification (with the divine). It is a system of meditation and self-discipline that utilizes exercise and breathing control. Yoga improves flexibility, aids in relaxation, improves circulation, and increases energy. Certain styles of yoga can also improve muscular strength and endurance. Yoga classes are easy to find; you just need to find the appropriate level. Remember to leave your walkman at home; yoga classes require your full attention.

• • •

Definition

Midline of the body: The midline of the body is an imaginary line that starts from between your eyes and runs the length of your body, which would effectively create two halves of you.

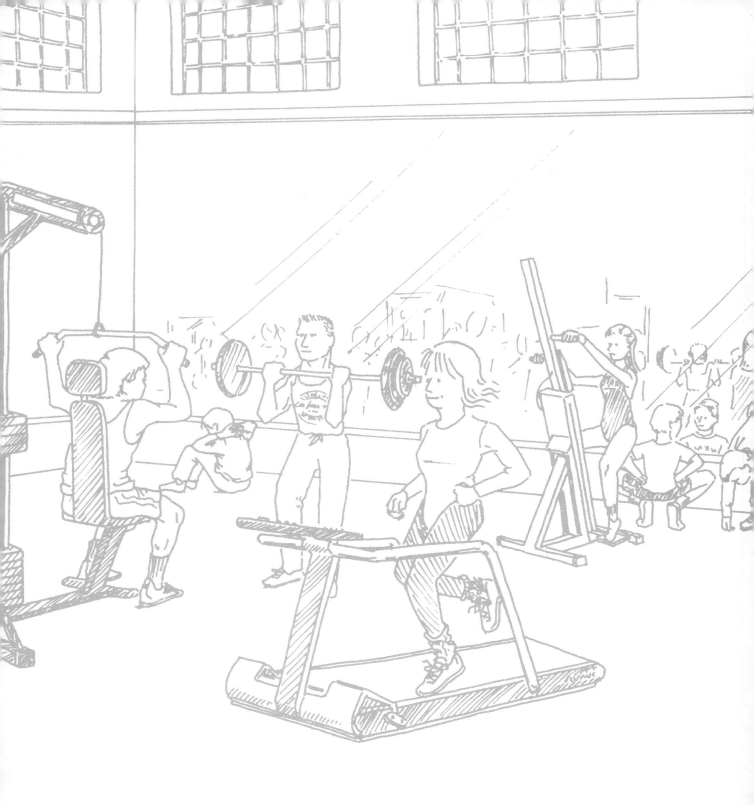

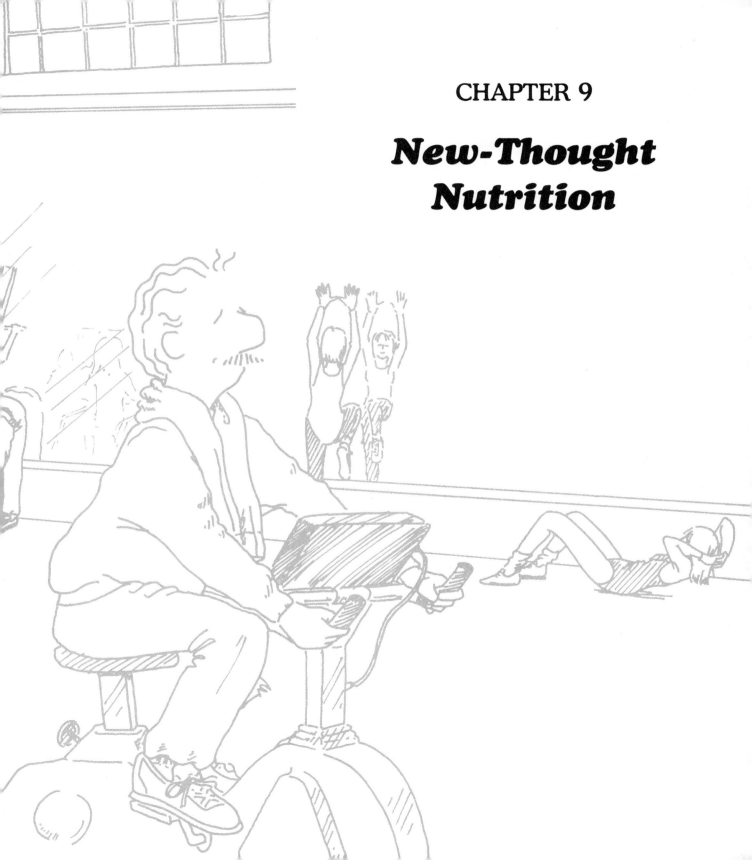

CHAPTER 9

New-Thought Nutrition

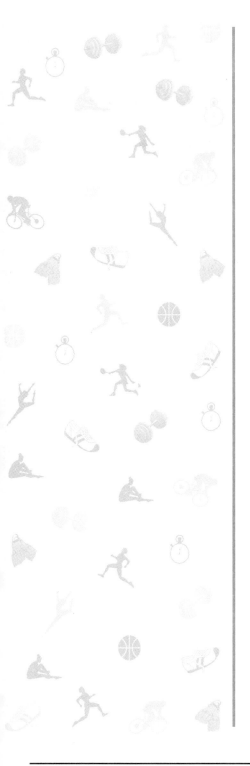

What do you think about when you have lots of energy? Do you think about the many things you want to do, places where you want to go, people you want to see? How do you feel when you don't have energy? Do you think about staying in bed, lying around the house, closing out the rest of the world? The truth is that when we have energy, we say yes to life, and when we have little or no energy, we say no to life.

This chapter is an instruction guide on how to eat for optimum energy and nutrition and a plan for how to use it for your good health for the rest of your life. Whereas the word *diet* has always meant "the foods a person habitually eats," its meaning has become blurred such that it has become synonymous with the word *restriction*. It is time to regroup and recall what and how we need to be eating to optimize our energy and maintain our health.

So far you have learned how exercise, especially exercise that utilizes oxygen, can feed your energy supply. But exercise alone cannot carry the energy load. Eating with the purpose of feeding your cells and fueling your system is one of the simplest ways to build your energy and invest in your health. Learning and applying some basic knowledge about how your body is best fueled is as simple to implement as knowing that you don't put oil in your gas tank and that your car uses more gasoline than oil on a regular basis. You need to know which and how much of the major fuel types you need to put in your machine.

Purposeful eating doesn't mean depriving your taste buds or losing your enjoyment of food. And it doesn't mean exiling certain foods altogether. But if the foods that are regulars in your weekly intake are not contributing to the type of energy or overall health you want, then it might be helpful to find a new point of view about the foods in your life.

The powerful tools of marketing and advertising have caused a lot of confusion about what foods are nutritionally good, bad, and fad. We as a nation are obsessed with weight issues. Fad diet books and fast weight loss schemes entice us because they make weight management seem so easy. And yet, with all of this focus on dieting and losing weight, doesn't it seem crazy that we are still becoming fatter and losing our leanness? A large part of the obesity problem has to do with sedentary lifestyles. However, the nutritional part of the issue is that in our quest for short-cuts for losing weight, we have strayed so far away from the basics of nutrition that we are lost. This is why we need to regroup and refresh ourselves with the basic principles of our energy and nutritional needs. Wouldn't you like to never go on a diet again? After reading about your fat cell activity and other sources of energy, you will never want to diet again; you will see how dieting only makes you fatter. Once that foundation is in place, it is much easier and simpler to make adjustments to accomplish personal body goals. Feeding your body the nutrients it needs is important and can be done in conjunction with changing your body composition. The first place to start is by getting in touch with your energy. When you have energy, you will feel up to doing those activities that will help you to change your body composition.

Energy Perspective. Hippocrates' famous quote, "Let food be your medicine and medicine be your food," reminds us that we want the foods we eat to contribute to our good health and that we should include those things that are good for us abundantly and regularly in our lives. Eating for energy gives you a new way of looking at food and new foods to look at (and eat!). You are about to learn some new perspectives about food and eating that might help change your attitudes about how you eat. You will learn about the major energy sources for the body and how to use them for the type of energy you desire. You will learn how to determine how much energy you need on a regular basis, how to manipulate your intake and output for changes in your body composition (fat and weight), and how to use the Food Guide Pyramid to your advantage. In that spirit, here are some new thoughts to digest about your nutrition.

New Thought—Food Perspectives
Energy-Driven Choices

Imagine that you can determine your energy by the foods you eat; well, the truth is you can. Of course, exercise and sleep have a lot to do with your energy level too, but let's assume that all things are equal. Eating well starts with a question. While you make your grocery list, or decide which restaurant to go to, or order from the menu, ask yourself this question: What type of energy do I want to have as an outcome of this eating/food experience? Put this question in along with the others that run through your mind, such as, Now what sounds good or looks good? Then make your selections accordingly.

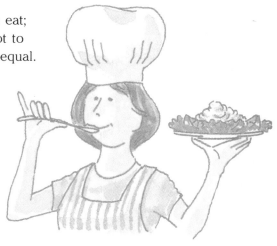

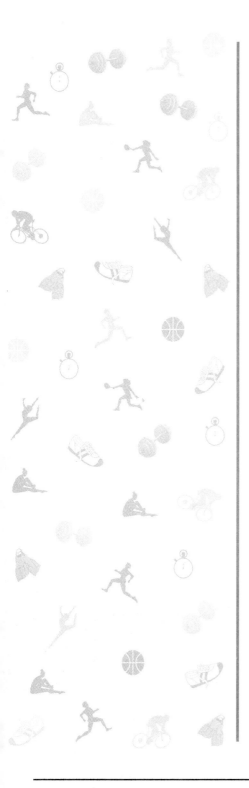

In just a moment, you will learn in useful detail the role of carbohydrates, fat, and protein in your nutrition and how they affect your energy. Equipped with these basic facts, you can control your own energy by the foods you eat. Without realizing it, you may already apply this type of thinking to other areas of your life, such as when you choose to consume alcohol, caffeine, or heavily sugared foods. Either you have personal experience with them or you are educated about how they affect your energy. This makes you more selective about when you have them. We are going to use this same approach and apply it to the food and energy element of your life.

Suppose you asked yourself these questions before making any selections: What type of energy do I want to have? How is this going to affect my energy now and later? Is eating *this* consistent with what I want for myself? It is possible to enjoy eating and to come out of the experience feeling satisfied, good about yourself, and energized. Eating with the idea of "I dictate my energy" is one idea that you can enjoy and live with!

Energy Control

When you make food choices, you are, to a large degree, the controller of your energy. If you want to feel sleepy and lethargic after eating, then eat a high fat meal; you are nearly guaranteed to get that result. If you want to feel energized, eat a meal that has more than half (55 to 60 percent) of the total calories from carbohydrates, less than 25 percent from fat, and the rest (15 percent) from protein. Are you someone who likes control over how you feel? What kind of energy do you want, starting now? You are in charge.

Emerging Independence

As children we learn some basic rules of nutrition, and as adults we can even recite the nutritional words of advice our parents preached to us: **Eat your vegetables. It's good for you. Just try it; if you don't like it, you don't have to finish it. You're not a food coward are you? Don't you want to grow up to be big and strong?** As we mature from children to free-thinking young adults, we act out our independence in many areas of our lives, including our eating habits. For some, skipping a family meal at the age of 16 may be as great an act of independence as getting the first set of keys to the family car. After high school, this desire to express independence can become even more pronounced. Many young adults covet their new freedom to eat what and when they please and demonstrate it in many ways. Eliminating breakfast, grazing on sodas and snacks throughout the day, and splurging on pizza, burgers, and the like at midnight for dinner are just some of the ways young adults express their nutritional independence. But for many, this newfound freedom is short lived; they start to notice that their energy isn't what it used to be. Or for the first time in their lives, they are experiencing a weight management problem. So they look for answers, quick ones.

The irony in these situations is that with each attempted shortcut, the very prize the person longed for, independence, is lost. They become dependent on shortcuts such as the newest diet, old diets resurrected, pills, deprivation, and the like. This leads to a long journey of dependence and frustration. It is a vicious cycle full of dietary lures and unsubstantiated promises.

If you seek independence from poor eating, poor weight management, marketing ploys, and low energy, seek to understand nutrition. Just as in exercise there are no shortcuts, the same is true for nutrition and optimum energy. Feeding your body with a healthy energy plan in mind gives you real independence and more opportunities for saying yes to life.

The Impact of Nutrition on Cellular You

We are energy beings made up of microscopic cells that have their own intelligence. These intelligent cells carry out an agenda that directs our bodily functions toward life and good health. This cellular scenario is a foundation for our life experience.

Just for a moment, imagine these cells as employees of your small business, your health. When they have the right work environment, they are very happy and produce a great product, your optimum energy and health. Although they prefer the best conditions possible, the employees do not expect perfect working conditions and are flexible enough to produce a good product in less than perfect working conditions. But when they are asked to work in poor conditions or without the proper resources, a series of negative events takes place. First, morale suffers. This causes the entire work environment to become stressed. Next,

Life Olympics

There is nothing like a goal to bring out the best in you and to motivate you for improvement. Imagine that next week you will be competing in the Life Olympics. Your event is the Iron-distance quadrathlon, the long-course combination of four events or "legs": the first leg is your spiritual connection, the second is your relationships with family/friends/pets, the third is your short- and long-term health, and the fourth leg is your professional work. In order to train and compete for your personal best, how would you fuel your energy system?

their ability to work suffers. The overall effect is a decline in productivity (a decline in your energy and health). And if these poor conditions go unchanged for a prolonged period of time, the employees eventually reach a breaking point at which they can no longer tolerate them. They resort to drastic measures. They either produce inferior products or they go on strike and shut down completely. This breaking point can manifest in many forms with minor or major consequences to your business (your health).

As the owner of this business, you have a choice about how you want to treat your cellular employees. The beauty of these employees is that most of them are forgiving and remarkably resilient. So when you are ready to correct the poor conditions of the past, they respond with vigor. The smart business owner knows that in this health business, the bottom line is best served by giving the cellular employees the best work environment possible. Doing so improves your chances for feeling good and staying healthy.

Nutrition is one very important working condition that has a positive impact on your cellular environment and daily energy. And as the owner of the business, you have a choice about the type of environment you provide for your cellular employees. Do you want to feel good or better? A good place to start is by creating a nutritional environment that gives your cells the best working conditions possible. You can do that by feeding them the right combination of nutrients in the proper intervals and quantities. Then you become the happy and prosperous business owner.

Our Physical History and Design

The human body is designed for survival. The desire to sustain life is strong, even among the ill and elderly. When we peek back at the origins of our physical history, we can see that many thousands of years ago, the human body was capable of surviving long periods without food. Flood, drought, fire, pest infestation, and plague were all harsh realities that created periods of famine. These certainly make today's reasons for not eating (such as not enough time, interest, importance) seem trivial now, don't they? Scientists believe that males were able to survive for 2 months without food and females for up to 9 months. These lengthy survival periods have been attributed to the brain's ability to detect famine and to respond appropriately by sending out a lifesaving message: Conserve energy. Store fat. Slow down all bodily processes.

Even though your chances of encountering a famine are less likely today than during the life of your ancestors, you are still well equipped with those survival capabilities. One of the reasons for the rampant obesity in this country is that many people's nutritional habits activate these metabolic survival activities, which during nonfamine conditions cause them to become very proficient at storing fat. Combine this with a sedentary lifestyle, and the health consequences are multiplied.

If we want to prevent and reverse obesity, we need to get more active and eat better. When we are active and eat well, the body adapts by releasing fat and increasing metabolic function. But first we have to convince the brain that the famine is gone. How do we do that? By eating properly and regularly.

Facts of Nutritional Life

Your body is an energy system, dependent upon outside sources of energy in order to sustain energy production and growth /life. *Metabolism* is the term used to describe all the chemical processes that occur within your body. Even though your metabolism adjusts/acts like a heating and air conditioning thermostat, you do not have a metabolism switch anywhere in your body.

Your body is dependent upon *nutrients*, substances that provide essential nourishment for the maintenance of life. It needs a variety of fuels and requires more than fifty known nutrients. Each has specific roles in the body. The six essential nutrients necessary for life are carbohydrate, fat, protein, water, vitamins, and minerals. The recommended amounts or proportions are as follows:

Carbohydrates

Carbohydrates (1 gram = 4 calories) should make up 55 to 60 percent of the total calories consumed. The majority come from complex carbohydrates. Carbohydrates are sugars, starches, and cellulose that fuel our brain and muscles. Their primary function is to supply energy, quickly.

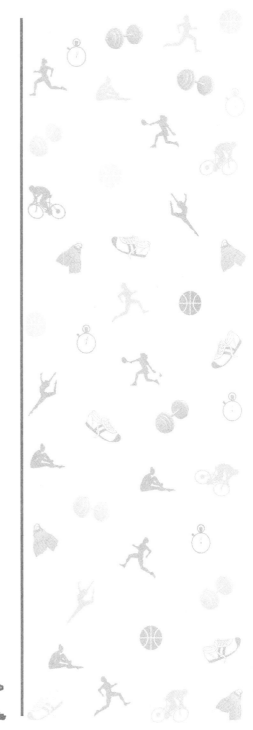

Complex carbohydrates (also called carbs, carbos) are long connected chains of molecules that are chemically more complex than simple carbohydrates. They are found in vegetables, beans, grains, and pasta. They take longer to enter the bloodstream because they are complex and take longer to break down. Complex carbohydrates are high in fiber, low in calories, and low in fat; they have a longer life span than simple carbs, which keeps energy level for lengthy periods of time, and give a contented feeling of fullness. They are stored in the liver and muscles as glycogen.

Simple carbohydrates are molecularly simple, with their single or double sugar molecules. This means they release quickly into the bloodstream but have a short life span. They are found in some fruits, processed sugar, and processed foods. They are usually lower in fiber and higher in calories than complex carbohydrates. They are absorbed quickly in the blood but have a relatively shorter life span than complex carbs. The "fireworks" of carbohydrates, simple carbs will shoot you up and drop you down.

Fats

Fats (1 gram = 9 calories) should make up less than 25 to 30 percent of total calories consumed, with no more than 10 percent from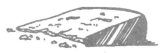
saturated fat. Even though you hear a lot of bad things about fat, it is a necessary nutrient—in the right amounts! Fat supplies essential fatty acids, an important source of energy for aerobic exercise. Free fatty acids make up the main fuel for muscles at rest and during light activity. Stored fat in the body is important for protecting vital organs, insulating against cold, and transporting the fat soluble vitamins (A, D, E, and K). There are two types, saturated and unsaturated.

Saturated fats cause much damage; they are known also as "artery blockers." Keep these well below 10 percent of your total calories consumed, or less than one-third of total fat consumed. Saturated fats are found in animal foods/products, dairy products, especially whole dairy products (whole milk, cheese, cream, ice cream), and oils. They are found in beef, pork, ham, sausage, coconut oil, cottonseed oil, and palm kernel oils. They are typically solid at room temperature.

*Trans Fatty Acids (TFAs)—alias hydrogenated vegetable oils—*although not officially considered saturated fats, are included with the saturated fats for a good reason. The body responds to TFAs as if they are saturated fats, the harmful kind that raises cholesterol and increases your risk of heart disease. When manufacturers recognized that they could improve the shelf life, flavor profile, and profit of their processed foods by hydrogenating (adding hydrogen to) polyunsaturated oils, they couldn't act fast enough. Hydrogenation turns polyunsaturated oils into solids. Read your packaged food labels carefully; if you eat foods that have TFAs, include them in your saturated fat count. Unfortunately, they are not yet accounted for on the nutrition facts panel along with the saturated fats, but will be in a few years. You have to look for them in the ingredients listing, where they are listed as partially hydrogenated vegetable (or other) oils. The most commonly hydrogenated oil is soybean oil. TFAs are found in manufactured cookies, crackers, and fried foods.

Unsaturated fats are the preferred fat, although not to be consumed above the recommended level. Two types are monounsaturated and polyunsaturated. Monounsaturated fats are found in olive and canola oils. They are touted as the healthiest of the oils. Polyunsaturated fats are found in corn, safflower, soybean, and sunflower oils.

Protein

Proteins (1 gram = 4 calories) are compounds derived from amino acids that provide basic structural properties of cells and are considered the building blocks for all tissues and cells in the body. The primary function of protein is to build and repair red blood cells, muscle, hair, and bodily tissue cells. A secondary function of protein is to be an energy provider, a backup to carbohydrates. Recommended intake is .4 gram per 1.1 (rounding off to 1.0 is close enough) pound of body weight, which is usually 12 to 15 percent of total calories. Athletes and vegetarians may figure up to 1.2 grams per 1.1 pounds of body weight. If you weigh 150 pounds, 150 times .4 equals 60 grams of protein or 240 calories of protein. Protein is found in meat, fish, dairy products (cheeses, milk, yogurt), and legumes (beans and peas). Legumes are excellent sources of protein; they are high in fiber and low in fat. Be aware that most nonvegetarian sources of protein have fat.

Vegetarian nutrition. Vegetable-based styles of eating, or vegetarianism, can be nutritious but require extra attention to ensure getting all

Legumes

What is a legume? A legume is the seed pod or edible part of leguminous plants (e.g., beans, peas, and lentils). Legumes are rich in protein, lecithin, vitamins C and E, and niacin.

of the nutrients, such as protein and calcium, that one would easily get from an animal product inclusive diet. Vegetarian based eating is high in fiber and water and as long as the foods are prepared without large amounts of added fat, such as the process of deep frying or sautéing in cream and butter sauces, it can be low in fat. So even though French fries, hush puppies, fried okra, broccoli in cheese sauce, and battered zucchini are vegetarian, they are hardly low in fat.

There are many degrees of vegetarianism (see sidebar) ranging from semi-vegetarians, those that include certain animal based foods, to vegans, those that exclude all animal or animal-derived foods. Some vegetarians start eating at one end of the vegetarian ladder (semi-vegetarian) and stay there, while others may start in the middle (lacto-ovo) and either climb or descend the rungs to stricter or lesser degrees. Or they may start out strict (vegan) and eventually descend a few rungs, relaxing their restrictions and ending somewhere near the middle of the spectrum (lacto-ovo). Regardless of the type of vegetarian eating one chooses, each warrant thoughtfulness for including a variety of nutrient rich foods.

Vegetarian sources of protein include legumes and bean-derived foods (such as tofu). Aside from protein, other nutritional qualities found in legumes are lecithin, Vitamins C and E, and niacin. Beans, one type of legume, come in many varieties and offer many excellent sources for protein and other nutrients. For vegetarian eaters, variety is especially important to ensure that they get as many of the more than 50 nutrients as possible. Here is a list of various types of beans:

- Adzuki beans are small tender red beans from China and Japan; they are often added to brown rice dishes.
- Anasazi means "the Ancient Ones" in Navajo language. These beans are generally sweeter and meatier than other beans.
- Black Turtle beans are found in Spanish-style foods, frequently seasoned with garlic, bay leaves, cumin, and tomato sauces. They also are made into soup.
- Chickpeas, or Garbanzo beans, have a nutty flavor that makes them perfect for salads. They are also famous for being turned into hummus spread and dips.
- Favas are lima-shaped beans that are good alone or added to soups.
- Great Northern beans are large white beans, useful for soups. They mix well with other beans.

Five Degrees of Vegetarianism

Semi-vegetarian—dairy foods, eggs, chicken, and fish (no other animal flesh)

Pesco-vegetarian—dairy foods, eggs, and fish (no other animal flesh)

Lacto-ovo-vegetarian—dairy foods and eggs (no animal flesh)

Ovo-vegetarian—eggs (no dairy foods or animal flesh)

Vegan—no animal or animal-derived food of any type

Food Technology, July 1991, Institute of Food Technologists.

- Lentils are a member of the pea family; they are one of the few beans that do not need presoaking.
- Lima beans have a distinctive flavor; they are known in the South as "butter" beans.
- Navy—the second most popular bean in America found primarily in soups and stews.
- Pinto beans are light brown in color; they lose their black spots when cooked. They are often used in burritos and stews and to make refried beans.
- Red Kidney beans are the most popular bean in America; they are found in chili, salads, and soups. They are the richest in fiber of all beans.
- Soybeans have the highest protein content of all the beans and are used in tempeh, tofu, tamari sauces, miso, and soy flour.

Water

Water is perhaps the least forgiving of the six essential nutrients. You may be able to survive for many days and even weeks without food, but not so with water. Drinking water because it is a vital nutrient is reason enough to consume it regularly. But it is also an exceptionally talented medium because of its ability to soothe, moisten, and cool and/or heat you. Water is found in food and fluids. The human body is approximately 60 to 70 percent water. It is one of the major ingredients of your anatomy and is necessary for an optimum physiological environment. Water has many jobs in the body, including the transportation of nutrients, gases, and waste products, and regulation of heat.

How do you know if you are getting enough water? Daily, you want to drink a minimum of 64 ounces (more than five 12-ounce glasses) of water, plus other hydrating fluids. Hydrating fluids are nonalcoholic, noncaffeinated, and noncarbonated fluids. If you drink 64 ounces daily and do not have the signs listed below, you probably are getting enough water. But when you notice these signs, add some water to your diet. Water is a very simple remedy to some pretty unpleasant conditions.

Alcohol

Alcohol is a depressant (drug). If you consume alcoholic beverages, be thoughtful and selective *before* you consume them. Remember, alcohol slows your reaction time (NEVER DRIVE when consuming alcohol!), packs a caloric punch (7 calories per gram; fat has 9 calories per gram), and dehydrates you.

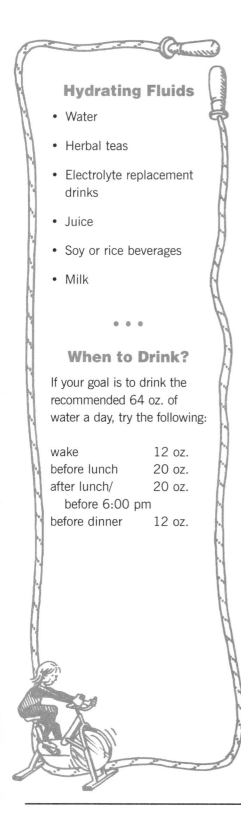

Hydrating Fluids

- Water

- Herbal teas

- Electrolyte replacement drinks

- Juice

- Soy or rice beverages

- Milk

• • •

When to Drink?

If your goal is to drink the recommended 64 oz. of water a day, try the following:

wake	12 oz.
before lunch	20 oz.
after lunch/ before 6:00 pm	20 oz.
before dinner	12 oz.

Signs that you may not be drinking enough water include the following:

1. Bad breath
2. Pasty mouth/tongue
3. Dark colored/smelly urine
4. Intestinal cramping
5. Difficult bowels
6. Dry skin
7. Headaches

Even though they are made with water, alcoholic, caffeinated, and carbonated beverages dehydrate the body, or cause it to lose fluid. If you consume those beverages, compensate with a 1:1 ratio of water for each one of those you consume. If you consume those beverages habitually, you might consider replacing them with water and a variety of the other hydrating beverages.

Fluid Plan

One of the simplest actions you can take toward improving your nutrition is to drink plenty of fluids. Having a conscious plan will help you to drink the recommended amount. Start your day with a 12- to 20-ounce water wake-up call. If you are a coffee/tea drinker, have the water first. It sets you up to be hydrated from the beginning of the day, gently wakes up your body, and helps stimulate your bowels, naturally. Secure a favorite water bottle and prefill it with water so that you have a visual reminder. Plan to drink it before lunchtime or before you leave the office. Keep a full bottle in your car, on your bike, or in your backpack and drink it before you reach your destination. If you work in an office, keep refilling the bottle at the water cooler. Have a cutoff time, typically a couple of hours prior to sleep, so your bladder will not be vying for your attention while you are sleeping.

Vitamins

Vitamins are the support crew or catalysts that enable other important functions to take place in your body. The best source of vitamins is from wholesome food sources. Vitamins from these sources are effective in part because of their synergistic effect. Plant and animal tissues contain a variety of compounds, and this group energy enhances their effectiveness. Many experts point out that vitamin supplements, which are isolated compounds, are incomplete and not as effective because they lack the supporting compounds that are found in the natural food source.

It is clear that vitamin supplementation is not intended to be a substitute for poor nutritional practices. The important emphasis here is upon the word *supplementation*, which means, in addition to. Vitamin supplements are best taken in addition to the natural source and are not advised as replacements for bad eating.

Too Much Can Be Dangerous

Even though they may look like cute, colorful pieces of candy, vitamins have serious effects upon the body. Before taking supplements, check with a health care provider to ensure you are not taking an inappropriate or dangerous dose.

Anti-oxidants

One group of supplements that have been proven to be effective and necessary are anti-oxidants. These counteract a phenomenon in the body known as free radical activity. Free radicals are nomadic type cells/molecules that float around in the body looking for a place to land. They can be dangerous and have been linked to causing immune function disorders and cancer.

Vitamins and Their Functions

Vitamins are compounds that help the body perform many functions. Here are just some of the highlights and good reasons why you want to eat a variety of wholesome foods:

- Vitamin A is a moisturizer for your skin and mucous membranes. It also aids vision. Sources include carrots, sweet potatoes, margarine, butter, and liver.
- Vitamin B_1 (thiamin) works with other enzymes to help you extract energy from carbohydrate. Sources include whole grains, nuts, and lean pork.
- Vitamin B_2 (riboflavin) is a coenzyme and does similar work as Vitamins A and B_1. Sources include milk, yogurt, and cheese.
- Vitamin B_3 (niacin) facilitates energy production in cells. Sources include lean meat, fish, poultry, and grains.

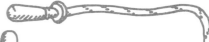

Suggestions for Drinking Your Daily Water/Fluid Quota

1. Drink water upon waking, 12 to 20 ounces.

2. Plan ahead. Drink half of your daily fluids before lunchtime and half before dinnertime.

3. Designate your "bottle size." Try two 32-ounce bottles or four 16-ounce bottles.

4. Fill the bottle and use it as a visual reminder.

5. Keep the bottle in your vehicle or on your bike.

6. Avoid large quantities at night to avoid interrupted sleep.

Note: When you are involved in athletic activities, consider drinking electrolyte replacement drinks (Gatorade, Powerade, etc.) for electrolyte balance.

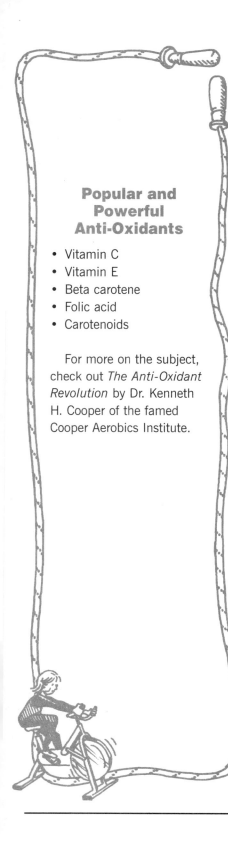

Popular and Powerful Anti-Oxidants

- Vitamin C
- Vitamin E
- Beta carotene
- Folic acid
- Carotenoids

For more on the subject, check out *The Anti-Oxidant Revolution* by Dr. Kenneth H. Cooper of the famed Cooper Aerobics Institute.

- Vitamin B_6 (pyroxdine) absorbs and metabolizes protein and aids in red blood cell formation. Sources include lean meat, vegetables, and whole grains.
- Vitamin B_{12} (cobalamin) is involved in synthesis of nucleic acids and red blood cell formation. Sources include meats, milk products, and eggs.
- Biotin is a coenzyme in the synthesis of fatty acids and glycogen formation. Sources include egg yolk and dark green vegetables.
- Folic acid (folacin) functions as a coenzyme in synthesis of nucleic acids and protein. Sources include green vegetables, beans, and whole wheat products.
- Vitamin C is responsible for intracellular maintenance of bone, capillaries, and teeth. Sources include citrus fruits, green peppers, and tomatoes.
- Vitamin D aids in growth and formation of bones and teeth; it promotes calcium absorption. Sources include eggs, tuna, liver, and fortified milk.
- Vitamin E protects polyunsaturated fats and prevents cell membrane damage. Sources include vegetable oils, whole-grain cereal and bread, and leafy green vegetables.
- Vitamin K is important in blood clotting. Sources include leafy green vegetables, peas, and potatoes.

Minerals

Minerals are inorganic substances that help the body perform many functions. Here are some highlights:

- Calcium aids bones, teeth, blood clotting, and nerve and muscle function. Sources include milk, sardines, dark green vegetables, nuts.
- Chloride aids nerve and muscle function and water balance (with sodium). Sources include table salt.
- Chromium aids glucose metabolism. Sources include meats, liver, whole grains, and dried beans.
- Copper aids in enzyme function and energy production. Sources include meats, seafood, nuts, and grains.
- Iodine aids thyroid hormone formation. Sources include iodized salt and seafood.

- Iron helps oxygen transport in red blood cells and enzyme function. Sources include red meat, liver, eggs, beans, leafy vegetables, and shellfish.
- Magnesium aids bone growth and nerve, muscle, and enzyme function. Sources include nuts, seafood, whole grains, and leafy green vegetables.
- Manganese aids enzyme function. Sources include whole grains, nuts, fruits, and vegetables.
- Phosphorus aids bone, teeth, and energy transfer. Sources include meats, poultry, seafood, eggs, milk, and beans.
- Potassium aids nerve and muscle function. Sources include fresh vegetables, bananas, cantaloupe, citrus fruits, milk, meats, and fish.
- Selenium works with vitamin E. Sources include meat, fish, whole grains, and eggs.
- Sodium aids nerve and muscle function and water balance. Sources include table salt.
- Zinc aids enzyme function and growth. Sources include meat, shellfish, yeast, and whole grains.

Calcium

The disease osteoporosis, a softening of the bones, has shed the spotlight on the need for adequate daily calcium intake. This important mineral helps keep your bones strong. The daily recommended intake for calcium is 1000 milligrams per day. When eating dairy products, use the low-fat or nonfat varieties. Even though most of the fat has been removed from low-fat skim milk and yogurt (not frozen), they retain all the calcium and protein. If you plan to take a calcium supplement (calcium citrate is recommended), you will want to get at least half of your calcium from food sources.

Caffeine

One of the world's most popular drugs, caffeine is a stimulant that affects the central nervous system, the digestive tract, and the body's metabolism. Caffeine is found in coffee beans, tea leaves, cocoa beans, and products derived from these sources. It is absorbed quickly in the body and can raise blood pressure, heart rate, and brain serotonin levels (low levels of serotonin cause drowsiness). The body adapts to

Vitamin Advice

Question: What's the best way to get your vitamins?

Answer: Eating your vitamins (in food) versus *taking* your vitamins (in pill form) is always recommended.

caffeine with an addictive quality such that withdrawal from caffeine can cause headaches and drowsiness. The pharmacological active dose of caffeine is defined as 200 milligrams, and the daily recommended "not to exceed" intake level is the equivalent of one to three cups of coffee per day (139 to 417 milligrams).

Dietary Fiber

Dietary fiber is from substances found in the walls of plant cells that the body cannot digest. There are two types of fiber, insoluble and soluble. The recommendation for daily dietary fiber intake is 25 to 35 grams, and if you currently eat less, you should increase your fiber intake gradually. You will notice the difference between having more fiber in your diet. The indigestibility of fiber, especially insoluble fiber, aids in overeating because it gives you a feeling of fullness. But even more importantly, it works wonders on your digestive tract.

Fiber is lost during food processing, so when possible, eat the less-processed version of a food. Juicing fruits, pureeing vegetables, and removing edible skins off fruits and vegetables are all processes that reduce fiber. It is also recommended that you eat a variety of fiber-rich foods so that you get enough of the two types of fiber, insoluble and soluble.

Insoluble fiber traveling through the digestive tract acts like a low-grade magnet-sponge, attracting and absorbing water and digested food to form fecal matter. This attraction and absorption softens and adds weight to stool, which helps facilitate transit time. Insoluble fibers such as those found in wheat bran and other grains, fruits, and vegetables help to prevent hemorrhoids, diverticulitis, colon cancer, and varicose veins. When adding insoluble fiber to your intake, remember to drink plenty of fluid so that it can do its softening job.

Soluble fiber has magnet-sponge traits similar to those of insoluble fiber. The difference is that soluble fiber such as oat bran, attracts and absorbs cholesterol, which helps prevent heart and gall bladder disease. Soluble fiber also slows glucose absorption from the small intestine. The best way to get enough soluble fiber is to eat a variety of whole grains, fruits, and vegetables. Too much fiber can exacerbate GI problems, so again, if you increase the fiber in your diet, do so gradually.

How Many Milligrams of Caffeine?

- Brewed cup of coffee
  139 mg of caffeine

- Brewed cup of tea
  (not herbal)
  48 mg of caffeine

- 1 cup chocolate chips,
  semisweet
  92 mg

- 1 ounce bittersweet
  chocolate
  18–30 mg

Cholesterol

You mostly hear how bad it is, but cholesterol provides the starting material for the synthesis of sex hormones, adrenal hormones, vitamin D, and bile. But the liver makes cholesterol, so there is no need for additional dietary sources. In excess, cholesterol deposits itself on the walls of the arteries, which can interfere with blood flow. Cholesterol is found in food products that come from animals, such as meat, fish, poultry, eggs, and dairy products. It is recommended that less than 300 milligrams be consumed per day.

A blood profile will report total cholesterol, *HDL* and *LDL*. These are cholesterol designations that refer to the type of protein carriers involved in the transport of cholesterol in blood.

HDL—High Density Lipoprotein (the good guys)

HDL collects cholesterol residues and transports them to the liver for reprocessing and excretion. High levels of HDL work to keep the arteries clear of deposits and reduce the risk of coronary artery disease. The best way to elevate HDL cholesterol is through exercise; some research suggests that reducing body fat will also elevate HDL.

LDL—Low Density Lipoprotein (the bad guys)

LDL brings cholesterol into the bloodstream to be used for cell building, but it can leave residues of cholesterol on artery walls. Eating foods high in saturated fat stimulates the liver to produce cholesterol, so reducing saturated fat intake is as important as reducing dietary cholesterol.

Metabolic Maintenance

Metabolic maintenance is the balance between energy (calories) consumed and energy expended. *Calories* are the unit of measure for expressing energy value. We take energy into the body in the form of food. We expend a great deal of energy to fuel daily living processes, as well as other activities.

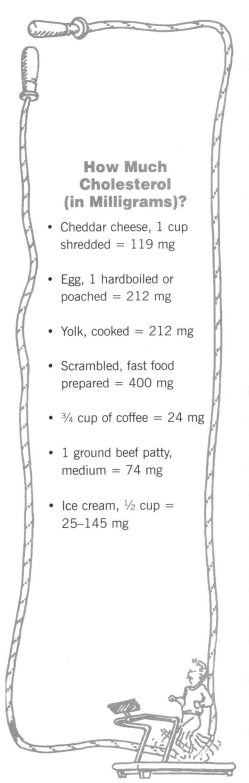

How Much Cholesterol (in Milligrams)?

- Cheddar cheese, 1 cup shredded = 119 mg

- Egg, 1 hardboiled or poached = 212 mg

- Yolk, cooked = 212 mg

- Scrambled, fast food prepared = 400 mg

- ¾ cup of coffee = 24 mg

- 1 ground beef patty, medium = 74 mg

- Ice cream, ½ cup = 25–145 mg

Fuel and Energy Sources

In *Fit or Fat*, Covert Bailey uses the example of firewood in a fireplace to describe how the body uses glucose and fat for energy. Here is an adapted and expanded use of the fire in the fireplace, to demonstrate energy metabolism.

• • •

Once upon a time, no just kidding . . . One cold wintry day in the mountains, Lisa ventured outside for a run. Near the end of her run, the cold began to penetrate her body. All she could think about was finishing and warming up beside a cozy fire in the fireplace, a fire that she would have to start.

She looked in the woodpile and found mostly big fat logs. She knew it would be impossible to start a fire with fat logs. They were too big and too dense. As Lisa looked near the back of the woodpile, she spotted some small pieces of kindling wood. She took the kindling pieces and stacked them in the fireplace so that some air (oxygen) would flow between them. Then she lit them. The kindling pieces lit easily, and in just a few moments, she had a small fire. She noticed how quickly the kindling pieces burned and how she had to continuously feed the fire more kindling. Gradually, she increased the size of the kindling, and the fire grew in strength and size. Within a short period of time and progressing from very small to larger pieces of kindling, she built a strong, lively fire.

As much as Lisa wanted the fire to keep burning to heat the cabin, she did not want to have to stand there and continuously feed it. So, she put a big log on top of the kindling pieces. The big log caught fire and burned slowly, steadily—differently from the kindling. Lisa now felt confident that she could leave the burning to the big logs and that she could go on with her other business.

Later, when she returned, she saw that where the kindling had once been piled, it was now burned to ash. She also noticed that the big log was engulfed in warm, orange flames. The fire was burning steadily and did not need kindling or logs added to it for a while. Feeling contented, Lisa made herself a cup of hot tea, parked herself in front of the fireplace, and basked in the glow of her fire.

• • •

What does Lisa's story have to do with our discussion of the body's fuel? The fire, kindling, and fat logs are symbolic of how your body uses fuel for energy. The fire represents your energy, how you feel. The kindling wood is similar to glucose. It can ignite and provide energy quickly but also burns quickly and needs to be restocked frequently. The log is similar to fat. It is too big and too dense to start a fire, but when added to a base of kindling or glucose, it can provide steady, sustainable energy for a long time.

Just as a fire needs the right combination and proportion of wood types for a healthy stable fire, your body needs the right combination and proportion of fuels to provide energy for all types of activities (thinking, moving, metabolic processes). It needs a solid base of kindling (glucose), and it needs comparatively fewer logs (fat) to provide for energy for basic human existence as well as for leisure time physical activities.

A fire fueled predominantly by kindling (glucose) or a fire fueled predominantly by logs (fat) has limited energy production. The former will burn quickly; the latter will smoke and smolder, and neither will be very effective in producing optimum heat (energy). You can see that eating a high fat meal is essentially like throwing big fat logs on a struggling flame. What do you think happens to your energy? It is likely to die out.

What types and combinations of wood are you putting in your fire? Are you producing reliable, lasting heat, or are you smoking?

What about Protein?

But wait. Barely a word was mentioned about protein. Why? Protein's full-time, number one priority job is to provide the building blocks for cellular repair production and tissue growth. Its role as energy provider is its *secondary role*; it does the job when the total number of calories is inadequate. Protein by choice would rather not be an energy provider. This is, in part, why high-protein and/or low-carbohydrate diets (discussed later in this chapter) are not good for the body. They distract protein from its full-time job.

"The Feel" Factor—Blood Glucose and Energy

In addition to the *types* of fuel you put into your body, your energy can be directly linked to the *amount* of energy you put (or don't put) into your body and the *timing* of it. *Nutrition is about fueling the body*

The Elimination Dance

Have you noticed what your pets do immediately after eliminating? Happily they thrust their legs behind them and bounce and sprint around the house or yard. Voiding your body of waste products feels good and is good for you too, but is a subject that many would rather not think or talk about. But think about how you can include natural fiber, through fruits, grains, and vegetables in your diet. A high fiber, low fat diet aids your digestive and elimination systems. Eat your 25–35 grams of daily fiber combined with plenty of fluids and who knows, you may feel like dancing after eliminating too.

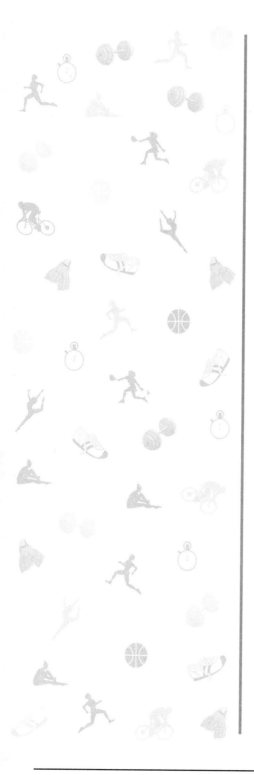

for optimum function. Many Americans have become so preoccupied with weight loss that they have lost sight of the main event.

A basic fact of physiology is that your brain absolutely must have its glucose, period! And if glucose is not adequately provided, the brain sends messages disguised as symptoms in an effort to get your attention. Even though the muscles may be able to continue their work for a while, the brain is not as accommodating. Low or sinking blood glucose will activate brain-originated messages like dizziness, weakness, or blurred vision. Think of these symptoms as your blood glucose barometer. If you experience these symptoms, you will want to raise the blood glucose soon by eating. Symptoms of low blood sugar include the following:

1. Lack of energy, lethargy
2. Difficulty concentrating, indecisiveness
3. Irritability
4. Headache
5. Shakiness
6. Stomach growling

If you delay your response by waiting to eat (perhaps you're thinking, "It's really not a convenient time for me to break away from . . . "), you set yourself up for indiscriminate eating. And if you ignore your response to the brain's initial messages (remember, at this point you are not thinking clearly anyway), the brain will send an even more powerful message; you will eventually faint.

Drowning Blood Sugar. For just a moment, imagine yourself drowning. Panic sets in; clear, logical thinking goes out. Your survival instinct takes over. You do not think; you merely react. In desperation, you grab onto the first "life preserver" you can find that will save you.

The desperation of this situation is very similar to a low-blood sugar scenario played out in your body. If your blood sugar falls uncomfortably low, you start looking for "life preservers" to rescue you. Your survival instinct takes over; clear logical thinking goes out. The brain sends you a message in the form of a craving. The craving is for food that will elevate the blood sugar quickly. And because your clear logical thinking abilities are unavailable, you devour the first foods you see. You are also more likely to eat quickly and in great volume because all you care about at that point is feeling better by rescuing your blood sugar.

When you eat quickly, you override the built-in "I'm full" mechanism that the stomach sends out to the brain. This causes you to overeat, to feel overfull and sometimes ill. You also have taken in more energy (calories) than your body needed. Then in frustration, you chastise yourself: "Why did I do that?" So, you proclaim, "Okay, I'll skip the next meal to make up for it." This cycle is physically undesirable and emotionally draining. But you can avoid it.

Eating for Energy—How to Eat

You can avoid the drowning blood sugar scenario. With a basic plan about how to eat, you can avoid the negative scenarios that will drag your energy down. You can maximize your energy and your body's ability to use the energy that comes in. The plan for eating to maximize your energy and achieve metabolic maintenance is interval eating, manipulating your fat cell storage, eating breakfast, snacking, and eating 2 to 3 hours before going to sleep.

Interval Eating

Interval eating means eating in regular frequent time periods. There are several good reasons why you should eat frequently. It can be stabilizing to your blood sugar to eat every 3 to 6 hours that you are awake. This keeps your blood sugar within adequate levels and prevents the activation of that desperate "send-me-a-life-preserver" scenario. Another good reason to eat in frequent intervals is to keep your fat storing enzymes quiet. So eat three meals every day and include wholesome snacks in between those meals so that you have fresh energy supplies coming in every 3 to 6 hours.

Fat Cell Storage

Your body has an adaptability response to starvation and perceptions of starvation. When your brain senses famine, it responds by activating fat enzymes to protect and store the energy inside your fat cells. Imagine these enzymes as troops who surround the cell as they would a fortress. They remain at their post until the famine passes and the flow of energy is once again regularly available.

Eating irregularly, skipping meals, and not getting enough energy (calories) rallies more of these fat-storing enzyme troops, which means that fat will be stored and not released. If you eat irregularly, skip

Coffee Break: A False Positive

Do you know anyone who enjoys coffee to wake up or perk up in place of breakfast or a light snack? Coffee is popular because it gives an energy boost and is calorie free. The only problem with using caffeinated coffee to boost energy is that it masks what is happening to the blood sugar when it is consumed in place of food. Meals and snacks stabilize blood sugar and keep it from sinking too low. When coffee alone is used to boost energy, the blood sugar continues to plummet. When the effects of the caffeine eventually wear off, it can leave you feeling very low. So if you want to enjoy your coffee break but avoid the plummeting blood sugar syndrome, eat some complex carbohydrate (banana, kiwi, crackers) during your coffee break.

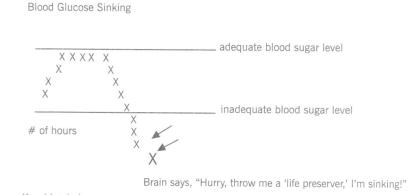

Blood Glucose Sinking

—————————————————————————— adequate blood sugar level

X X X X X
X   X
X   X
X   X
—————————————————— X ——————— inadequate blood sugar level
X
\# of hours   X
X
X

Brain says, "Hurry, throw me a 'life preserver,' I'm sinking!"

X = blood glucose

Blood Glucose Sinking
When blood glucose falls uncomfortably low, the brain sends out progressively stronger pleas for help.

meals, and do not get enough energy for your metabolic need (see section on Dieting later in this chapter), this may explain why your body has become very proficient at storing fat. By eating at regular intervals, you not only stabilize your blood sugar but you also convince your brain that all is well and there is no threat of famine. This allows the fat-storing enzyme troops to go on leave and allow the energy stored in the fat cells to be used.

Now that you understand how important it is to eat frequently, let's be clear about where to start.

Eating Breakfast

When you awaken each morning, you are coming out of a fasting state. Eating breakfast (break fast) breaks the fast. Its effect is like putting gasoline in your fuel tank, air in your bicycle tires, or shoes on your feet, *before* you take the trip. Without those essentials, you will not get very far. Such is true for breakfast and energy for your "day trip." Eating breakfast activates your energy and eating patterns for the day. When you skip breakfast, you send famine-like messages to the brain (you know what happens next), and you start the day in an energy deficit.

As you may have experienced in your personal finances, it is always harder to start anything from a deficit

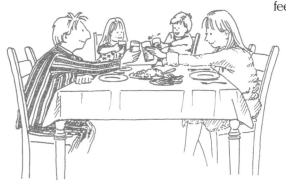

than it is from level or zero balance. Remember the blood sugar scenario from above? When you skip breakfast, you are essentially preparing your body for the low blood sugar/rescuing routine. Because you skipped breakfast (or any meal), you feel entitled to overindulge at other times, rationalizing, "Well, I skipped breakfast" (as if that is something to brag about). You end up chasing your nutritional imbalance all day long. Skipping breakfast, or any meal, usually sets up a negative pattern of nutrition to come.

Snacking

Second to eating breakfast, it is good to include snacks in your daily eating plan. A snack is a small amount of food eaten between meals. Snacks should bridge the gap between your main meals. Eating snacks that are complex carbohydrates (fruit, vegetables, and grains), high fiber, or low in fat between meals will help prevent plummeting blood sugar. If you eat breakfast at 7:00 A.M., then plan for a snack sometime between 10:30 and 11:30 A.M. Light snacks can be just enough to energize you until your next meal and can help take off the ravenous edge that can cause you to overeat.

Eat First, Sleep Later

It is 4:55 P.M., Friday afternoon, and you are at work. You just returned to your desk from a short meeting. You start thinking about all the fun things that you are going to do during the weekend. And it all starts in only 5 minutes. But out of the corner of your eye, you notice something sitting in your "in box" that wasn't there only moments earlier. It is a memo from your boss, which reads, "I'm really sorry about this, but I need you to read through this report *now* and respond to me within the next 3 hours." How do you feel?

Just as you were psyched up for the weekend, the refreshing "time off" you'll have from work, your body gets psyched up for its own "nightlife," in this case, the maintenance and repair activities of the body. You may not be consciously aware of it, but while you are sleeping, your body is very busy. The kidneys and liver are busy filtering toxins, blood is busy circulating, digestive enzymes are fast at work, elimination is getting in order, and your immune system is in high gear. And those are only the highlighted activities.

Extra, Extra, Read All about It

For more about getting your fat cells to work for you, check out the national bestseller by Debra Waterhouse, *Outsmarting the Female Fat Cell*.

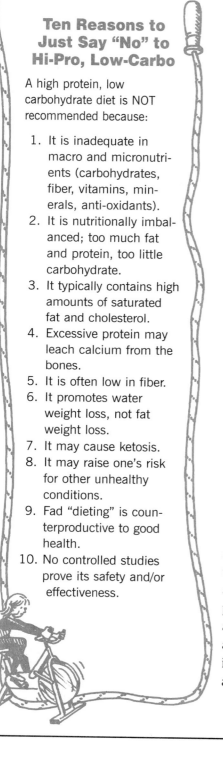

Ten Reasons to Just Say "No" to Hi-Pro, Low-Carbo

A high protein, low carbohydrate diet is NOT recommended because:

1. It is inadequate in macro and micronutrients (carbohydrates, fiber, vitamins, minerals, anti-oxidants).
2. It is nutritionally imbalanced; too much fat and protein, too little carbohydrate.
3. It typically contains high amounts of saturated fat and cholesterol.
4. Excessive protein may leach calcium from the bones.
5. It is often low in fiber.
6. It promotes water weight loss, not fat weight loss.
7. It may cause ketosis.
8. It may raise one's risk for other unhealthy conditions.
9. Fad "dieting" is counterproductive to good health.
10. No controlled studies prove its safety and/or effectiveness.

If you eat either a lot of food or high caloric food close to the time when you will be sleeping, you have essentially put more work in the body's "in box" during a time when the body was planning on something else. It is the equivalent of receiving that last minute memo from your boss.

Eating heavily close to the time when you will be sleeping can also contribute to heartburn and poor sleep cycles. If you experience these conditions, try eating 2 to 3 hours before going to bed.

Caloric Value—How Much?

Remember the firewood story? Would you like to know how much wood/energy you need to fuel your daily fire/energy? There are many reputable, scientifically based guidelines to help you determine daily caloric expenditure. One easy-to-use guideline for estimating your daily caloric need is provided later in this chapter. It will help you to estimate your daily total caloric need. Keep in mind that your caloric or energy need may change from day to day. Adjust your intake accordingly.

BMT—Basal Metabolic Testing

For $195, you can have BMT performed to determine exactly how many calories your body burns during inactivity. This information gives you an exact number of calories to work with and can be helpful if you have difficulty establishing just how many calories you need on a regular basis. It is quick, easy, and painless and measures your inspired and expired gases. (For details, see the Appendix resources.)

Establish a Benchmark

Do you know what percentage of your current intake is from fat, carbohydrate, and protein? Do you know how much calcium, sodium, and potassium you take in on a regular basis? If you want to understand and competently change your nutrition, start by having a nutritional analysis. It will tell you the objective story of your nutrition. In addition to the valuable information that comes from the analysis, the process of writing down what you eat is awareness building. It focuses attention on your eating patterns and will help you identify the good areas that you want to keep and the other areas that you may want to improve. A nutritional analysis takes the guesswork out of your eating and gives you the facts.

Nutritional Analysis

There are many inexpensive paperback books ($6.95 to $10.95) you can pick up that will help you to analyze your intake. If you have the time but not the money, this is the way to go. If you are short on time and have between $45 to $75, you can have your nutrition analyzed professionally by a nutritionist or other qualified consultant. There are also software programs that will perform this function.

A good analysis requires you to keep a food diary for a total of 3 days. You write down everything that you ingest for 2 typical weekdays and 1 typical weekend day. This helps you identify differences between the two types of days. If you are saying to yourself, "But I don't have 2 or 3 typical eating days," that alone is an important finding and may be the first opportunity for improvement.

It is also worthwhile to write down the time of day that you ate or drank so that you can identify the intervals of time between eating. Recording where you were when you ate/drank can help you become more aware of eating without thinking. Eating the candy off the desk of a coworker may seem insignificant at the time, but it can add up. In addition to writing down what you eat, you also write down the approximate serving sizes. This helps you in two ways: You get a more accurate appraisal of your intake, and it makes you more aware of quantities that you eat.

Calculating Your Intake

A good nutritional analysis should at least include your total number of calories and the percentages of the three macronutrients (carbohydrate, fat, and protein). You can also learn how much sodium, potassium, calcium, and other minerals you ingest on a regular basis. Later in this chapter, you will read about the desired levels for the nutrients, and when you have your analysis in hand, you can compare the two and begin making some small improvements.

Then what? Once you establish a benchmark for how you typically eat, you can compare it to your estimated need (see p. 199). It is not necessary that you count your caloric intake all the time, but it is important that you have a general idea of how many calories you take in on a regular basis. Remember, calories are units of energy. You need enough energy to "fund" the activities of your life, but not in excess. The overaccumulations will be stored on your frame. You need to have

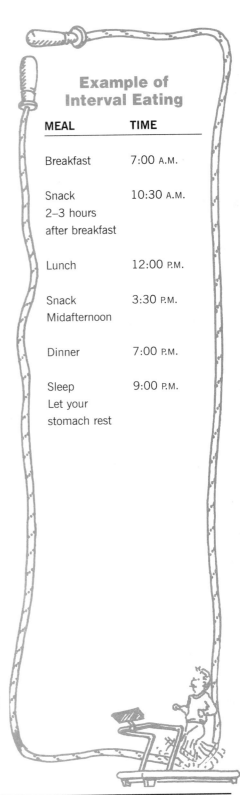

Example of Interval Eating

MEAL	TIME
Breakfast	7:00 A.M.
Snack 2–3 hours after breakfast	10:30 A.M.
Lunch	12:00 P.M.
Snack Midafternoon	3:30 P.M.
Dinner	7:00 P.M.
Sleep Let your stomach rest	9:00 P.M.

some idea of your eating income and expense patterns so that you can design a plan that suits your needs. If you have been unsuccessful managing a healthy weight, this exercise will help you.

The Depository System

The body's energy storage system operates much like a bank account. The only difference is that in one you want to amass accumulations and in the other you don't, but in terms of storage they are the same. When you accumulate a hundred pennies, you have the equivalent of a dollar, which you can either spend or save. Accumulations of pennies/dollars not spent are stored for future use in your savings account. A calorie is much like the penny or dollar. When your body's calorie bank accumulates calories, you can either spend them or save them. Accumulations of calories not spent are stored as fat in your body's savings account for future use. These fat accumulations can be measured by size and by weight. When we speak of the accumulations in terms of weight, we say you have gained a pound of body weight. When we speak of the accumulations in terms of size, we say you have gained inches.

Calorie Types and Body Weight

The body's calorie bank, or "depository," does not discriminate based upon the types or source of calories that cause it to gain. Whether calories consumed are high fat, low fat, or nonfat, they add to the sum of the caloric equation. When the body accumulates an excess of 3,500 calories (calories not being used), it will store them as 1 pound of fat regardless of whether they are from carbohydrate, fat, or protein. In terms of storage and weight gain or loss, a calorie is a calorie.

Where do calories come from? Calories only come from carbohydrate, fat, and protein, not from vitamins or minerals. And each of the three nutrients has its own energy value. Earlier we discussed how protein fills in for energy when needed. Look at the chart on p. 220 and notice that carbohydrate and protein have the same caloric value. Now *that* is a convenient coincidence! And notice that gram for gram, fat has more than twice the energy value as that of protein and carbohydrate. This energy density helps explain why we need fewer logs (fat) on our fire as compared to kindling (carbohydrate). Fantastic design!

Some Complex Carbohydrates

- All whole grains: brown rice, barley
- All vegetables: artichokes, avocados, banana squash, corn
- Dried peas, beans, and lentils
- Fresh and dried fruits
- Hubbard squash
- Pastas
- Potatoes, yams, pumpkin
- Sweet potatoes
- Water chestnuts

U.S. Dietary Guidelines—Reputable Supporters

Once you have established how many calories your body needs, the next step is to apply the recommended percentages from the three primary fuel sources: carbohydrate, fat, and protein. They are given as a percentage of total calories consumed, which takes into account the variability in total caloric intake from person to person. **The U.S. Dietary Guidelines are** carbohydrate, 55 to 60 percent; fat, 20 to 30 percent (no more than 10 percent from saturated fat); and protein, 10 to 15 percent. These guidelines are recommended by the American Dietetic Association, American College of Sports Medicine, American Heart Association, American Cancer Society, and the surgeon general. They are based upon the biological, nutritional needs of the body and will best fuel your cells, keeping them happy and positively productive. And you can use them to manage your weight too.

You may want to consider eating these recommended amounts at each meal. Remember the fire and energy analogy? If you ate only carbohydrates at a meal, that would be similar to burning only kindling in your fire. Your carbohydrates would burn up quickly, and you would very likely feel hungry sooner than expected. And if you ate only protein at a meal or fat at a meal, you would be depriving your body of the igniting energy that kindling/carbohydrate provides. Eating a balanced variety of the three fuels keeps your cells well fed and your energy balanced.

With a little knowledge of which foods are carbohydrates, fats, and proteins you can then categorize the foods you eat by their nutrient identity.

CARBOHYDRATES	FATS	PROTEINS
Fruits	Oils	Fish
Vegetables	Cheeses	Poultry
Grains	Nuts	Lean Meat

Now it is time to take the total caloric and nutrient information and apply it to your daily nutrition.

*Guidelines for protein vary for vegetarians, body builders, etc.

A Good Eating Schedule

To feel good and optimize your energy, follow these tips:

1. Eat breakfast.

2. Eat every 3 to 6 hours throughout the day.

3. Stop eating 2 to 3 hours before bedtime.

Daily Nutrition by Percent and by Volume

Percentage Approach

Figure 1 illustrates the recommended percentages of total calories. These percentages can be applied to each meal to ensure balanced nutrition and energy supply. Total calories from carbohydrate, 55 to 60 percent, total calories from protein, 15 percent, and total calories from fat, 20 to 30 percent, with no more than 10 percent from saturated fat.

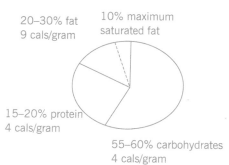

20–30% fat
9 cals/gram

10% maximum
saturated fat

15–20% protein
4 cals/gram

55–60% carbohydrates
4 cals/gram

Figure 1: USDA Recommended percentages
Calorie values and source of calories by percent of total calories

Volume Approach

Figure 2 illustrates the recommended percent of total calories but with a practical application, as if it were your plate. Because fat has more than twice the caloric value as carbohydrate (Fat yields 9 calories per gram, carbohydrate and protein yield 4.) and protein (gram for gram), the volume or amount on your plate needs to be comparatively small. Even though the recommended percentage of fat is higher than that of protein (fat, 20 to 30 percent, protein, 15 percent), you need less of it by volume (size) because it is calorie dense.

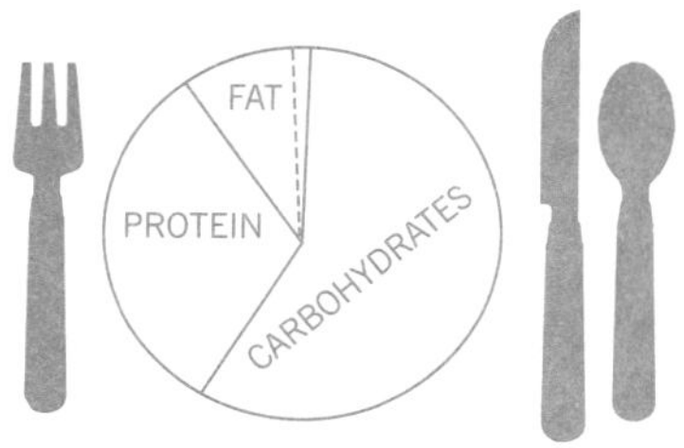

FAT

PROTEIN

CARBOHYDRATES

Figure 2: Recommended percentages as applied to your plate
Source of calories by food volume

Percentages by Volume Approach

Applying these percentages (approximately 60 percent, 25 percent, 15 percent) by volume makes meal planning and eating simpler than by counting calories. Think about how much space each of the three nutrients are taking up on your plate. When you grocery shop, look in your basket and think, "I want more than half of my food coming from carbohydrates. Is what is in my cart consistent with that guideline?"

With a little knowledge of which foods are carbohydrates, fats, and proteins, you can generically categorize what you eat and apply the percent by volume approach to your intake. For example, what if you ate the following for dinner: one average-sized chicken breast without the skin, a cup of steamed brown rice (no butter), a cup of steamed broccoli with a touch of olive oil with balsamic vinegar, and an apple raisin salad made with celery, low-fat yogurt, and cinnamon?

Once again, we will use your plate as a model for what you actually ate. Is more than half of the space on your plate taken up by carbohydrate? Is protein a significantly smaller portion relative to the amount of carbohydrates? Is fat even smaller than the amount of space protein occupies? If so, you are probably close to the recommended percentages based on eyeball volume. However, if the chicken is taking up most of the space on your plate, the broccoli can barely squeeze on, and you have about a tablespoon of rice, then you probably ate more protein and less carbohydrate than your goal (60 percent carbohydrates, 15 percent protein, 25 percent fat (no more than 10 percent from saturated fat). If the plate view does not help, try listing the foods you ate by their respective category. The chicken dinner we described above would look like this:

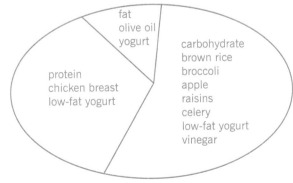

Estimating Total Calories

1. Determine the caloric value to cover your resting metabolic rate (RMR), the number of calories you need to live, by taking your body weight (or healthy body weight) and multiplying it by 10.
2. Determine how many calories you need for today's purposeful exercise (see Calories Burned During Exercise).
3. Determine how many calories you need for your daily activity level aside from purposeful exercise. If you are sedentary, add 20 to 40 percent RMR; moderately active, add 40 to 60 percent RMR; very active, add 60 to 80 percent RMR.
4. Add the answers to the steps above to determine today's total calorie requirement.

Adapted from *Nancy Clark's Sports Nutrition Guidebook*, Second Edition, 1997.

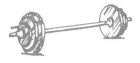
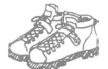
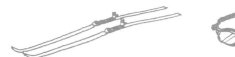

Calories Burned During Exercise

You can use this information to determine a reasonable estimate of the amount of calories you burn when exercising at a comfortable pace. If you are pushing yourself hard, add more calories. Multiply your body weight times the calories per hour times the increments of an hour for an estimate of the calories you burn during that activity.

ACTIVITY	CALORIES PER HOUR PER POUND OF BODY WEIGHT	ACTIVITY	CALORIES PER HOUR PER POUND OF BODY WEIGHT
Badminton	2.6	Sawing, by hand	3.3
Bicycling, 10 mph*	2.7	Scrubbing floors	2.9
Chopping wood, ax	2.3	Scuba diving	3.8
Dancing, ballroom	1.6	Skating, ice	2.6
Dancing, modern	2.6	Snow shoveling, light	2.9
Farming, light	2.3	Skiing, cross-country	3.7
Farming, heavy	3.2	Skiing, alpine (downhill)	2.6
Gardening, hoe, dig	3.2	Snowshoe, walking	4.5
Golf, walking	2.3	Squash	4.3
Horse grooming	3.5	Swimming, slow crawl	3.5
House cleaning	1.6	Soccer	3.7
Hiking, hilly	3.6	Table tennis	1.9
Horseback riding, trot	2.8	Tennis, singles	2.9
Jogging, 6 mph/10 min/mile*	4.2	Tennis, doubles	1.8
Jumping rope	3.8	Volleyball	2.2
Mopping	1.7	Walking, 3.5 mph*•	2.4
Painting, outside	2.1	Water skiing	3.0
Racquetball	4.1	Weight training	1.9
Rowing machine	3.1		

Example: Your weight = 150 pounds; activity—walk 3.5 mph; time walked = 1 hour*

If you weigh 150 pounds and walk at 3.5 mph for 1 hour, you would multiply 150 x 2.4 (the number of calories burned at that speed) x 1 hour = 360 calories burned per hour.

*For increments less than an hour, multiply by the decimal equivalent of an hour: 1/2 hour = .5, ¼ hour = .25, etc.

*See Pace versus Miles Per Hour for information on how to convert miles per hour to pace and pace to miles per hour.

Adapted from B. Stamford and P. Shimer, 1990, *Fitness Without Exercise* (New York, NY: Warner Books).

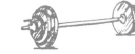

Just looking at the breakdown gives you an idea that you have a meal whose percentages and volume are close to the recommended 60-25-15.

As long as we are discussing food tracking and accountability, we need to include the *gram*. Sometimes nutrient value is expressed in grams; for example, someone on a, say, 2,000 intake plan should consume no more than 55 grams of fat per day. If you are more familiar with caloric value, simply convert the gram value to calories by multiplying the number of grams by the per-gram value. In the case of fat, you know that 1 gram equals 9 calories. Therefore, a recommendation to consume no more than 55 grams of daily fat translates to 495 fat calories, which by the way is 25 percent of the total 2,000 calories. The benefit in performing these calculations is that you will develop a reference value for foods that you regularly consume. It will also help you use the nutrition facts information to your advantage. Here is an example:

Given: This average adult needs 2,000 calories a day.

STEP 1: Multiply the total calories desired per day (2,000) by the percentage for each of the three nutrients above to determine total calories from each.

Total caloric need:	2,000
Carbohydrate—60%; fat—25%; protein—15%	
Total number of calories from carbohydrate:	2,000 x .60 = 1,200
Total number of calories from fat:	2,000 x .25 = 500
Total number of calories from protein	2,000 x .15 = 300
Total calories	2,000

STEP 2: Using the per gram caloric value for each nutrient, you can establish the number of grams for each fuel using information from Step 1. To convert calories of nutrients (from step 1) to grams desired, follow these steps:

1 gram of carbohydrate has a value of 4 calories.
1 gram of fat has a value of 9 calories.
1 gram of protein has a value of 4 calories.

Use the figures from Step 1 above to answer these questions:

Question: What is the gram equivalent of 1,200 carbohydrate calories?

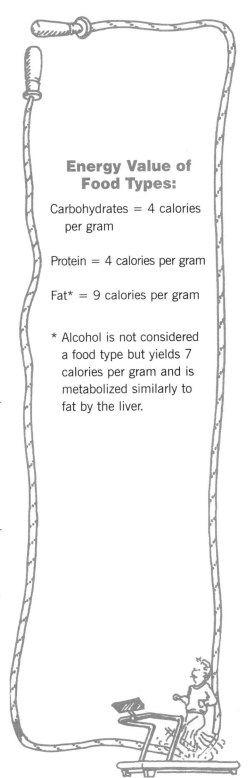

Energy Value of Food Types:

Carbohydrates = 4 calories per gram

Protein = 4 calories per gram

Fat* = 9 calories per gram

* Alcohol is not considered a food type but yields 7 calories per gram and is metabolized similarly to fat by the liver.

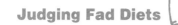

Judging Fad Diets

The next time you read about another fad diet, use this criteria to help you decide whether it is safe or not.

1. Check for clinical studies that validate the claims in reasonable numbers.
2. Is it an enduring diet, one that if you stayed with it for your lifetime, you would be healthy? No harmful side effects?
3. What other *reputable* organizations support it (if any)?
4. Use common sense. Do you think it is sound nutritional practice to eat, for example, just grapefruit, carrots, cabbage? Is the diet "narrow," directing you to limit the variety of foods you eat? If you're using the diet, is your skin turning colors? Is your breath "off" and awful?

Total calories from carbohydrate = 1,200.

Divide 1,200 calories by 4 calories per gram to get the total number of grams.

Answer: 1,200/4 calories per gram = 300 grams of carbohydrate.

Question: What is the gram equivalent of 500 fat calories?

Total calories from fat = 500.

Divide 500 fat calories by 9 to get the total number of grams.

Answer: 55.55 grams of fat = 500 fat calories.

Question: What is the gram equivalent of 300 protein calories?

Divide 300 protein calories by 4 to get the total number of grams.

Answer: 75 grams of protein = 300 protein calories.

So, the nutritional profile for this individual would look like this:

Total daily caloric need: 2000 divided as 60% carbohydrate, 25% fat, 15% protein.

Carbohydrate: 1,200 calories or 300 grams

Fat: 500 calories or 55.55 grams

Protein: 300 calories or 75 grams.

The next step can be fun. Liken it to planning a road trip with a map. Using a food reference guide book/Web site, or other books for food values, look up some of the foods that you regularly consume and familiarize yourself with their portion size and caloric and nutritional value. Determine what type of fuel they are, carbohydrate, fat, or protein (many foods are combinations of two or all three). You can do this yourself or you can work with a nutritionist, dietitian, or related consultant.

Another useful tool for steering you toward healthy eating is the USDA Food Guide Pyramid. In 1992 the federal government released the Food Guide Pyramid, which was the new and improved eating plan for Americans, replacing the outdated Basic Four Food Groups. The pyramid classifies and recommends numbers of servings for specific groups of foods, for example, fruit group, 2 to 4 servings per day; vegetable group, 3 to 5 servings per day. As mentioned earlier, the body needs more than fifty nutrients to function normally. The USDA Food

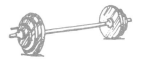
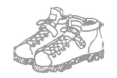

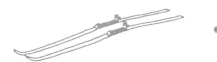

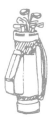

10 Calcium-Rich Foods

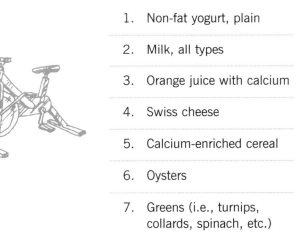

	ITEM	SERVING SIZE	CALCIUM (MG)
1.	Non-fat yogurt, plain	1 cup	350
2.	Milk, all types	1 cup	300
3.	Orange juice with calcium	1 cup	300
4.	Swiss cheese	1 oz.	260
5.	Calcium-enriched cereal	1 cup	200
6.	Oysters	¾ cup	170
7.	Greens (i.e., turnips, collards, spinach, etc.)	½ cup	145
8.	Ice cream or ice milk	½ cup	100
9.	Beans, cooked	1 cup	90
10.	Broccoli, cooked	½ cup	70

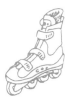

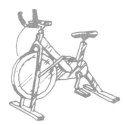

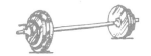
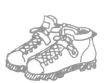

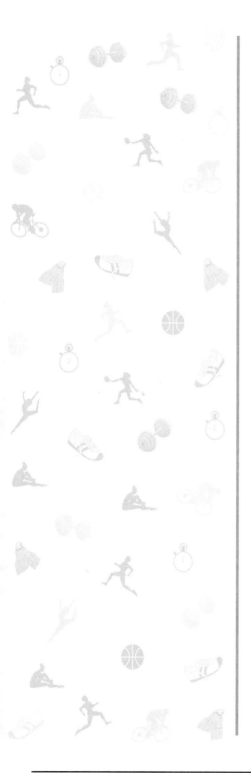

Guide Pyramid is designed to guide you toward a variety of foods that will help you consume as many of those 50 nutrients as possible.

Although the Food Guide Pyramid does not mention the food types by nutrient category, it can be very helpful to recognize them. Look at the pyramid and read the bottom two tiers: tier one lists the "bread, cereal, rice, and pasta group," and tier two lists the "fruit group" and "vegetable group." These are all carbohydrates. The tier above, "milk, yogurt, and cheese group" and "meat, poultry, fish, dry beans, eggs, and nuts group," are predominantly protein and fat sources. And, the top tier, "fats, oils, and sweets," are fat and sugar dense.

When asked to name carbohydrates, many say, "Pasta, grains, and rice," and those are indeed carbohydrates. But fruits and vegetables are also carbohydrates, and they are the foods you want to include heavily into your meal and snack agenda.

Serving Sizes—Simplification and Familiarization

The Food Guide Pyramid recommends numbers of servings for each group. Here are two useful suggestions for defining what is a serving. First of all, plan to set aside only 10 to 15 minutes of your time. Read through a list of foods and their serving sizes and narrow them down, highlighting those you frequently eat or plan to eat (a small sample is provided below). Then, one by one, take a moment to visualize what they look like. Or if you want to have some fun in the kitchen, take out a ½ cup measuring cup and scoop out the serving size (of rice, or pasta, etc.) so that you get a visual picture. Even though you may not, for example, have a half cup of spaghetti sauce readily available, you can improvise by measuring some other comparable thick liquid. The visual association is memorable and transferable for when you actually get ready to eat.

Variety

The importance of eating a variety of foods is twofold. There is no one food that has all the nutrients needed by the body, and some foods have more of one type of nutrient than another. As the body regenerates on a cellular level, it wants the full package of nutrients in the appropriate quantities. If you want those cellular employees to turn

COMMON SOURCES OF CARBOHYDRATE, PROTEIN, AND FAT

Macronutrient	Food sources
Carbohydrate	
Starches	Pasta, rice, grains, breads, cereals, potatoes, dried beans and peas
Sugars	Fruits, candy, cookies, cakes, jelly, sugar, honey, syrup, molasses, soda pop
Protein	Meats, fish, poultry, eggs, milk, yogurt, cheese, nuts, dried beans
Fat	
Saturated	Animal fats, butter, cheese, whole milk, mayonnaise, egg yolks, ice cream, chocolate, lard, hydrogenated oils, coconut and palm oils
Polyunsaturated	Some margarines, nuts, and oils (i.e., corn, safflower, soybean, cottonseed, sesame, and sunflower oils)
Monounsaturated	Olive, canola, and peanut oils

Note: From "The Food Guide Pyramid" by U.S. Department of Agriculture, Human Nutrition Information Service, 1992, Leaflet No. 572, U.S. Government Printing Office, Washington, D.C.

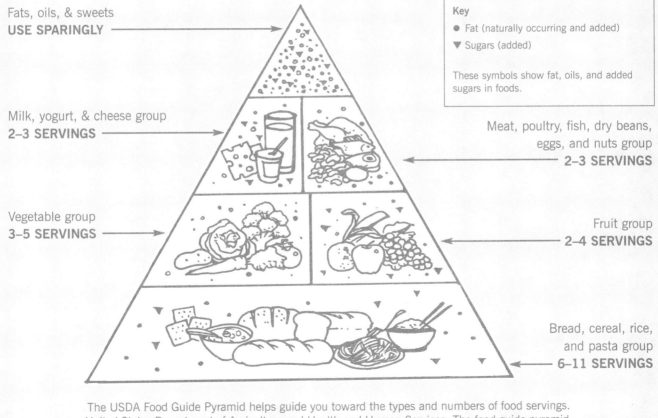

Fats, oils, & sweets
USE SPARINGLY

Key
● Fat (naturally occurring and added)
▼ Sugars (added)

These symbols show fat, oils, and added sugars in foods.

Milk, yogurt, & cheese group
2–3 SERVINGS

Meat, poultry, fish, dry beans, eggs, and nuts group
2–3 SERVINGS

Vegetable group
3–5 SERVINGS

Fruit group
2–4 SERVINGS

Bread, cereal, rice, and pasta group
6–11 SERVINGS

The USDA Food Guide Pyramid helps guide you toward the types and numbers of food servings.
United States Department of Agriculture and Health and Human Services: The food guide pyramid.

out the superior product (your energy and health), feeding them a variety of nutrients is the equivalent of giving them the best supplies to do the job.

The other reason to eat a variety of foods is the human, psychological factor. Variety *is* the spice of life, and eating a variety of foods will help you avoid food ruts, burnout, and boredom. Mother Nature's change of seasons is a timely reminder to eat the fresh fruits and vegetables of the season. It is a satisfying way to feel connected to the earth and to stay "fresh" mentally with your food.

Items You Should Reduce or Avoid— Processed Foods

Snack Food Syndrome

A large part of the obesity problem in this country is lack of activity and the overconsumption of calories. *Manufactured edible products*, better known as processed, packaged foods, are partly to blame for the overconsumption part of the scenario.

Manufactured food products originate as food from nature but are subjected to processing by humans. Many of these foods start out as complex carbohydrates, low in fat (such as whole wheat flour, potatoes, rice, and corn), but end up as high-fat human-made snacks such as chips, cookies, and cakes. In processing, they are stripped of their fiber, their original nutrients, and frequently are bleached, heavily sugared, and/or salted. In an attempt to revive their nutritional content, manufacturers fortify them with manufactured vitamins and minerals. Although this is a thoughtful effort, the fortification levels are often less than the levels that were intact in the original form.

These products are targeted strictly to consumers' taste buds, and consumers are biting the bait. The term *empty calories* refers to edible products that have caloric value without much nutritional benefit. The other calorie-packing factor to consider when eating processed snacks like chips is the number of calories consumed when other ingredients are added to them. For example, dipping (and eating) a chip in a sour

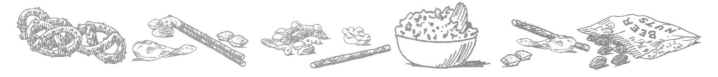

cream dip adds saturated fat and numerous calories on top of the already empty calories of the chip. And it is easy to overeat them. When you eat these snacks, consider their low- or nonexistent nutritional value and their high contribution to your total caloric intake.

Snack products are typically high in calories (even low fat can be high calorie), low in fiber, and high in salt/sodium. They have little to no fiber, so rarely do you feel full from eating just a few, or even a whole bag. Plus, the salty flavor keeps you coming back for more. After eating a bag of snack products, you have ingested many calories, but you do not have the satisfaction of feeling full. So you eat more, or again, and take in more calories, very likely an excess of calories, which are then stored as fat. The overconsumption of processed foods and the snack food syndrome is a significant contributor to the obesity problem in this country.

White Flour

White flour, whose origin is the wonderful wheat plant, is the end product of a dismantling process that removes the endosperm and outer bran casing (fiber) in order to deliver a soft, white, clean-looking flour. White flour is less expensive and easier to manipulate than whole wheat flour (less gluten) and explains why it is the preferred choice of manufacturers. They can produce less-expensive, uniform-looking snacks and breads. Due to the processing, white flour is a very distant relative of its healthy ancestor, the whole wheat plant. This is one reason why white flour is marketed as "fortified, enriched," and so on. It is an effort to make up for what processing took away from its natural state. These foods in their original form were complex carbohydrates, but manufacturing and processing changed everything.

Bad Advice about Carbohydrates— Wrongly Accused

There are several different types of carbohydrates, including starches, sugars, and fibers; all make valuable nutritious contributions to your energy and health. Bread, cereal, rice, pasta, vegetables (including potatoes), and fruit are all carbohydrates and the foods that should constitute the majority of your intake. So why do carbohydrates get such bad

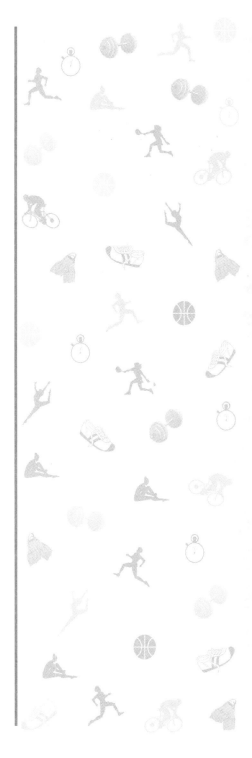

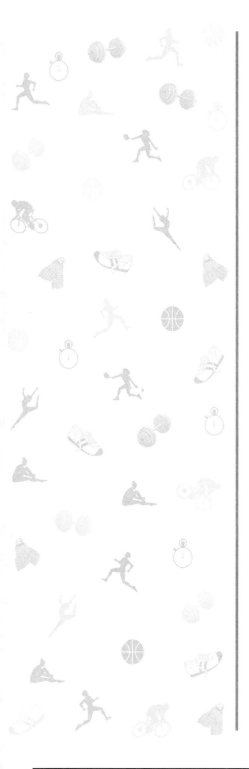

publicity, and why are they blamed for much of the obesity problem in this country?

There are a few reasons. One is that cooks and manufacturers turn them into high-fat, high-caloric taste thrills that people find irresistibly delicious. A simple truth about cooking is that fat adds flavor. (However, fat isn't the only flavor! See flavorful hints later in this chapter.) But this practice of eating foods that have been prepared strictly for the flavor objective is what leads to the obesity problem. If you want to truly test the ability of creative cooks, ask them to prepare your food for flavor minus the flood of fat. It can be and is done every day by many cooks.

Another reason why carbohydrates are the scapegoat for obesity involves what people do to them and the quantity in which they eat them. For example, you may complain that eating potatoes or bread makes you fat. What you may not know or be paying attention to is the impact of the glob of butter you put on the bread. Or did you not know that the cheese and sour cream swimming atop your potatoes is high in fat and calories or that eating the entire loaf of bread and the entire potato cheese casserole will make you fat if it is in excess of the calories you typically burn? Anything you eat in excess will make you fat, be it apples or cheese. But when you eat fat in excess, it has double the caloric impact. In situations like these, people blame carbohydrates as the culprit that made them fat. But the poor carbohydrate didn't have a fair chance, especially when overrun with saturated fat. You will get fat if you eat an excess of fat or an excess of calories—period.

The claim that "Americans are eating too many carbohydrates . . . they are getting fat on carbohydrates . . . they need more protein," etc., is a misdirected attack upon a very healthy nutrient category. The consumption of carbohydrate is not to blame. A more appropriate assignment is the overconsumption of high-caloric manufactured and processed foods. To blame and dismiss carbohydrate from your nutritional plan is like throwing out the baby with the bathwater. Keep the baby; throw out the bathwater!

Eat 55 to 60 percent of your total calories from carbohydrates, those that come from the earth and have been unscathed by processing and manufacturing. And if food volume is important to you, remember that in terms of caloric equality (gram for gram), you can eat twice as much carbohydrate as fat.

Name Those Carbohydrates

As mentioned earlier, *fruits and vegetables are carbohydrates.* Many people mistakenly think fruits and vegetables are their own nutrient category, but that is not true. When nutritionists recommend carbohydrates, they are *recommending fruits, vegetables, and whole unprocessed grains.*

Blood Sugar and Insulin Response

Insulin is a hormone that has many functions including regulating rising blood sugar and promoting fat storage. When blood sugar is elevated, insulin is secreted by the pancreas in order to bring down blood sugar levels. It is a sort of checks and balance system. When insulin levels are low, the body supposedly burns more stored fat for energy. Some argue that for weight reduction, it is best to keep blood sugar low in order to keep insulin levels low. The flaw in that argument is that when you have low blood sugar, you have no energy to do anything, and that means you are more likely to be sedentary, which is what makes you fat. Regular exercise and weight control automatically keep insulin levels in line. So be clear about the role of insulin. Insulin does not make you fat. Overeating and underexercising do.

Dieting versus Solid Nutrition Practices

Dieting in America has become a phenomenon, a past time, and a lucrative business. Dieting is typically associated with short-term bouts of trying different ways and combinations of eating in an effort to lose weight. But dieting is actually making dieters fatter than before they "dieted." Many people who diet erroneously declare, "I lack willpower." In reality, people who diet and restrict food work harder, not smarter; it takes hard work to understand and implement sound nutrition. Following are some excellent reasons why you never want to go on a diet, a restriction plan of eating, again.

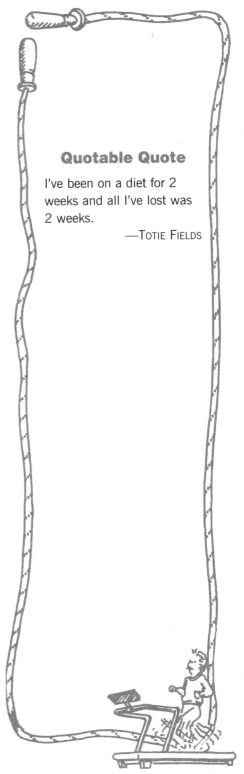

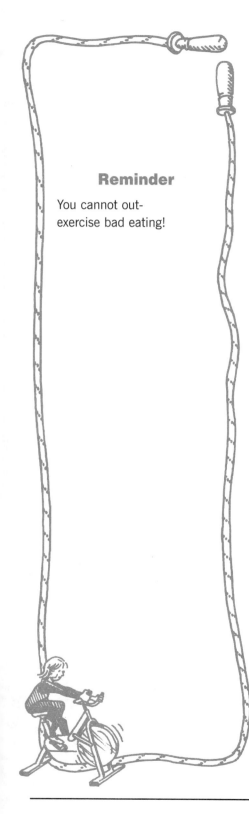

Reminder

You cannot out-exercise bad eating!

Short-Term Speculating versus Long-Term Investing

Going on a diet and looking for a quick fix for your weight problem is the equivalent of putting your financial savings into the stock market for a short period of time and expecting to make a fortune. Even if you know little about investing, you certainly have heard that the most successful investors are those who invest using prudent, sound investing techniques and are committed for the long term. Unfortunately, many people go from diet to diet, speculating that this time it will be the right one. It is impractical, and it is dangerous! Are you someone who is more prudent about your money than your health? If so, reconsider and try to get a realistic, healthy perspective about your health. Your health is far more important than your finances. So allow yourself to take a new attitude, a healthy, sustainable attitude about how you are investing in your health. Most everyone would agree that wealth without health is meaningless.

Genetics and History

As described by Deborah Waterhouse in *Outsmarting the Female Fat Cell*, the human body has adapted to survive famine and other disaster periods. One adaptation has to do with fat enzyme activity. Fat enzymes determine how fat cells store and release energy. Whenever the brain detected signs of famine, such as inadequate food quantity and irregular eating periods, it sent a "message" to the fat enzymes that said, "Hey, it feels like a famine; start conserving to preserve." And with that message, lipogenic (fat storing enzymes) enzymes multiplied and surrounded the fat cells doing their best to preserve and ration the release of stored energy.

Once the famine was over and the body received more frequent/regular energy, the lipogenic enzymes could "relax" and allow the partner, lipolytic enzymes, to enter the scene and allow fat cells to release energy more quickly.

So what does this fat enzyme activity have to do with you now? Although at this time the threat of famine appears unlikely, your body still has the innate intelligence to respond to famine and to do its best to conserve to preserve. When you "diet" or restrict calories to levels below the amount needed to perform regular metabolic function, or when you are inconsistent about when you supply your body with calories, your brain senses and interprets that as "Uh oh, there may be a famine approaching." In response, the brain calls up the fat enzyme team to prepare for the possibility of a famine. This recruits even more of the lipogenic (fat storing enzymes) team, who in turn begin to control tightly the energy inside every fat cell. The result is that your body becomes efficient and well trained at producing fat enzymes, which keep the fat cell intact. The bottom line is that it makes it even harder for you to lose fat.

Slowed Metabolism

The irony about dieting is that the very goal dieters are striving for, to lose fat/weight, is further delayed by dieting. When the brain is deprived of its glucose and regular energy income, it slows down other metabolic events in the body too. Since it does not know when or how many calories it is going to be receiving, it wants to make the most of what it gets. The effect of this dieting restriction is that the dieter actually has trained the body to store calories better than before. That is why dieters get fatter from eating too few calories and nutrients.

Rebound Effect

The other reason to avoid dieting is because of the rebound effect it has upon the psyche. When we feel deprived of something, it seems to motivate us to want it even more. How many times have you been told you couldn't have something only to find your-self wanting it more than ever? Self-imposed deprivation is even more difficult to endure. Periods of self-imposed deprivation are often followed by periods of overindulgence. This rebound effect only demonstrates the importance of learning how to eat for nour-ishment and for nurture-ment. When you relax and allow yourself to eat and nourish your body machine, you can avoid the impending rebound effect.

Appealing Snacks

When was the last time you ate a bag of apples for a snack? Probably never; you would have become full from the water and fiber content. Plus, apples do not have the levels of salt that lure your taste buds to come back for more and more and more . . .

Nothing to Come Off of

Some very savvy marketing efforts are driving many Americans to go on "quick and easy" diets, high-protein diets, low-carbohydrate diets, appetite suppressants, spot reducing, and so on. These are medically and nutritionally unsound, potentially dangerous, ineffective for long-term practice, and expensive. Going on a diet implies coming off the diet. Dieting is emotionally draining and physiologically confusing. When you learn to eat for energy and health, there is nothing to come off of. When you practice eating with your energy and health in mind, you can lose fat and weight by eating well. And if you want to maintain or gain weight, you can do that too. The principles are the same; the details will vary. There will always be someone writing a new theory about how to lose weight. But the questions you need to ask yourself are, What effect will it have upon me (the risk) if I stay on it for too long, and What do I do when I come off of it? Learn how to eat for the rest of your life now; your energy and health will be all the better for it.

Overeating

Whereas dieting is one extreme of the eating spectrum, overeating is at the other end. Overeating is also an unhealthy practice that can usurp your energy and lead to heart disease. One of the biggest challenges for many Americans is eating in moderation. There are many reasons why we overeat. Frequently we do so because we get too hungry or because we aren't paying attention while we are eating. And even though most of us enjoy food and love to eat, we are not always attentive to our food experiences. This can make us feel unsatisfied and lead us toward eating more than if we were paying attention at the time.

Overeating and the Fullness Scale

Developing a rating system to describe how you feel *while you are eating* can be just the tool to help you become more aware of when you need to eat and when it is time to stop eating. The idea is to eat before you become very hungry or irritable and certainly before you become dizzy. And, to quit eating when you feel very comfortable. A fullness rating scale can help you to check in with yourself, to slow down, to focus attention to your food, and to enjoy your eating experience. If you truly love food and the eating experience, then slow down, savor the experience, really taste your food, and when you still feel comfortable, stop! This may help you realize that "more is not always better" and that sometimes "less is best"!

A Food Connoisseur

Do you love to eat but sometimes eat too much? If we borrow a concept from wine connoisseurs we can enhance our eating experience and also eliminate useless calories.

A wine connoisseur slowly sips and savors her wine and uses many senses to fully appreciate the wine experience. Once the wine is poured she lets it breathe in the wineglass, and as she does so, her anticipation grows. She studies the wine's appearance for body, clarity, and color in the reflection of the wineglass. Then *slowly*, she sips it. She then allows this "fruit of the grape" to rest in her mouth, feels it rolling along the tongue, awaking the taste buds along the way, making for a full tasting experience. Then the wine must be judged and rated. Your food is truly a blessing to be appreciated; it gives you energy for life. So try something new, like eating with the appreciation of a connoisseur, a food connoisseur.

In its attempt to define balanced nutrition, the U.S. government came out in the early 1990s with the Food Guide Pyramid and later with the new guidelines for food labeling of packaged foods. These tools can help you make more informed choices about the foods you eat and the nutritional effects to expect from them. Whereas the information listed is pretty straightforward, here are a few tips that will help you to use it all to your advantage.

Nutrition Facts: The "Confessional"—The Ingredients Listing

Set apart from the enticing packaging of the product, the nutrition facts panel can be thought of as the confessional section of the packaging, the place where the manufacturers have to get honest about everything that is in their products. Ingredients are listed in order by *weight*, from most to least, so you want to pay close attention to the first few ingredients listed. If the first few are fat, sugar, or various

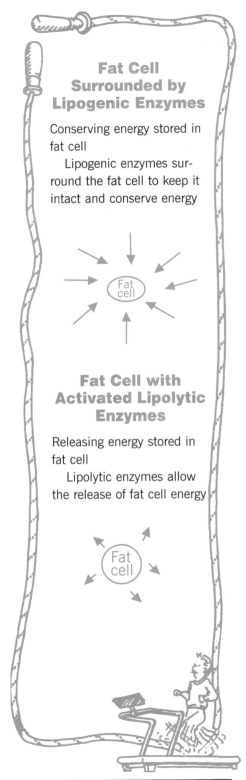

Fat Cell Surrounded by Lipogenic Enzymes

Conserving energy stored in fat cell

Lipogenic enzymes surround the fat cell to keep it intact and conserve energy

Fat cell

Fat Cell with Activated Lipolytic Enzymes

Releasing energy stored in fat cell

Lipolytic enzymes allow the release of fat cell energy

Fat cell

forms of fat or sugar, you know that those are the predominant ingredients. You can then decide if that food is consistent with how and what you want to be eating. For example, your breakfast cereal may have an ingredient listing like this: oat bran, unsulphured molasses, whole wheat flour, yellow corn flour, salt, baking soda, natural vitamin E, vitamin C. Such a listing tells you that by weight there is more oat bran than any other ingredient in this cereal. The second heaviest ingredient would be unsulphured molasses (a form of sugar), followed by the whole wheat flour, yellow corn flour, and so on.

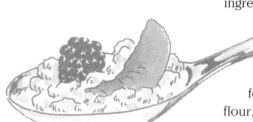

Judgment Time

Although the facts are presented on the label, you still have to sort through them and make your own judgments about how they fit into your nutrition goals. For instance, some ingredients do not necessarily weigh a lot, but they can make a powerful nutritional impact. Such is the case with some frozen dinner entrees marketed as "healthy." Let's pretend that you are on a sodium-restricted diet and that you need to consume no more than 1,000 milligrams of sodium daily. The ingredients listing may list salt and flavorings as the very last ingredients, and that may lead you to believe that there is not much sodium in the product. But all it really means is that the salt and flavorings weigh less than the other ingredients. It is very possible that the sodium value could be very high, in some cases equal to or more than the total daily value and certainly more than your 1,000-milligram total daily value.

In such a case you would next want to read the information on the nutrition facts panel about the amount of sodium in each serving of the product. If the total sodium count per serving was 1,200 milligrams, then you would know it was too high for your personal needs. And you can compare that number to the percent daily values based upon a 2,000-calorie diet (also on the nutrition facts panel). Once you have the information, you can make your own decision about whether you want to include that product in your diet.

Serving Size

As mentioned earlier, your "calorie bank" fluctuates based on the total calories consumed regardless of the type of calories consumed. Even foods that are "nonfat" or "low fat" can be high in calories, which can quickly inflate your total caloric intake. The serving size helps you to understand specifically how many calories you are consuming per food serving. Read these with a watchful eye, some serving sizes can be smaller than you might expect. For example, a label might read *Nutrition Facts: Serving Size ¾ Cup (32g), Servings per Container about 14.*

Calories and Calories from Fat

The label lists the *total number of calories* and *calories from fat.* But the label does not tell you the total percentage of fat for that item. Since you want approximately 25 percent of your total calories from fat (and no more than 10 percent of those from saturated fat), you need to divide the total calories by the calories from fat to arrive at a total percentage of fat for the product. This is a very important piece of information; it can have a healthy impact on your food selections. Do not shy away from it just because it involves some mathematical thinking on your part. If the math is too much effort for you, use a little handheld calculator or make an estimate.

Room for Improvement

It is hoped that in the future, the USDA will make the *fat* and *calories from fat* listings more meaningful and convenient by requiring manufacturers to "do the math" and print it on the food label. But until that day, the consumer will have to do the math. So think of it as an opportunity to practice your division/mathematical skills.

Here is the math: If a particular food has 120 calories, 15 of which are from fat, simply divide the calories from fat by the total calories (15 ÷ 120 = .125 or 12 percent).

% Daily Value

The figures listed below are the percentage of the total daily value of various nutrients based on a 2,000-calorie diet. Once you have estimated your daily recommended caloric intake (discussed earlier), you can adjust these numbers accordingly.

Approximations Will Work

If the math is too challenging, try estimating. If there are 100 calories and 15 are from fat, you could easily estimate the percentage of fat to be 15 percent. But since 120 is larger than 100, you can simply estimate that it is even less than 15 percent fat.

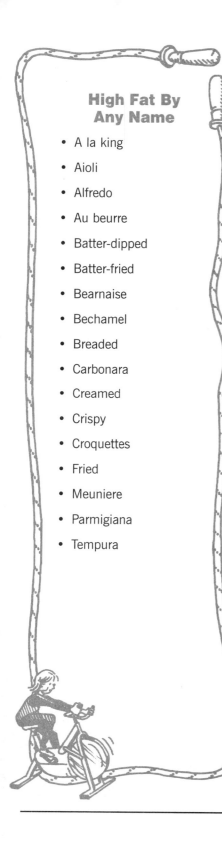

High Fat By Any Name

- A la king
- Aioli
- Alfredo
- Au beurre
- Batter-dipped
- Batter-fried
- Bearnaise
- Bechamel
- Breaded
- Carbonara
- Creamed
- Crispy
- Croquettes
- Fried
- Meuniere
- Parmigiana
- Tempura

AMOUNT PER SERVING	% DAILY VALUE
Total Fat 1g	2%
Sodium 0 mg	0%
Total Carbohydrate 47g	16%
Cholesterol	less than 300 mg per day
Sodium	less than 2400 mg per day
Total Carbohydrate	300 g
Dietary Fiber	25 g
Potassium	3750 mg per day

The percent of daily values is based on a 2,000 calorie diet. Your daily values may be higher or lower depending on your calorie needs.

Flavorful Fat Replacements

The plain fat truth is that because fat is plentiful, cheap, textured, and flavorful, most Americans eat too much of it. The consequences are proving to be costly to our energy, health, and pocketbooks.

The expression "it's to die for" is frequently used in jest to describe foods with exceptional flavor, but it seems to be coming true for many Americans who eat too much fat. If you eat more fat than is recommended, you can reduce the amount of fat you eat without sacrificing flavor. Fat is not the only food that tastes and feels good in the mouth. There are numerous ways to cut fat in your diet and add other tasty, textured, more nutritious alternatives. If you need to reduce the amount of fat that you eat, try some of these tips.

1. Use nonfat yogurt in place of sour cream. It has the creamy feel and tartness but substantially less fat. Use it on potatoes and in sauces, dressings, dips, and cakes.
2. For sautéing and sauces, use minimal amounts of butter/margarine and use low-sodium chicken or vegetable broths.
3. Remove the skin from poultry and you reduce the fat content by three-quarters and the calories by half. Eat the white meat (breast) instead of the dark meat (thigh). Skinless dark meat has twice as much fat as skinless white meat.

4. Read and interpret restaurant menus for more than what sounds good. Learn to recognize cooking styles that are synonymous with high fat and low fat.
5. To enhance flavor, use fresh minced garlic, onion, ginger, and fresh or dried herbs such as basil, cilantro, rosemary, tarragon, sage, and dill.
6. Use an oil spraying device (Misto brand is a good one) for recipes that call for oil, rather than dabbling oil.
7. Buy low-fat or nonfat dairy products.
8. Buy quality cheese; it's more expensive but generally more flavorful. Use it sparingly.
9. Avoid fried foods, and if you miss the crispiness, try overbaking or broiling until crispy (without charring).
10. When eating pizza, make it or order without cheese or with half the normal portion.
11. Use orange, pineapple, and apple juices to replace some of the oil in homemade salad dressings.

Good nutrition is not about perfection; it is about making choices that will enhance and improve your overall energy and health. Think of your daily nutrition choices as opportunities to cast yes votes for feeling good. But start gradually. Try just one new nutrition idea and give it a decent trial period (more than a few days). You will notice how much better you feel! And feeling good is the best motivation of all. Fueling your body at the right times, in the right amounts, and with the right types of food will boost your daily energy and overall health. And when good nutrition is combined with exercise as part of an overall fitness plan, you will experience many more "yes to life" days than "no, I don't have the energy for it" days.

Helpful Food Hints

For convenience . . .

1. Make large enough dinners at home and plan to eat leftovers for next day's lunch or dinner.
2. Take a cooler to work, or if you spend your workday in your car, keep it in the car with fruits and vegetables.

Rating Scale for Discriminating Calories

If overeating is something you would like to reduce in your life, try this rating tip. To reduce the amount of excess or "not worth it" calories that you consume, taste, judge, and rate *the very first taste* of any high fat, high caloric foods. Rate it on a scale of 1 to 10 (1 = not worth eating the calories and 10 = absolutely heavenly delicious). If the taste doesn't rate at least an "8" or better, be the discriminating connoisseur. Just say "no" to having any more of it. Save your calories for the 8s, 9s, and 10s; savor them slowly like the food connoisseur you are. You will have greater enjoyment and overall fewer calories from your eating experience.

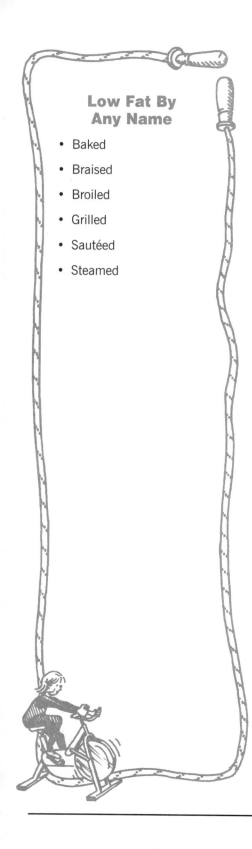

Low Fat By Any Name

- Baked
- Braised
- Broiled
- Grilled
- Sautéed
- Steamed

3. Make friends and eat lunch with others who care about their health.

4. When planning an extended motor trip, stock up ahead of time with fruit and vegetables.

5. At work, make a map or mental note of nearby food establishments with healthy alternatives.

6. If there are certain foods that you eat frequently, measure their serving size out once so that you can grasp the mental picture of that serving size. This will give you an idea of what you are eating.

7. One helpful practice for keeping your fat intake at or below 25 percent is to eat foods that are 25 percent or less fat and not to eat foods that are 25 percent or more fat. Or when you do eat higher fat foods, compensate for them by eating less fat at another meal that same day.

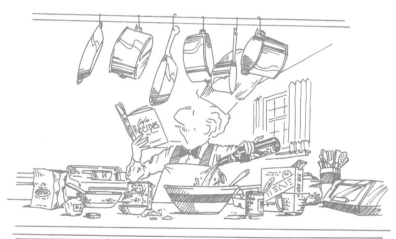

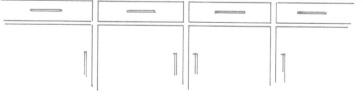

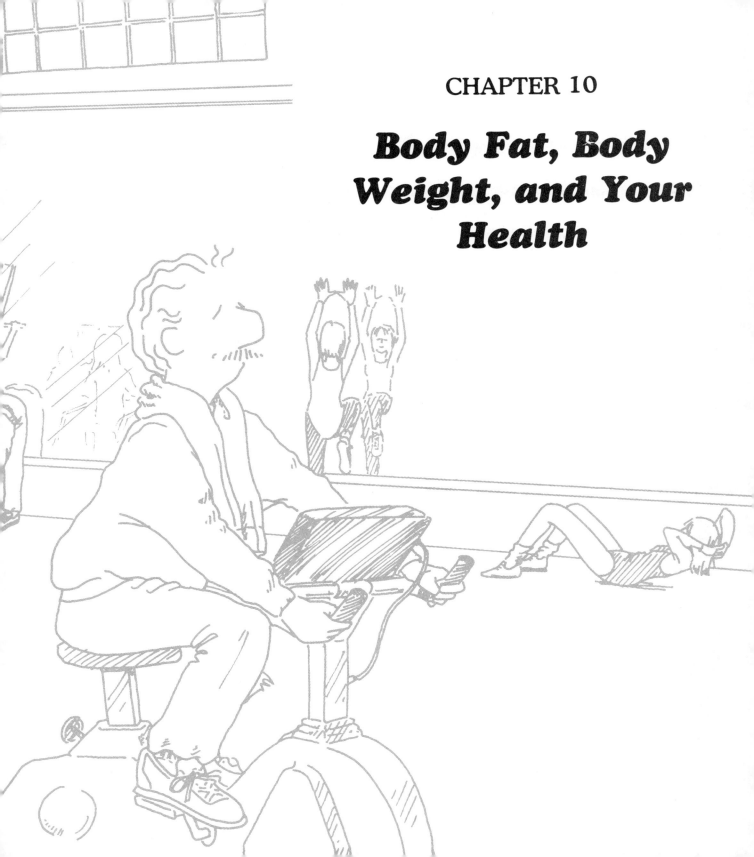

CHAPTER 10

Body Fat, Body Weight, and Your Health

Is maintaining a healthy weight difficult for you? Do you even know what a healthy weight is for you? Although you hear a lot about body weight when it comes to health, your body composition is of greater importance. The amount of lean mass (everything but fat) and body fat are collectively referred to as body composition. Healthy body composition is an important part of your health because serious conditions arise from having either too much or too little body fat, not necessarily from being overweight or underweight.

According to the Public Health Service in 1988, obesity is an excess of body fat at which health risks begin to increase. Obese individuals have a higher risk of cardiovascular disease, high cholesterol, high blood pressure, diabetes mellitus, obstructive pulmonary disease, osteoarthritis, and certain cancers.

Statistically speaking, obesity is a prevalent and rising problem in the American population. Approximately one of every three adults and one of every four children and adolescents are overweight, and those rates have accelerated over the past 15 years.

Too Little Body Fat

At the other end of the spectrum are persons with too little body fat. Those individuals tend to be malnourished, have a relatively higher risk of fluid-electrolyte imbalances, osteoporosis and osteopenia, bone fractures, muscle wasting, cardiac arrhythmias, and sudden death, edema, and renal and reproductive disorders.

A disease called anorexia nervosa is an eating disorder associated with extremely low body fat and excessive weight loss. If left untreated, it can cause permanent bodily damage and death. The disease is associated with psychological factors, so it is strongly suggested that persons with symptoms of anorexia nervosa seek medical and psychological help.

Body Weight Versus Body Composition

There are important distinctions between body weight and body composition and what they reflect about your health. Body weight is the force experienced by a body as a result of the earth's gravity and includes

Fat As Limiting

Overfat and overweight = extra effort. Find either a 10-pound weight or 2- to 5-pound weights and carry them around with you for 10 minutes. Did you notice how tiring it was to carry that extra weight with you?

all bodily tissues, organs, and fluids. Body composition refers to the type of matter that composes that weight. In terms of health, it's fat not weight that increases your risk for health problems. Body weight alone does not provide an accurate assessment of health.

Overweight, Underweight, and Overfat

A body hosting too much fat could be either overweight or underweight. The terms overweight and underweight have traditionally been used in reference to tables derived from skeletal frame size, height, and weight. But these are not accurate assessments of health. You can be heavy but lean and healthy, and you can be light, yet fat and unhealthy. For example, the fact that muscle weighs more than fat means that very fit, muscled individuals who have small amounts of fat would be considered overweight according to those tables. And individuals who are underweight according to height and weight tables could still have too much fat as a percentage of their body composition. When assessing your health, body composition, the amount of lean mass versus fat, is significantly more important than how much you weigh.

The conditions related to obesity and excess body fat are life-limiting and life-threatening. Seemingly simple physical acts such as walking up a flight of stairs, raking leaves, or playing with a child can be very laborious. Many obese people avoid activities that most would consider normal and basic experiences. What is causing all this obesity? For most Americans, the obesity problem is related to too much energy taken into the body and too little energy expended. Basically, eating more than is needed and not exercising as much as needed.

Impact of Too Much Fat

To better understand the impact of too much fat on your skeletal system, consider the following. Your skeleton is like the foundation of a building, your body mass like the contents of the building. The foundation is engineered to comfortably withstand relative amounts of weight and mass. When the weight and mass become too great for the foundation, the entire structure can suffer. Extra weight from fat, which is nonfunctional tissue, stresses the foundation. And even though muscle

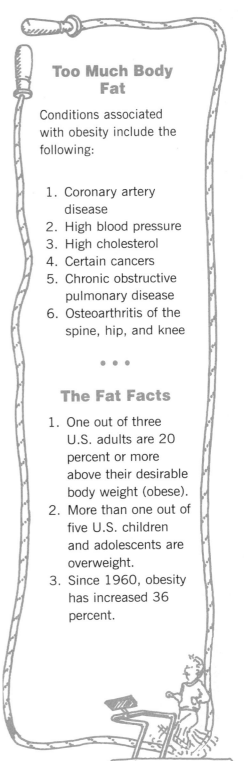

Too Much Body Fat

Conditions associated with obesity include the following:

1. Coronary artery disease
2. High blood pressure
3. High cholesterol
4. Certain cancers
5. Chronic obstructive pulmonary disease
6. Osteoarthritis of the spine, hip, and knee

• • •

The Fat Facts

1. One out of three U.S. adults are 20 percent or more above their desirable body weight (obese).
2. More than one out of five U.S. children and adolescents are overweight.
3. Since 1960, obesity has increased 36 percent.

tissue weighs more than fat, it is active tissue, which means it pulls its own weight (plus that of other tissues) and adds to the foundation with additional support. Skeletal and joint systems are susceptible to breakdowns when overloaded with fat weight. These breakdowns can appear in the form of osteoarthritis and other joint-related conditions.

Other uncomfortable and devastating physical disorders stemming from obesity are coronary artery disease, high blood pressure, and certain cancers. And then there are the psychological and emotional consequences of obesity, which often include depression, withdrawal, and poor self-concept.

Fat Standards

Percentage of body fat standards have been established to help guide men and women toward healthy levels. Note that men are considered obese when more than 25 percent of their body mass is fat and women when more than 32 percent of their body mass is fat.

There are many methods for measuring your body fat. A summary of them follows. First, let's make sure you understand how to use body composition measurements to your advantage.

Body Fat Measurements—Periodically and Consistently

Decide which method you will use and have your body fat assessed now. Use this result as your benchmark or starting point measurement. Then in approximately 6 months, after you have put into practice some of what you have learned about exercise and nutrition (from *The Everything Total Fitness Book*), have another body fat measurement *using the same method you used the first time*. Try to duplicate as many of the original assessment conditions as possible, such as same time of day/month, same administering personnel, same pre- or post-eating and hydration conditions, and so on. Duplicating as many of the assessment conditions as the original measurement eliminates some inconsistencies that can slightly affect your result.

Useful Tool

Knowing your percentage body fat is useful; it's best to have it measured as accurately as possible. But even if you are not measured by the most precise method, you can still gain valuable information. The relative result, whether your body fat increased, decreased, or stayed the same, is the important indicator that lets you know how you are progressing. If your goal is to lose body fat and after exercising consistently for 6 months your body fat has decreased, then you know you are on the right track. Periodic (6 months to a year) results about body fat are useful in helping you determine which components of your exercise and nutrition program are or are not working to help you meet your health goals.

Measuring Methods

There are many methods being used to determine your percentage of body fat. None are perfected, and each allows for some margin of error. For most individuals, the comparison of multiple and periodic measurements are more important and meaningful than the accuracy of the measurement.

Methods administered in laboratory and clinical settings are typically more accurate and expensive than those performed outside of a laboratory. These methods include hydrostatic or underwater weighing, DEXA (dual energy X-ray absorptiometry), and Plysmography (Bod Pod). Nonlaboratory methods administered by trained personnel may be accurate within 1 to 3 percent of laboratory methods and are typically not expensive. They include the skinfold caliper method and bioelectrical impedance analysis (BIA).

There are also anthropometric measurements. They are the simplest to administer and typically the least expensive. They cannot measure body fat, but they can measure other useful indicators of health status, including waist-to-hip circumference ratio and body mass index (discussed later in this chapter).

Here is a summary of each of the measurements to help you determine which you may prefer.

Body Fat Norms Based on Percentage of Body Weight That Is Fat

CLASSIFICATION	MALE	FEMALE*
Essential fat	3–5%	11–14%
Athletes	5–13%	12–22%
Fitness	12–18%	16–25%
Potential risk	19–24%	26–31%
Obese	25% +	32% +

*Females before puberty use the male scale. There is no health reason for increased body fat with age; thus the same standards are applied to all ages.

Adapted from G.E. Doxey, B. Fairbanks, T.H. Housh, G.O. Johnson, F. Datch, and T. Lohman, "Body composition roundtable: Part 1. Scientific considerations," *National Strength and Conditioning Association Journal* 9 (1987):14–15.

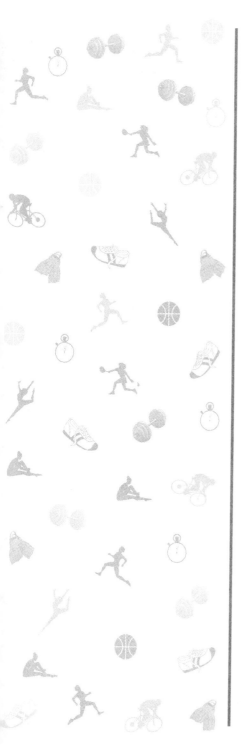

Hydrostatic Weighing

This is an underwater weighing technique that utilizes Archimedes' principle that an object's loss of weight under water is directly proportional to the volume of water displaced by the body volume.

Hydrostatic weighing requires individuals to sit with legs crossed in the weighing chair and to exhale as much air as possible from their lungs *before and while* totally submerging their body under water for just a few seconds. Mathematical corrections are made for residual air volume and the weighing equipment. Hydrostatic weighing is the most accurate, statistically reliable, and most widely used laboratory method for assessing body composition. However, for some individuals, it is too uncomfortable to exhale completely and remain under water even for a few seconds. In such cases, another method would be suggested.

Dual Energy X-ray Absorptiometry

DEXA is a relatively new method that estimates bone mineral, fat, and lean soft-tissue mass. The individual lies on a table while the X-ray scans the length of the body. There is a high degree of agreement between percentage of body fat obtained by hydrostatic weighting and by DEXA. As compared to other methods, it is highly reliable and more expensive.

Plysmography—Air Displacement Plethysmograph (Bod Pod)

The Bod Pod is a method that requires the individual to sit inside an oxygenated capsule. It works on the same principle as that of hydrostatic weighing except that the medium used with the Bod Pod is air displacement rather than water displacement.

Skinfold Caliper

This method is a common, less-expensive method that requires individuals to have their skin slightly pulled and pinched by the technician's hand and caliper. Skinfold method indirectly measures the thickness of subcutaneous adipose tissue. Certain general assumptions must be made in order to calculate the results. Assumptions such as age, gender, and population subgroup affect the validity of this method. Skinfold caliper results can be very useful as relative values (whether you have lost, gained, or stayed the same) when measured in similar conditions.

Bioelectrical Impedance Analysis

BIA is a fast, noninvasive, and relatively inexpensive method that requires the individual to be in contact with electrodes applied to the individual's hand, wrist, foot and/or ankle. A low-level electrical current is passed through the individual's body, and the impedance or opposition to the flow of current is measured with a BIA analyzer. BIA is extremely sensitive to factors such as the individual's food and fluid intake, exercise, medication, and bladder fullness. Consumer methods have been developed, such as handheld and scale-style devices. BIA is a reliable technique, which means the results are consistent in the same person. However, the results are not as valid or accurate as compared to the standard criterion technique (hydrostatic weighing). Persons with low-fat measurements in hydrostatic weighing show high measures in BIA and vice versa.

From Percentage of Fat to Weight in Pounds

Once you know your percentage of body fat, you can calculate a desirable body weight based on the present lean body weight. With the percentage of body fat in hand, you can then make judgments about whether you are overfat versus overweight or both.

Here is an example of how to calculate desirable weight and the amount of weight one would need to lose: Pretend that you are a 150-pound woman with 30 percent body fat and you want to sensibly lose 5 percent body fat by exercising and improving your nutritional intake. Based upon your goal of losing 5% body fat, what is your new desirable body weight? And how much weight would you need to lose to attain that 5 percent reduction goal?

Step 1. From your current percentage body fat (30%), calculate both fat and lean weight (pounds).

A. .30 x 150 lbs. = 45 lbs. of fat weight
B. .70 x 150 lbs. = 105 lbs. of lean weight*

Step 2. Enter current body weight: 150 lbs.

Step 3. Enter current percentage body fat: 30%

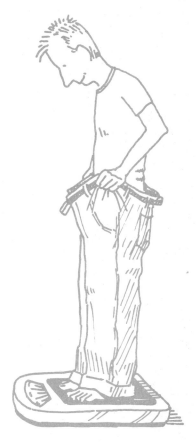

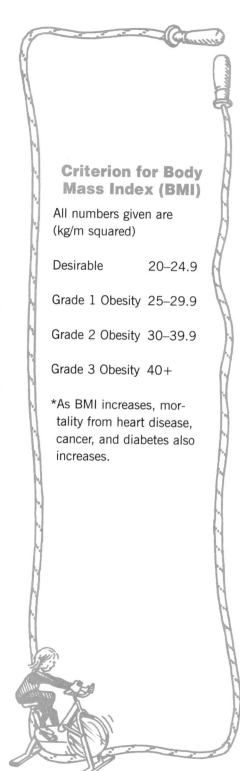

Step 4. Enter fat weight (1A above) or current body weight x % fat weight: 45 lbs.

Step 5. Calculate lean body weight* (1B above) or current body weight minus fat weight: 105 lbs.

Step 6. Select goal body fat percentage: 25%

Step 7. To calculate goal body weight and weight change, plug in the figures from above to the formula below.

Formula:
$$\text{Desirable weight} = \frac{\text{Lean body weight}}{1.0 - \text{Goal body fat \% in decimal form}}$$

Formula:
$$\text{Desirable weight} = \frac{\text{Lean body weight (\# 4 above)} = 105 \text{ lbs.}}{1 - \text{Goal body fat \%} = 1 - .25}$$

Convert % body fat to decimal i.e. 25% = .25
25/100 = .25
1 – .25 = .75

Formula:
$$\frac{\text{Lean body weight} = 105}{.75} = 140 \text{ lbs.}$$

Body Mass Index

Body mass index (BMI) and waist-to-hip circumference ratio are used to identify individuals at risk for disease. BMI is a rough estimate of total body fatness but is not accurately used to estimate body composition. The BMI is the ratio of body weight in kilograms to height squared in meters.

To figure your BMI, use the following formula:

Step 1. Convert body weight in pounds to kilograms by dividing your weight in pounds by 2.2.

Step 2. Convert height in inches to centimeters by multiplying total inches by 2.54. Then convert centimeters to meters, by dividing by 100.

Step 3. Square your height in meters (multiply the number by itself).

Step 4. Divide weight in kilograms by the height squared.

Waist-to-Hip Circumference Ratio

The **waist-to-hip circumference ratio** is an index of body fat distribution and is used to determine the degree of risk for cardiovascular disease, Type II diabetes, and high blood pressure. Excess fat in the abdominal area is associated with these diseases.

To determine your risk, first take your waist and hip measurements. Use a flexible but nonelastic tape measure. Measurements are best made on bare skin. Pull and hold the tape snugly around the body part but not tightly enough to indent or compress the skin. A waist measurement is taken at the level of the narrowest part of the torso. A hip measurement is taken at the maximum circumference of the hips/buttocks.

Next calculate the waist-to-hip circumference ratio by dividing the waist circumference (in centimeters) by the hip circumference (in centimeters). This will tell you the ratio. Find your ratio as applies to your age and gender on the waist-to-hip ratio chart on p. 231.

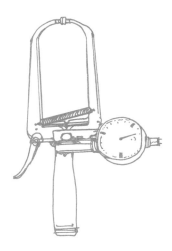

Skinfold Caliper
Skinfold caliper method for measuring body composition. A common, convenient, and affordable method for measuring body composition. A trained technician pinches designated areas on the body and uses the calipers to measure the thickness of subcutaneous adipose tissue (fat).

Weight Management
Body Business

If you decided to start a small business, what would you need to get it going? Aside from proper planning and marketing, you would need the lifeblood of business—money. First you would need money to pay for opening expenses, that is, *before* you opened. You would need money to pay for overhead expenses such as an office, storefront, Web site, post office box, and telephone. You would need money to pay for insurance, taxes, inventory, and employee wages. To be successful in business, you need to spend/invest money to get started, and then you would need to reinvest money in the business to keep it up to date and competitive. It takes money to make money.

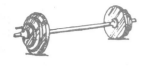
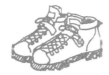
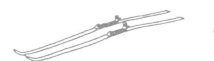

Waist-to-Hip Ratio Chart

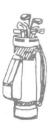

	Age	Low	Moderate	High	Very High
			RISK		
Men	20–29	<0.83	0.83–0.88	0.89–0.94	>0.94
	30–39	<0.84	0.84–0.91	0.92–0.96	>0.96
	40–49	<0.88	0.88–0.95	0.96–1.00	>1.00
	50–59	<0.90	0.90–0.96	0.97–1.02	>1.02
	60–69	<0.91	0.91–0.98	0.99–1.03	>1.03
Women					
	20–29	<0.71	0.71–0.77	0.78–0.82	>0.82
	30–39	<0.72	0.72–0.78	0.79–0.84	>0.84
	40–49	<0.73	0.73–0.79	0.80–0.87	>0.87
	50–59	<0.74	0.74–0.81	0.82–0.88	>0.88
	60–69	<0.76	0.76–0.83	0.84–0.90	>0.90

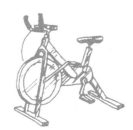

Adapted from Bray and Gray, "Obesity: Part I. Pathogenesis." *Western Journal of Medicine* 149 (1988): 432.

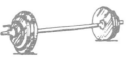
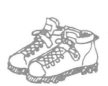

How often have you heard and read about businesses that failed because they were "undercapitalized"? How many failed because they did not invest enough in areas that would keep them competitive, by paying better wages or buying newer equipment? What does this have to do with weight and body composition management? Eating and exercising are the income and expense of weight management. And calories are to your body what money is to business—the life force. You have to spend money to make money, and you have to take in calories to expend calories. When you balance the income and expense of your calories, you are investing wisely in the "business" of calorie expenditure. By "investing," you can successfully manage the weight component of your health.

A Plan—Putting Exercise and Nutrition Together

How can you put a healthy eating and exercise plan together to achieve and maintain healthy body weight and composition goals? Here is an example that you can adapt to your specific situation. This example (utilizing what you have learned from previous chapters) will show you how to eat sensibly, moderately, and comfortably and help you to progressively and steadily achieve your goals.

Use steps 1 and 3 of "Estimating Total Calories, page 201, to establish how many calories you need. Do not include the calories for your purposeful exercise yet. Next, use the table (page 202) on Calories Burned During Exercise to estimate how many calories you expend through exercise.

Recall that 1 pound equals 3,500 calories. Then, 10 pounds equal 35,000 calories. Your goal is to create a minor caloric deficit but supply yourself with enough energy to perform your regular activities and to exercise several days each week. A slight deficit allows you to continue eating without feeling deprived but to still make a difference in changing your body composition as desired. Note the significant effect exercise has on caloric expenditure. Such a plan may look like the one on the next page:

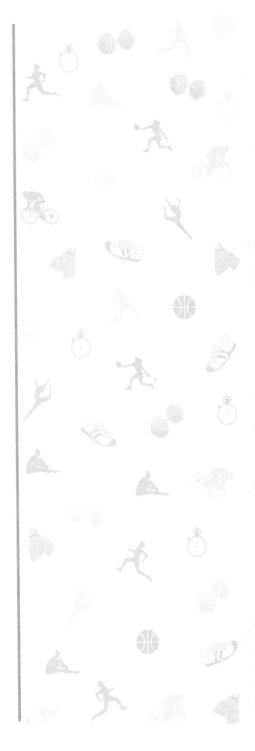

	SUN	MON	TUE	WED	THURS	FRI	SAT	WEEKLY TOTAL
Metabolic need in calories	2000	2000	2000	2000	2000	2000	2000	14,000 calories
Energy/ caloric intake	2000	1800	1800	1800	1800	1800	2000	13,000 calories
Net caloric effect from food	0	-200	-200	-200	-200	-200	0	-1,000 calories
Exercise caloric expenditure	-250	rest day	-250	-250	-250	rest day	-250	-1,250 calories
Daily net caloric expenditure	-250	-200	-450	-450	-450	-200	-250	-2,250 calories

Again, pretend you are the 150-pound woman who wanted to lose 5 percent body fat, the equivalent of 10 pounds. Following this plan, you would meet your ultimate goal in 15.5 weeks. Initially that may sound like a long time, but consider this: It probably took you longer than that to gain it. Now you have not only stopped the increase, you are reversing that unhealthy direction and reaping the numerous improvements along the way. You will have increased energy, you will be exercising and getting more physically fit, and you will be losing body fat and making some nutritional improvements. Most noticeably, you will feel better! Once your weight and fat loss goals are met, you can maintain your fitness and healthy weight/composition by adjusting the caloric intake slightly higher. You will want to maintain exercise as a healthy fixture in your life. Notice that unlike dieting, there is nothing to "come off of."

Perspective

Certainly every best plan and intention occasionally has to yield to the surprises of daily life. If you miss a day or two of exercise when you planned for it or took in more calories than you expected, do not worry. Keep your overall goal in mind, look upon the progress that you have made, and pick up where you left off.

Review your plan weekly:

Energy need =	14,000 cals
Energy intake =	13,000 cals
Net caloric effect	-1,000 cals deficit through nutrition
Exercise expenditure	-1250 cals
Total deficit	-1,000 cals through eating/nutrition
Created	-1,250 cals through exercise
Grand total	-2,250 calorie deficit
	(2,250 = 64% or 2/3 of I lb. in 1 week).

Week 1	-2,250
Week 2	-2,250
Week 3	-2,250
Week 4	-2,250 (after 4 weeks, 2.57 lbs.)
Week 5	-2,250 etc.
Week 10	-2,250 (after 10 weeks, 6.43 lbs.)
Week 15	-2,250 (after 15½ weeks, 10 lbs.)

If you maintain this plan for 4 weeks, you will burn 2.5 pounds worth of calories, lose fat, gain muscle, increase your metabolism, and develop good lifelong habits of healthy eating and exercise.

Your Weight and the Scale

As discussed previously, body weight alone is a poor indicator of your health. But the bathroom scale is very common in American households, and many individuals habitually weigh themselves. If you are someone who habitually weighs yourself, consider the following:

"Scale Back"

Unlike body weight, where changes are seen frequently, real changes in body composition (from less fat to more muscle) take time, definitely more than a few days. And they show up first in places other than on your bathroom scale. Muscle weighs more than fat, so the

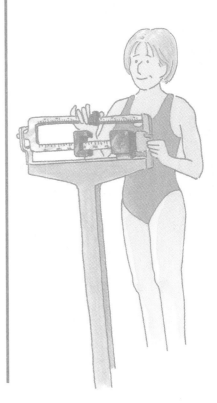

weight scale will not reflect this healthy change. Plus, body weight can fluctuate daily in response to many factors, including hormonal and fluid changes. Because muscle takes up less space than fat, the changes you may notice are that you feel stronger and more energetic and/or that your clothes fit a bit looser than before. Yet neither of these healthy changes are displayed on the bathroom scale. A traditional weight scale cannot distinguish between high energy, body fat, or muscle. Be attentive to the other changes and scale back the emphasis you have been giving to your scale. It tells a one-sided story.

You Are More Than Your Weight

Many individuals experience emotional yo-yoing as a result of what their scales tell them they weigh. If they read the number they desire, they are happy, and if not, they are disappointed. If your mood is determined by the reading on your weight scale, you could benefit from the following advice: **Scale back the scale!** If you must weigh yourself, do so only periodically. If you want to be happy, go live your life and make a plan about how to include exercise and moderate nutritious eating as a part of your quality assurance plan. But do not let a scale dictate how you feel or let it be your measure of happiness or sadness for the day. You are so much more than what you weigh.

Conclusion

Managing your body composition and weight are important health issues that affect the quality and quantity of your life. You have the ability to improve and maintain them. Get your body fat tested. Determine your long-term and short-term goals. Make a plan about how to gradually achieve them. Focus your attention on your energy and how you feel throughout your days. Start and keep exercising regularly. This is how to manage the body weight and body composition component of your health.

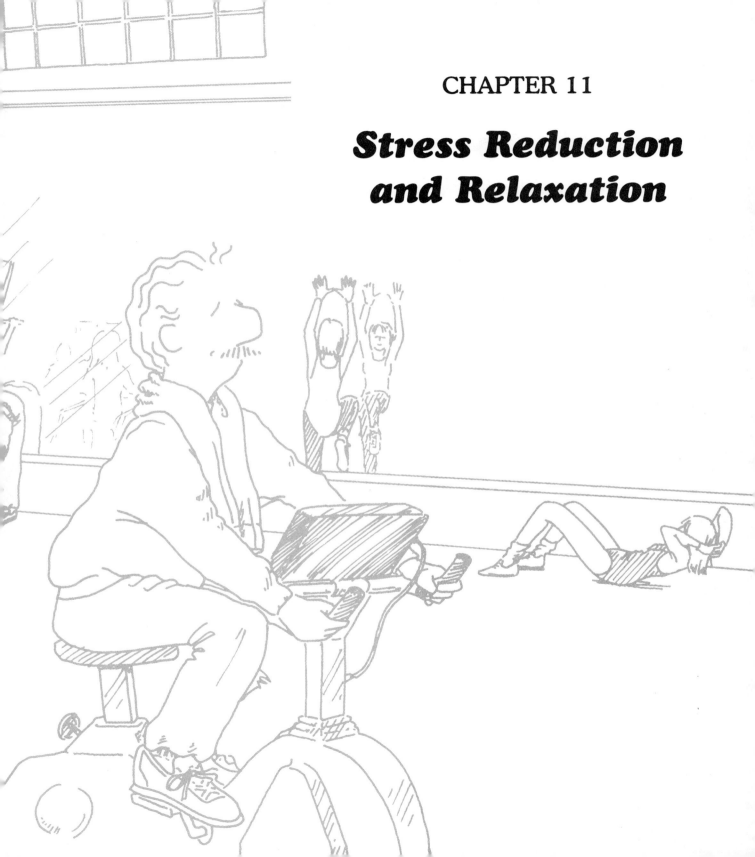

CHAPTER 11

Stress Reduction and Relaxation

Stress Detectors

1. Irritability
2. Shallow breathing
3. Jumpiness/inability to sit still
4. Muscular tension
5. Intestinal abnormality
6. Cold extremities
7. Weakened voice
8. Headache
9. Mindless eating
10. Loss of appetite

Stress is pressure, tension, or demand on physical or mental energy. "Hurry up you're late!" "Your flight has been cancelled." "Your test results show . . . " "I need that report in 5 minutes!" "The estimate is $4,000." "It won't be ready until . . . " Would any of these bring about stress for you? Even persons who exercise regularly and eat appropriately can succumb to the deleterious effects of uncontrolled chronic stress. Taking care of yourself and being fit includes managing stress in your life.

Scientific Proof

In 1956 scientist Hans Selye demonstrated that when mice were repeatedly stressed (they were dropped), they developed ulcers. When those same mice were stroked and hugged, their ulcers reversed. That finding ignited interest and led the way for more studies about the effects of stress. Dr. Tiffany Fields at the University of Miami studied the effects of massage upon premature babies. Those who were massaged gained weight more quickly and were happier, calmer, and healthier than those who were not. These two findings suggest that perceived stress has negative effects on the body but can be reversed if treated. Hiding from life and stress is not the solution; learning how to cope with it is.

Stress Reaction

When your body is stressed, it reacts by prioritizing and shutting down less important bodily functions (reproduction is one) to focus on quickly remedying the situation. This response is best known as the "fight or flight" syndrome. Survival responses to stress include increased heart rate, respiration, blood pressure, body temperature, blood sugar levels, blood flow to muscles, sweating, and muscular tension, and decreased rate of digestion. Once the stress is alleviated, your body's physiology returns to its normal levels of function.

These lifesaving responses were designed for short-term survival, not for long-term living. When these intense responses continue over time, they can be harmful to your health. What can you do about stress in your life? As Hans Selye wrote, "Life is stress. Stress is life." Your best choice is to learn and practice coping skills that will help you adapt to the stress in your life.

It is the inability to cope with stress that makes it a secondary risk factor for coronary heart disease and a powerfully negative influence on other areas of health. Many of the stress-related conditions today are, as stress physiology expert Dr. Pamela Peeke says, a result of "uncontrolled, unrelenting stress."

Control Concept

Common among stressful situations is the feeling of being out of control. The idea of gaining control of your life is important in coping with stress. Getting in control of your health through exercise and nutrition can be stress relieving. Letting go of unhealthy behaviors and habits, becoming more competent in a subject, setting and asserting your limits, and learning how to relax are ways to reduce stress in your life.

Hormone to the Rescue

A great strategy for relieving the effects of stress are to produce endorphins. Endorphins are the "feel good" hormone you commonly hear associated with endurance athletics. There are many ways to produce endorphins, many of which begin with relaxing your mind.

Learning How to Relax

Activities that give your mind a rest from negative stress can help you relax. Activities often associated with relieving stress include sports, games, yoga, tai chi, meditation, guided progressive relaxation, and sleep. During stressful times, we need to insert healthy relaxing corrections. Often we are quick to medicate stress with alcohol and/or drugs, which can lead to and exacerbate already stressful situations. Try some healthy stress relievers instead.

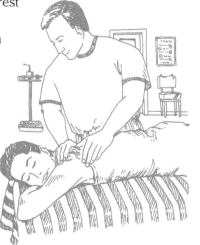

Stress Is Not Aerobic

"When I am stressed at my workstation, my heart rate is higher. Isn't that good? Doesn't that mean I am aerobic?" You are aerobic when major muscle groups are performing work that cause an increase in the use of oxygen, which causes heart rate to increase. When your heart rate increases in response to a nonexercising stressful situation, it is because of a constriction of blood vessels, which builds pressure in the cardiovascular system causing the heart rate to increase. No, it is not good, and no, you are not aerobic.

Stress Relieving Activities

Exercise
Listening to music
Prayer
Meditation
Watching a movie
Reading
Talking with a friend
Laughing
Crying
Sports/games
Family time
Singing
Nature
Writing
Guided progressive
    relaxation
Massage
Sleeping
Yoga
Tai chi

Stress Detector

Does being late or unprepared for important events make you stressed? Does being in traffic or missing connecting airplane flights make you stressed? When things do not go your way, how do you react? What do you notice about yourself when you become stressed? Does being stressed improve the situation? What effect does your behavior have on the situation? Does it make others want to be around you, to help you, or to avoid you?

How many stress detectors do you experience? Those listed in the chart are some, but certainly not all, of the reactions your body can have to stress. You can use them to your advantage to turn the situation around. The next time you notice stress symptoms flaring up in your body, use them as "stress detectors," and let them be a reminder for you to put in healthy stress corrections. Identify the situations that make you stressed, then think about how you can respond differently.

Laughter Heals

Studies show that endorphins are released from laughing and other sources of enjoyment and have a positive effect upon the body. In *Anatomy of an Illness*, Norman Cousins wrote how laughter helped him deal with the stress of a serious illness. He watched old, funny movies that made him happy and affected him in a positive way. His way of dealing with a stressful situation is a model for many. Laughter is a powerful tool in reducing stressful situations; it is also a healing medium. Include laughter as part of your daily diet, and while you are at it, share it with others (see Chapter 5 for laughing exercises).

Are you Z Z Z Z Z Z Z ing? Now Wake Up and Read This

Sleep is the condition of body and mind that normally recurs for several hours every night. During sleep, the nervous system is inactive, the eyes are closed, the postural muscles are relaxed, and consciousness is practically suspended. Sleep is one of the most taken-for-granted components of health and, for many, is regarded as a luxury rather than a necessity. But the truth is that sleep is vital to your health. While you are asleep, your body is engaged in its highest level of immune func-

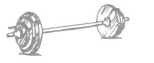
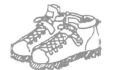
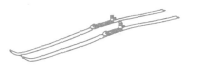

"Is This Worth It?" In-the-Moment Stress Reduction

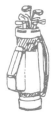

A man with a heart condition complained that following phone calls from one of his important business associates, he felt stressed. But he could not figure out how to better handle the situation. It was suggested that he become more aware of his body's stressful reactions to the situation *in the moment* when they occurred. He decided that he would wear his heart rate monitor. The next time this associate called, he became stressed. He watched his resting heart rate surge from 80 beats per minute to 110 beats per minute—a 30-beats-per-minute increase! He also noticed that he was clenching his fist and tightening his jaw. Being aware of his response to this situation helped him to understand that he needed to get better control of the situation.

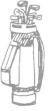

Are you interested in improving your response to stress? (Awareness is the first step.) If so, wear your heart rate monitor in the environment where your stressful situation appears. When that stressful moment

happens, look at your heart rate monitor and see whether your heart rate is elevated. Notice any other bodily responses you may be experiencing. Then, use the following tips to instantly de-stress.

1. Focus on your breath. Inhale and exhale fully and slowly.
2. Take a time-out. Close your eyes. Walk away from the situation for a moment.
3. Cry, release your tension, and then move on to the solution.
4. Focus on the solution rather than the problem.
5. Think of something funny. Find some humor in the current situation.
6. Keep it in perspective. Nearby photographs of your loved ones can remind you that life is for loving and that you will get through the situation.
7. Pray and meditate.
8. Write about it; talk about it.

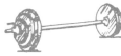
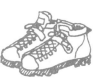
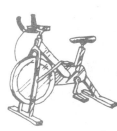

tions and is recovering from stress. Sleep nourishes the body by allowing it to relax and unwind. When you continuously sleep less than you need, you compromise your immune system by depriving your body of the time and opportunity to heal itself. During stressful, overly busy times, we often sacrifice our sleep, yet those are the times when we need it the most. If that is the case for you, wake up and start making sleep a priority in your day. Sleep is not a luxury; it is an important component of your health.

How Much Sleep?

Sleep needs vary from person to person, but the general requirement is 5 to 9 hours per day/night, and most people have a sense of the number of hours that makes them feel refreshed. Sleep can have very powerful effects upon your mood and health. When you are rested, you are less irritable and more energetic. Even persons who exercise appropriately and eat nutritiously can feel poorly if they do not get enough sleep. If you turn back to Chapter 2 and review the components of a complete exercise, you will see that "rest" is one of the four. If you pride yourself on being fit and healthy but do not regularly get enough sleep, start including sleep as another of the important elements of your health and fitness that needs attention.

Sleep Record

A helpful exercise for increasing your awareness about sleep is to record on your workout calendar the number of hours of sleep for each day. This will help you develop awareness about your sleep. You may also see some relationships or patterns that can help you plan for sleep more successfully.

Sample Sleep Record

	SUN	MON	TUE	WED	THU	FRI	SAT
sleep	9 hours	6 hours	7 hours	6 hours	7 hours	6 hours	9 hours

From this sleep pattern, it appears that the individual doesn't get enough sleep during the week and tries to make up for it on the weekend.

Conclusion

Stress can be a positive influence and a motivating factor in your life. And stress can be a devastating experience never to be forgotten. Chronic stress that is considered uncontrolled and unrelenting can overwhelm even the fittest of folk. Just as you cannot out-exercise poor nutrition, you cannot out-exercise chronic stress. Gain control over the stress in your life by identifying your stressors, putting in healthy corrections, performing endorphin-secreting activities, and getting plenty of sleep. Everyone experiences stress. Learning how to adapt and respond to it will make life happier and healthier for you and your loved ones.

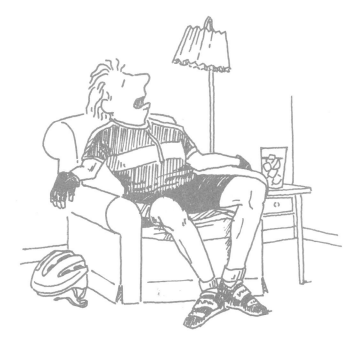

Sleep Insurance: An Alarm for Bedtime

Do you have a wake-up time? Just as you decide approximately what time you want to awaken most days, setting a bedtime goal can be useful too. Give yourself a designated bedtime, enough to satisfy your body's needs, and observe it. To ensure that you "call it a night before it is too late," set your alarm to remind you it is time to go to sleep and hang out your "closed" sign for the day. A bedtime goal will help you get the sleep you need.

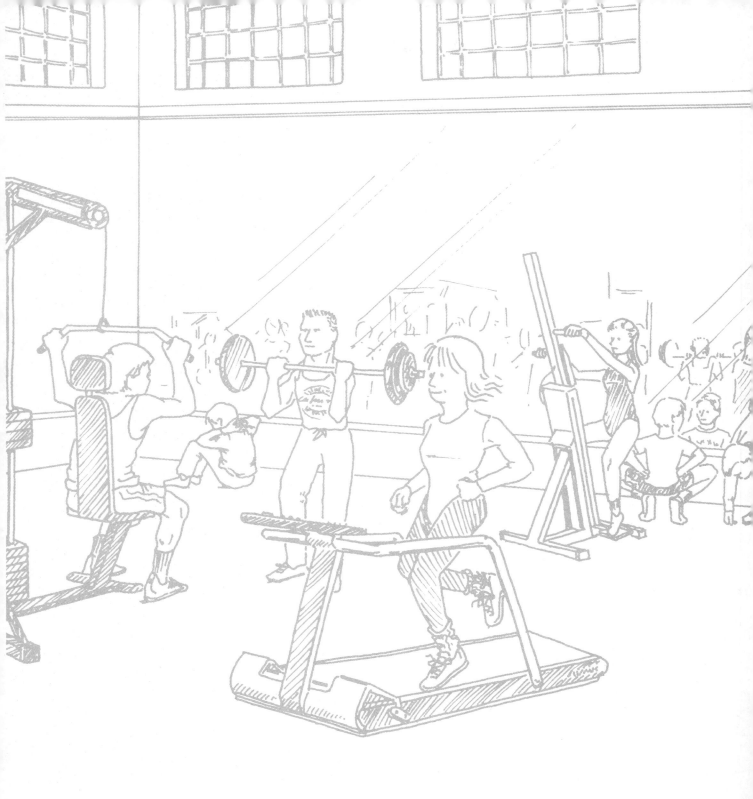

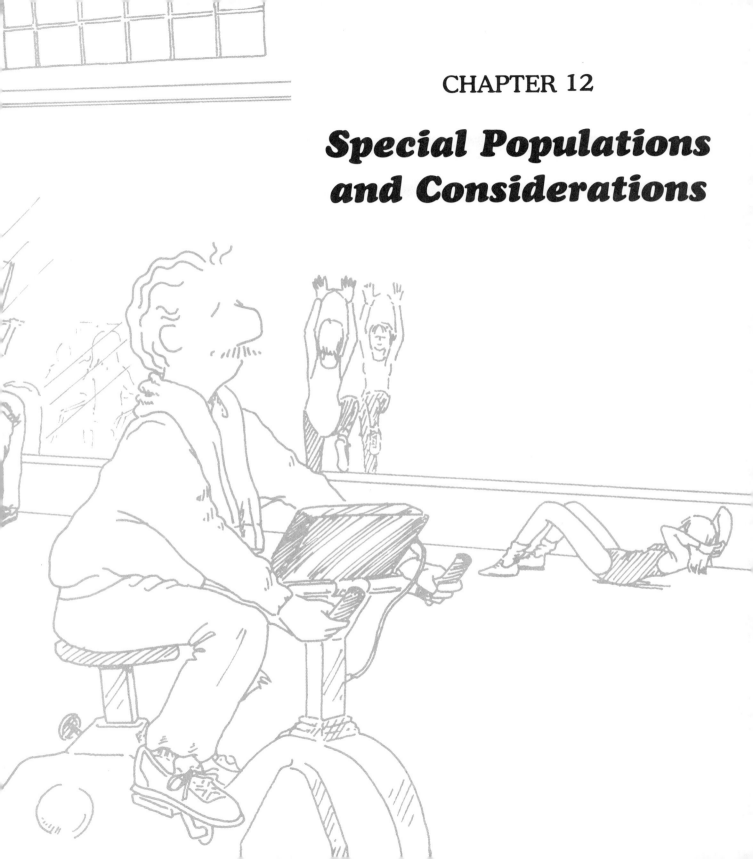

CHAPTER 12

Special Populations and Considerations

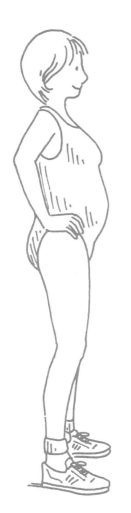

This chapter concerns special populations: prenatal and postnatal women, children, and older adults. There are sections on diabetes and hypertension (high blood pressure). In addition, it includes information about exercise and travel, as well as exercise and environmental factors. It is most likely that at some point in your exercising life, you will encounter one or more of these conditions. When you do, apply the following guidelines and recommendations to keep healthy and feeling your best.

Fitness for Prenatal Women

It is beginning to sound like exercise is a panacea for most conditions . . . well, if not a cure-all, it certainly seems to improve most conditions, including pregnancy. According to the American College of Obstetricians and Gynecologists (ACOG), "regular exercise improves a woman's physical and mental health at a time when she may feel tired, overweight, and moody . . . exercising and being fit help a woman during pregnancy and may improve her ability to cope with the pain of labor . . . exercise will also make it easier for a woman to get back in shape after the baby is born." Those certainly are motivating reasons to exercise while pregnant!

With more prenatal (before the birth) and postnatal (after the birth) women exercising, we continue to learn about the effects of exercise. In 1994, the ACOG revised its guidelines for exercise, during pregnancy and postpartum. One prior guideline *that has been dropped* concerned exercising at a limited heart rate. The guideline has been revised to reflect the more important issue of women exercising at a level that feels moderate and comfortable.

Approval First

It is important to consult with a physician or health care provider before beginning or continuing an exercise program and to get approval to do so. For most women, exercise during pregnancy is safe and recommended, but in some cases, it is not. Even in cases of gestational diabetes, exercise is helpful, but it is still essential to seek approval first. If the physician gives the go-ahead to start a fitness program, a woman should monitor herself during exercise for any changes that may be warning signs of a problem.

Moderate exercise (for women with a noncompromised pregnancy) does not appear to interfere with oxygen delivery to the fetus, and the heart rate response of the fetus shows no significant, long-term signs of distress. Catherine Cram, an exercise physiologist who specializes in prenatal and postnatal fitness, offers the following advice for a safe and effective prenatal exercise program:

1. Reassess fitness goals.
2. Listen to the body and respond.
3. Consider a supervised prenatal exercise class with a qualified instructor.

Even if a woman regularly exercised before becoming pregnant, she may not be able to continue the same activities at the same intensity as before. Reassess the fitness goals and use the body's signals to set exercise limits. This is not the time to be striving for personal records in frequency, intensity, or time. If a woman has not exercised regularly before becoming pregnant, she is advised to learn to listen to her body and become familiar with what feels normal. This "body awareness" will be helpful both during and after pregnancy.

Prenatal Exercise Class

For some women, taking part in a supervised exercise class can provide assurance and support. Before enrolling in any prenatal program, find out whether the program meets the following criteria:

- The instructor has a fitness or health-related degree and experience or training in obstetrics.
- The instructor is competent to answer fitness- and pregnancy-related questions.
- The instructor incorporates ACOG guidelines and knows warning signs and symptoms with regard to pregnancy.
- A health history and physician's consent are required before joining the class.
- There is an established procedure for management of injuries or emergencies.
- The facility is appropriate for prenatal exercise—it has a supportive floor, mats, and nearby rest rooms, and the exercise room is kept cool.

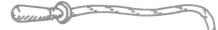

Warning Signs and Symptoms for Prenatal Women

Stop exercising and call the doctor if these symptoms are present:

- Absent fetal movement
- Severe pain
- Difficulty walking
- Dizziness, faintness, or extreme shortness of breath
- Tachycardia
- Pubic pain
- Uterine contractions
- Vaginal bleeding or fluid loss

Pregnancy and Exercise

The following are contraindicated prenatal activities (NO!):

Sauna
Steam room
Hot tubs
Scuba diving
Waterskiing,

The following activities are not advised*:

High altitude or snow
　sports
Ice or in-line skating
Gymnastics
Horseback riding
Step aerobics

*Check with a physician
first.

- The safety and comfort of the participants are never sacrificed.
- The class accommodates varying levels of fitness
- The class provides frequent breaks to check level of exertion and to hydrate.
- The class includes a warm-up, aerobic exercise, strength and flexibility exercises, and a cool-down.
- The class includes pregnancy-specific needs such as low back flexibility and pelvic floor exercises.

Mode of Exercise

Aside from the contraindicated activities listed in the chart, a woman may use comfort to determine the form of exercise. If the activity becomes uncomfortable, she should either find a way to make it comfortable or find another activity.

The Pelvic Floor Muscles

A woman's pelvic floor muscles play an important role during pregnancy and throughout life. They maintain proper alignment of the spine and support the pelvic organs. Normally the pelvic floor muscles should be supportive and span in an upright curve from the pubic bone to the tailbone. Weakness in this area results in sagging and loss of support. Many of the problems associated with pregnancy that affect the pelvic area (uterine prolapse, urinary incontinence, bowel dysfunction, low back and pelvic pain) are actually the result of poor pelvic and abdominal strength. Pelvic floor muscle exercises are just the remedy and are simple to do.

Overheating

Keep cool by drinking cool fluids before, during, and after exercise. Use air conditioning or a fan to keep cool. Avoid brisk exercise in hot, humid weather or when sick with a fever. Pregnant women should avoid activities that cause an overheating effect. Prenatal and postnatal specialist Catherine Cram adds, "If a woman exercises in a cool dry environment and hydrates well she runs very little risk of overheating."

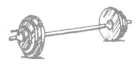
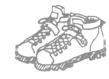
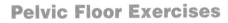

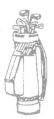
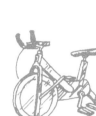

Pelvic Floor Exercises

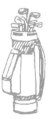

First it is important to locate the correct muscles. Here are two methods:

- Method 1: Movement of the pelvic floor muscles can be felt by coughing while placing the finger tips on the area that surrounds the urethra, vagina, and anus. Upon coughing, the muscles push downward toward the fingertips.
- Method 2: The muscles that contract when attempting to stop the flow of urine are the pelvic floor muscles. Use this method only to learn how to isolate the muscle group; repeated stopping and starting of urine flow may cause urinary tract infections.

And here are the exercises:

- Exercise 1: Contract the muscles and hold for 10 seconds.
- Exercise 2: Slowly contract and release the muscles; contract progressively tighter to a count of five and relax to a count of five.

The abdomen, buttocks, and thighs should not be tensed when doing these exercises. Lie (not after the first trimester), sit, or stand with legs slightly apart to isolate the correct area. Because of the internal nature of these exercises, they can be performed almost anywhere without anyone noticing.

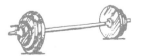
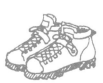
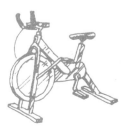

Shoes and Clothing

Wear shoes one-half to one size larger to allow room for foot swelling. Shoes with Velcro closures can make frequent adjustments easier. Clothing should be comfortable. If overheating is a problem, wear clothing that is nonconstricting, breathes, and wicks moisture away from the body to help stay cool. A sports bra with wide shoulder straps can provide good support, help protect the breasts, and ease or prevent shoulder discomfort. (See Exercise Clothing, Chapter 6.)

Duration of Pregnancy

Assuming that it is safe to do so (there are no complications), a woman should try to exercise throughout the duration of pregnancy. Some studies suggest that full benefits are not realized if women stop exercising partway through pregnancy.

Calories In!

A woman should never exercise to lose weight while pregnant and should not restrict calories for the purpose of preventing weight gain. Mother and fetus need an extra 300 calories a day (for multiple-birth pregnancies, add 300 calories per fetus). To determine whether a woman is eating enough, she should monitor her body weight regularly. Prenatal women can expect to gain 25 to 35 pounds. Lean, athletic women who had low levels of body fat before pregnancy may need to gain more. Women who fall into this category may take comfort in knowing that they will recover quickly. If a pregnant woman is not gaining weight (or is losing weight), she needs to increase her caloric intake from nutrient rich foods. Pregnancy may not be an athletic event, but it is very physically demanding. It is important to remember that the new life inside the womb needs nutrients and calories to grow and be healthy.

Fitness for Postnatal Women

During the postnatal (or postpartum) period, a woman's body works hard to return to its nonpregnant status. This process can take nearly as long as the pregnancy. Muscles and skin that stretched to allow for the baby's growth take time to return to their original tone and can

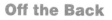

Off the Back

A woman should avoid performing exercise on her back *after the first trimester*. She may sit, stand, or squat, but she should stay off her back.

make fitting into prepregnancy clothes challenging. Although this can be emotionally discouraging, it is normal. This adjustment period is the time when a postnatal woman can make healthy progress by treating herself with patience.

Approval First

As in the prenatal stage, a woman in the postnatal period should get approval from her doctor or health care provider before engaging in exercise. If approval is given, the prenatal and postnatal fitness guidelines can be followed until the postnatal period ceases.

The new mother's postnatal condition will affect the time and type of exercise activities that can be resumed. Aside from the physiological adjustments, one of the biggest challenges to a new mother's fitness is time. But with a little planning, a new mother can carve out a piece of her busy day for exercise that will enhance her physical and emotional health.

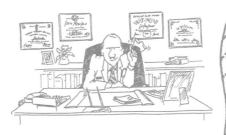

Creating (Creative) Support

Dad's Time

Designate Mom's exercise time as Dad's exclusive time with baby and vice versa. This can be a satisfying arrangement for everyone involved.

Rotating Family

A rotational schedule can work nicely for grandparents, aunts, uncles, and older siblings to have time with baby. Be considerate of others by scheduling a start and a finish time.

Friends, Neighbors

Friends, especially those with young children, can fill and share the need to watch baby while Mom exercises. Again, schedule the time as you would a class or an appointment. Designating a start and a finish time will help you to recruit others; it communicates a respect and appreciation for their time.

Prenatal and Postnatal Fitness Guidelines: F-I-T

- Frequency: Prenatal and postnatal women may exercise three to five times per week and even engage in some form of activity on a daily basis.
- Intensity: The highest recommended exercise intensity is at a level of 12 to 14 on the Borg RPE Scale or at the point where the woman's overall perceived effort feels "somewhat hard" to "hard."
- Time: If a woman is just starting an exercise program, she should start with 5 or 10 minutes at a time and always include a proper warm-up and cooldown. If a woman was fit prior to pregnancy, she can exercise for 20 to 45 minutes. The same warm-up and cool-down recommendation applies.

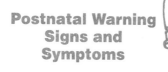

Postnatal Warning Signs and Symptoms

Contact your health care provider if you have any of the following symptoms:

- Fever of 100.2°F or higher for 24 hours or more

- Dizziness, nausea, faintness, or extreme shortness of breath

- A red, warm, painful area on either breast or excessive breast tenderness

- Inability to urinate or painful urination

- Loss of bladder control or leakage on exertion that continues 4 to 6 weeks postdelivery

- Opening or increased pain or drainage of Cesarean incision

- Red, warm tender or painful area on either leg

- Severe pain

Baby-sitters

Exercise is at least as important as going out for the evening for new mothers. Arrange a baby-sitter for regular days and times. Unless Mom is training for a marathon (and she is already living one!), as little as an hour of time can make a huge difference.

Baby Friendly Equipment

Baby friendly equipment makes it possible for baby to safely go along for Mom's and Dad's walks, jogs, runs, or bike rides. The baby jogger/runner is more stable and durable than a conventional stroller. For bicycling, there are numerous options for baby and child apparatus. There are screened-in trailers, child seats, and mount-on tandem attachments (see the Appendix for resources).

Indoor Activity

Find an indoor or at-home exercise activity to do in the event that other support is not available.

Postnatal Exercise Classes

With increased demand, these are popping up all over. Contact your local health clubs, YWCAs/YMCAs, community learning centers, and schools. Check to see whether the class instructor is educated and certified to instruct prenatal and postnatal women.

Children and Fitness

In a 1998 issue of the ACSM Health & Fitness Journal it was reported that "childhood obesity in the U.S. is at an all time high and the physical activity level of most boys and girls is down. There is evidence that 40% of five- to eight-year-olds in the US already have at least one risk factor for heart disease." These statistics reflect an unhealthy present and a not so great future. The time for change and improvement is now.

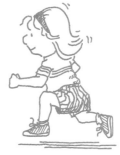

Before the omnipresence of television and computers, kids were more active. Many seem unable to break away from their televisions and computers, so we need to put some extra effort to ensure that kids get the activity they need. In a recent survey, it was reported that only 37 percent of high school students perform 20 minutes of vigorous physical activity three or more times per week. If you want to make a difference in the lives of your and other children, here are some ideas to keep in mind and put into action.

Activity—From the Very Beginning

The American Academy of Pediatrics (AAP) supports a "safe, nurturing, and minimally structured play environment for the infant," rather than structured infant exercise programs.

Fundamentals First

First and foremost, young children should be learning new skills and having fun. They should learn a variety of fundamental movement skills such as running, jumping, twisting, kicking, balancing, catching, and throwing. Many of kids' vigorous play activities, such as running, jumping rope, bicycling, and skating, fulfill the aerobic component. For strength training, kids should be encouraged to participate in climbing and hanging activities, such as those that can be performed on jungle gyms and other playground apparatus. Even climbing trees is very effective. For children under the age of 8 years, fitness should come in the form of active play. By age 8, a child should have activity as a regular part of life.

With physical education programs reduced in many school districts, it is wrong to assume that kids are learning these lifetime skills at school or getting enough activity. Parents can investigate the many youth programs offered at community and health club centers. With competent instruction and practice time, kids can learn the basic skills they need for success and enjoyment in recreational fitness activities and organized sports.

Puberty

Add "physical activity" to the list of challenges children (and parents) face during puberty. At this time, many kids sift themselves out of sports and exercise activities because they feel less competent or less skilled than other kids. It is an opportune time to encourage the concept of lifetime fitness and noncompetitive activities such as walking,

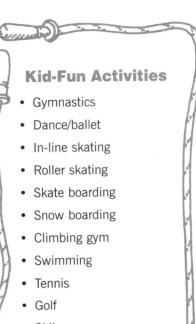

Kid-Fun Activities

- Gymnastics
- Dance/ballet
- In-line skating
- Roller skating
- Skate boarding
- Snow boarding
- Climbing gym
- Swimming
- Tennis
- Golf
- Skiing
- Biking
- Running
- Frisbee games
- Basketball
- Soccer
- Tag football
- Field games
- Golf

Components of a Kids' Exercise Program

1. Aerobic fitness

2. Muscular strength and endurance

3. Flexibility

4. Rest/recovery

bicycling, swimming, and jogging versus competitive sports activities. Parents make a tremendous impact on their child's fitness by example and by encouraging and participating in fitness activities with their children. If you know children who are not getting enough physical activity, here are three suggestions for inspiring them to get moving.

1. Make it fun. If you want kids to be active, healthy, and fit, one of the best ways is to find activities that are fun. When kids have fun, they are more likely to participate. If it is not fun or stops being fun, they will likely lose interest. Observe and listen to children to understand their idea of fun (not someone else's).

Competitive versus noncompetitive activities. In the 1970s and 1980s, little league baseball earned the reputation for being competitive to a fault. Many parents and coaches pressured little league kids by their "win at all costs" attitude. This is in part what led to the proliferation of soccer in the 1980s, 1990s, and into 2000. Soccer was the fresh, new sport that kids, especially those turned off by little league baseball, could play, without the pressures of little league.

Competitive fitness activities can be great learning grounds for kids, as long as the objectives for fitness and enjoyment do not become lost in the competition. Losing focus can happen in any sport, whether it is baseball, soccer, tennis, golf, or swimming. Competition is about being, doing, and giving the best effort possible; it is about striving for superiority. Through competition, kids learn how to perform under pressure, how to get along with others, how to gracefully win and lose, and that life goes on even after a loss. If your child is 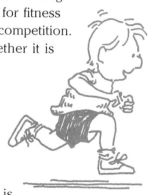 involved in competitive activities, check to see that fun and focus are alive and well.

2. Make it family time together. Engage in family activities that are physically active and fun. Make time for a yard game of basketball or shoot around, play H-O-R-S-E, or soccer, go in-line skating or swimming, play softball or baseball, take a walk down by the river, run around the park or lake, bike ride together, or go dancing. For some one-on-one time, have your child ride a bike alongside while you jog.

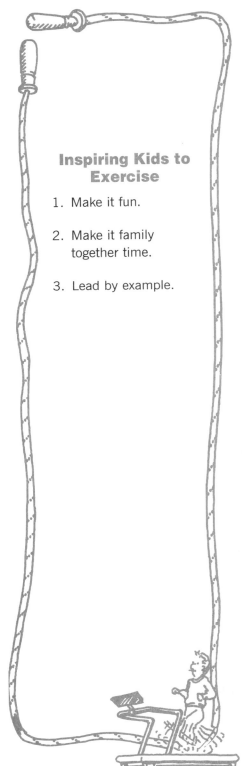

Make fun memories with kids by playing sports games or other activities. Kids learn from seeing that you are active and having fun.

Peripheral/related activities. Invest in peripheral physical activities. If you know a child who is interested in a particular sport, treat him or her to a higher level event, such as a high school, college, or professional game. Take the child to a hall of fame or a related museum or movie. How about a special event such as a nearby 10k, marathon, triathlon, tennis match, baseball game, ballet, or dance recital? These types of activities can be fun and very inspiring to young people (adults too!).

3. Lead by example. Another way to enhance the possibility that your kids will be active is by example. Making exercise a regular part of your life makes an impression on kids. When your child sees you carving out a piece of your busy day to exercise, she/he learns that it is important. Remember, children learn what they live and see!

What and How Much? A Kids' Exercise Program

The components of a complete exercise program are the same for children as for adults, the differences being how they are accomplished.

Strength Training

Some basic strength training exercises that are effective and can be safely practiced are push-ups, curl-ups, pull-ups, or chin-ups. The epiphysial plates of adolescents and teenagers are still forming and should not be overly stressed by heavy weight training or their growth and natural potential could be impaired. The American Academy of Pediatrics (AAP) supports strength training for kids over the age of 12 only if supervised by well-trained, knowledgeable adults and states that kids should avoid maximal lifting until they have reached full maturity.

Here are some guidelines for kids who weight train:

Start with extremely light weights.
Focus on safety and technique.
Do 10 to 15 repetitions, 1 to 3 sets, only two or three times
    per week.
Involve the major muscle groups.

Inspiring Kids to Exercise

1. Make it fun.

2. Make it family together time.

3. Lead by example.

Overheating

Children who have not yet reached puberty are at higher risk for excessively high body temperature (*hyper*thermia) during exercise than children who are pubescent. A child's natural cooling system, the sweat glands, are not fully developed, so the ability to dissipate heat is less efficient. Plus, a small child's body has less surface area than adults on which to throw off heat. Therefore, they are more sensitive to heat. Small children absorb heat faster in hot climates and lose heat faster in cold climates. These factors can be easily managed by drinking 8 to 16 ounces of cool water or electrolyte fluids (diluted is fine) during exercise. Diluted electrolyte fluids are recommended mostly for the flavor more than the need for electrolytes. Because these fluids are not harmful and most kids like the taste, it helps them to drink more fluids.

Diabetes

The primary fuel for the brain is blood glucose, and its concentration level needs to be within a certain range. Hormones that are secreted by the pancreas regulate this range. When blood glucose falls, the pancreas secretes glucagon, which helps bring the level back up to normal. When blood glucose is too high, the pancreas secretes insulin, which allows glucose to be taken up at a faster rate to be used as a fuel or stored for later use.

Diabetes is a disease in which blood glucose concentration is chronically elevated either by a lack of insulin (Type I) or by a resistance to insulin (Type II). Diabetes can cause blindness, kidney disease, heart disease, stroke, and peripheral vascular disease that can lead to the amputation of a leg or foot. Type I diabetes occurs mostly in young people, which explains why it is also known as juvenile-onset diabetes. It accounts for 10 percent of the (more than sixteen million) diabetes patients in this country. The remaining 90 percent have Type II diabetes as well as other CHD risk factors such as high blood pressure, high cholesterol, and obesity. Type II diabetes is linked to lifestyle, specifically obesity, and typically occurs in adults over age 40. The good news about Type II diabetes is that because it is a lifestyle disease, it is generally preventable.

Whereas exercise is recommended for both Type I and Type II diabetes, the greatest recommendation for a Type II diabetic is for regular exercise. Exercise helps deal with the obesity problem and can decrease or eliminate the need for insulin or oral medication typically taken to stimulate insulin production. Before beginning an exercise program, it is important for diabetic patients to follow certain recommendations. Two recommendations that should be foremost in the diabetic's mind pertain to foot care and glucose levels.

Foot Care

The shoes should have sufficient clearance between the top of the toes and the top of each shoe to prevent bruising or jamming of the toes. Socks should be clean, fresh, and fit without tightness or bunching. Because of a decrease of sensory function in the lower extremities, diabetic patients with peripheral neuropathy (disease of peripheral nerves) are at risk for traumatic injury and ulceration of the feet. Use of a lubricant on the feet can be helpful in reducing friction that can lead to ulcers.

Persons who are excessively overweight run the risk of developing foot injuries or orthopedic complications due to the added stress placed on the joints from weight bearing activity. In such situations, nonweight bearing activities (swimming, bicycling) may be appropriate.

Glucose Level Control

Blood glucose should be "under control" prior to exercise session. "Under control" means that prior to exercise, the diabetic has eaten the proper quantity of carbohydrates and injected the proper amount of insulin to keep blood glucose concentration close to normal values.

Diabetics and Diet

Diabetics have much higher risk for heart disease and are advised to follow the dietary recommendations from the American Diabetes Association (ADA). Whereas the recommendations are nearly the same as for nondiabetic persons, the need for compliance is greater because the health of a diabetic patient is more sensitive to dietary factors. The ADA dietary recommendations are as follows:

1. Caloric intake should be adjusted to achieve and maintain ideal weight.

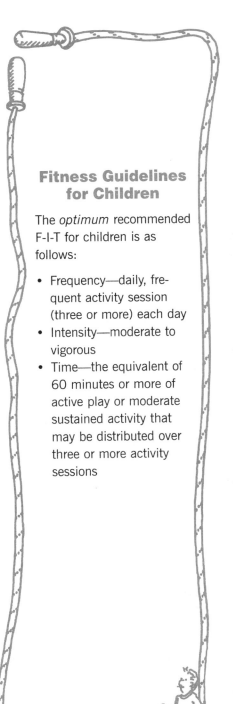

Fitness Guidelines for Children

The *optimum* recommended F-I-T for children is as follows:

- Frequency—daily, frequent activity session (three or more) each day
- Intensity—moderate to vigorous
- Time—the equivalent of 60 minutes or more of active play or moderate sustained activity that may be distributed over three or more activity sessions

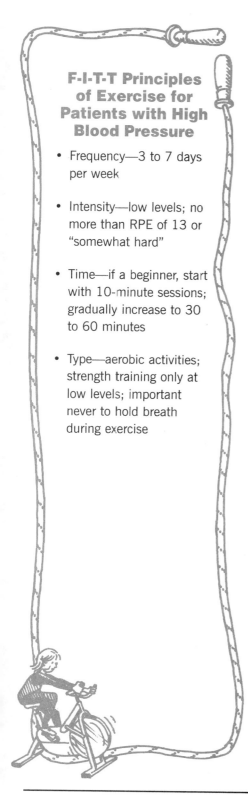

2. Carbohydrates should approach 55 to 60 percent of caloric intake.
3. Fiber should be increased and refined carbohydrates decreased.
4. Consume only 0.4 grams of protein per 1.1 pound of body weight.
5. Fat should be limited to 30 percent of caloric intake, saturated fats to 10 percent or less.
6. Sodium intake should be limited to 1 gram per 1,000 calories, not to exceed 3 grams per day.
7. Alcohol should be used only in moderation.

Contact the American Diabetes Association's national and local chapters for the latest information on treatment of the disease (see the Appendix).

Older Adults

We are learning more and more that age alone does *not* cause lack of or poor bodily function. Inactivity and weight gain are responsible for much of the "aging effect." Did you know that the fastest growing segment of our society is adults aged 80 or more? For older adults, the greatest reason to be fit is independence. Function is everything! More proof that it is never too late to exercise comes from a conditioning study of ten elderly men and women ranging in age from 87 to 96 years. It concluded that resistance exercise enables dramatic strength gains even in very old and frail persons. A balanced exercise program of moderate aerobic activity, strength training, and flexibility are especially important for older adults. Without these activities, older adults can lose strength, endurance, flexibility, and a capacity to perform daily function more quickly than those who perform them.

Osteoporosis—What Can You Do about It?

Osteoporosis is a disease that results in a loss of bone mass; hard bone becomes soft and sponge-like. It is responsible for over 1.2 million fractures each year. Hip fractures, prevalent in older adults, are generally related to osteoporosis. These are especially dangerous to older adults because they can trigger other events that lead to the end of an independent lifestyle. Two ways to combat the effects of osteoporosis are through exercise activities and adequate calcium intake (see Chapter 9). The beauty of strength training and weight bearing activity is that

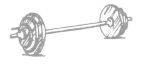
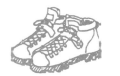
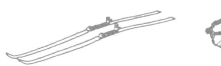

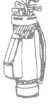

Recommendations for Exercise for Diabetes Patients

1. Before beginning an exercise program, have a thorough medical exam and share the exercise plan with the physician.
2. Always wear medical identification.
3. Make sure blood glucose is "under control" prior to exercise session.
4. Consume plenty of fluids before, during, and after exercise.*
5. Wear supportive shoes and cotton socks; check feet for blisters and cuts regularly.
6. Lubricate the feet to help prevent blisters and ulcers.
7. Carry a source of quickly absorbing carbohydrate (hard candy, sports drink, sports bar).
8. Let someone know you are exercising or exercise with someone.

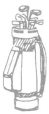

* Under control means prior to exercise the diabetic has eaten the proper quantity of carbohydrates and injected the proper amount of insulin to keep blood glucose concentration close to normal values.

• • •

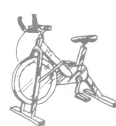

Reasons for Persons with Diabetes to Avoid Exercise

1. Retinal (eye) hemorrhages or recent eye surgery
2. Fever or infection
3. Blood glucose <80-100 mg/dl (Eat extra carbohydrate until blood glucose increases >120 mg/dl before exercising.)
4. Blood glucose >250-300 mg/dl and presence of urine ketones (Decrease blood glucose before beginning exercise.)

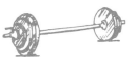
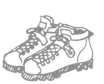

they stimulate muscular activity, which in turn stimulates production of bone density.

Socialization

The social benefits of attending exercise programs are another important component to life fitness for older adults. Being around others helps combat isolation that many seniors experience during their nonworking lives. If you are an older adult, get up, and get moving. Sign up for an exercise class, bring a friend, and get physical. Get involved! There are numerous exercise experiences offered specifically for older adults, from aerobics to yoga. Contact the religious, senior, and educational centers in your community.

Older Examples

There are many inspirational examples of older adults who have channeled their free time toward their health and other good causes. In July 1999, *NBC Nightly News* reported that an 89-year-old woman was so upset about campaign finance reform she decided to walk across America, over 3,000 miles, to raise awareness. She had never exercised before. Then there is Sister Madonna Buder, a competitor in the women's 65 to 69 age group, who just completed another of her many Ironman distance triathlons (2.4-mile swim, 112-mile bike ride, 26.2-mile marathon run) at the Ironman Canada race held in Penticton, British Columbia.

Older adults generally have fewer responsibilities, more time, and plenty of wisdom and experience to share with others. Exercise is a great opportunity to stay fit and enjoy life. Research shows that exercise is one vital component that can help older adults to be functional, independent, social, and happier. When it comes to regular activity and older adults, the message is clear: There is much to gain. Get going!

Hypertension (High Blood Pressure)

Hypertension exists when the systolic blood pressure is consistently above 140 mm Hg and/or the diastolic blood pressure is consistently above 90 mm Hg.

Foot Care Tip

A nonstaining, non-petroleum-based lubricant called Body Glide has been used successfully with diabetic patients in reducing foot irritation and ulcers. The product is successful because of its long-lasting lubricating properties without the staining and mess of petroleum-based lubes. Body Glide is sold in athletic stores and on the Web (see the Appendix).

What Is Blood Pressure?

Over fifty million Americans have high blood pressure, a major risk factor in the development of heart disease. Aside from knowing the levels for high blood pressure, let's get an understanding of what it is and what exercise can do for it.

The heart is a muscle that pumps blood throughout the body. When the heart contracts, it sends blood out to the body by way of our transportation system, better known as our vascular system. The vascular highway system is made up of our veins and arteries. As blood travels through the highway system, it creates pressure against the veins and arteries. When the heart contracts, causing a surge of blood, it creates a pressure known as systolic pressure. And when the heart relaxes, following the contraction phase, there is also pressure exerted against the veins and arteries, known as diastolic pressure. These two pressures constitute blood pressure. The top number indicates the systolic pressure, and the bottom number indicates the diastolic pressure (See the Blood Pressure classification table). If not relieved, high blood pressure can seriously damage the cardiovascular system.

Understanding Blood Pressure—Experiment or Visualization

Hook up a garden hose and grasp the hose (not the nozzle) in your hand. Next, turn on the water (open the valve) so that water comes out of the hose. Let it run for 10 seconds or so. Now, reduce the flow by turning the valve about halfway off. Repeat this one time, then shut it off.

Did you notice the surge of pressure in the hose when you turned it on? Did you notice how the pressure lessened when you turned it halfway off? This simulates blood pressure in the body. The surge of pressure from water traveling through the hose is similar to the surge of pressure in your vascular system when your heart contracts. This pressure is measured and known as systolic pressure. The lessening of pressure when you relaxed the flow of water is similar to the pressure exerted against your blood vessels during the heart's relaxation phase and is measured and known as diastolic pressure.

Lifetime Inspiration

A very fit woman shared a childhood memory: "I recall my father leaving early in the morning dressed in his running attire for his 3 mile jog, rain or shine. That's how he started his day. It was as regular as brushing his teeth, just something that he did. His commitment to exercise made a big impression on me. I grew up thinking that exercise must be important and that it was just one of those regular things adults did in life."

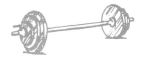
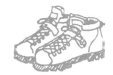
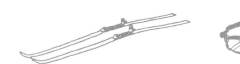

Classification of Blood Pressure
for Adults 18 Years or Older

SYSTOLIC BP	DIASTOLIC BP	CATEGORY
<130	<85	Normal
130 to 139	85 to 89	High normal
140 to 159	90 to 99	Mild hypertension—Stage I
160 to 179	100 to 109	Moderate hypertension—Stage II
180 to 209	110 to 119	Severe hypertension—Stage III
>210	>120	Very severe hypertension—Stage IV

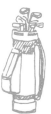

These measurements are for individuals not taking antihypertensive drugs and not acutely ill. Findings should be based on the average of two or more readings taken on two or more occasions. When systolic and diastolic pressures fall into different categories, use the higher category for classification.

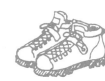
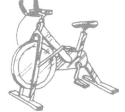

Exercise and High Blood Pressure

During exercise, certain elevations in blood pressure are normal. Because *rigorous* exercise causes steep increases in blood pressure, it should be avoided by persons with high blood pressure. But low to moderate intensity exercise is effective in reducing the incidence and severity of moderate high blood pressure. Here are exercise guidelines for individuals with high blood pressure:

1. Get physician approval to exercise before engaging in exercise activities.
2. Do not exercise if resting blood pressure is more than 200/115 mm Hg.
3. Report any weight gains, shortness of breath, or chest pain to the doctor immediately.
4. Stop exercising immediately if feelings of faintness, dizziness, or heart palpitations are present.
5. Warm up and cool down for at least 10 minutes at a comfortable intensity prior to exercising.

Exercise and Environmental Considerations

Being fit requires you to use your head as well as your body. Pay attention to the conditions that are constantly changing around you and consider how they can affect you during and after exercise. Adaptations are variable and specific for the exercise activity. Some environmental considerations are best modified by lessening the level of intensity; others, such as personal safety, warrant more creative adaptations (a partner, canine companion, light of day, new location). Be adaptable and seize the circumstances as a new experience. You might even enjoy the change.

Exercise and Travel Considerations
Exercise Tips for Travel

The word *travel* conjures up a variety of feelings. For some it is exciting, adventurous, and stimulating. For others it represents a lifestyle of packing suitcases, briefcases, and laptop computers, hustling to the next connection, and hoping transportation systems are running on

Fitness Guidelines for Older Adults

Older adults can utilize the F-I-T Principles of exercise but with greater emphasis on frequency of exercise, at lower intensity levels, and for shorter periods of time.

- Frequency—3 to 7 days per week; multiple times per day

- Intensity—low to moderate; 60 to 80% of HR; high intensities not suggested

- Time—10 to 60-minute sessions

- Type—activities that emphasize strength training and flexibility. Cardiorespiratory activities are also important and should be included, but not at high intensities.

Exercise Activities for Older Adults

- Aerobics
- Ballet
- Bicycling
- Bowling
- Calisthenics
- Croquet
- Contemporary dancing
- Golf
- Horseshoes
- Rowing
- Running
- Square dancing
- Stair climbing
- Strength training
- Swimming
- Tennis
- Triathlon
- Water aerobics
- Water exercise
- Yoga

time. In either case, travel can alter even the best plans for exercising and eating well. But that does not mean you have to sacrifice your health. A flexible and resourceful attitude can be a valuable travel "tool." *Before* your next trip, take just a few moments to think and plan for exercise and nutritious eating. Here are some ideas that will improve your chances for maintaining your exercise and nutrition program when travel is a must.

Inquire Ahead

1. Availability. *Before* selecting your accommodations, *inquire* about exercise facilities and equipment. Does the hotel have an on-site fitness center or swimming pool? Is there a nearby school track, a well-lighted, safe park or place to walk or run? Asking these questions can help you decide whether to stay there and what to pack. It also communicates to your service provider that fitness is important to you, their customer. If the hotel does not currently have any options for safe, convenient exercise, politely tell them you will consider staying there when they do. This is how customers educate suppliers about what is important to them. Your inquiry for facilities is essentially "casting a vote."

2. Reservations. Reservations are not just for tee times or dinner. Ask about the hours of operation for the fitness facility. Most will open early enough to accommodate early schedules. If the facility is small and equipment is limited (one treadmill, one stationary bike), ask how you can reserve a specific piece of equipment for a limited amount of time (i.e., treadmill at 6:00 A.M.). Be on time!

3. Friends and family. When staying with friends or family, *ask ahead* about nearby facilities or any in-home equipment you may use. You might motivate them as well.

4. Special events. Are you going to be in town when a special fitness/athletic participatory event (5k, 10k run, etc.) is happening? What a great way to take in the local flavor.

Plan Ahead

1. "Picture it, pack it." Before packing your suitcase, conduct a mental "dress rehearsal." See yourself putting on your shoes, socks, shorts, jog bra, jockstrap, heart rate monitor, hat, walkman, or whatever else you need. Pull out and put aside those items as well as a plastic bag (for soiled clothing). Or make a written list and pack them later.

2. Weather forecast. Prepare accordingly. One lightweight traveler's secret is a paper jacket. It is made from a material called Tyvek™. It weighs virtually nothing, takes up little space, and provides a lot of wind and warmth protection in moderate temperatures. Many bicycle stores sell them.

3. Healthy attitude and expectation. "Fit and healthy" are "in." You do not have to apologize for wanting to replicate your healthy behaviors while traveling. If your hotel tells you they "have not had this request before," you need not apologize. Remind them that accommodations for "fit and healthy" travel are standard practice among American hotels. If they are not accommodating, find another hotel.

4. Window of opportunity. Travel can result in erratic schedules. Do your best to find the window of opportunity for exercise time on a daily basis. Even a shorter than normal amount of exercise time can make you feel better. Some days might be impossible for exercise. If so, "count" them as your designated rest days and plan for the next exercise day. Keep the few missed days in perspective and don't be too hard on yourself.

5. "Don't just sit there . . . " Whether you're on a plane or in an important meeting, get up, stand, stretch, move your body, and plan breaks. You'll feel better for it (and others will thank you too!).

Be Flexible and Resourceful

1. Mode. If facilities or equipment are not available, try or create something new, such as jumping rope, "stepping" with your headset in the stairway, jogging, or dancing in place in your room. Remember that your objective is to make your body feel better and serve you better.

A "Back at You" Perspective!

An elementary school physical education teacher shared with his class a true story about an unfit, stressed 40ish-year-old businessman who had a heart attack while rushing through the airport. Student responses to the sad story were enlightening. They all said that they wished their parents took time to exercise regularly. Even if it meant spending less time with their parents, children said it would be worth it if their parents were healthier and happier on a daily basis. **The message to parents:** Your kids want you to be well. Make time for yourself and be the role model your kids need.

2. Adjust your F-I-T-T principles of exercise. Traveling can be tiring. Adjust (lower) your F-I-T-T (frequency, intensity, time, and type) levels accordingly. If you are tired from being in meetings all day, a little exercise "oxygen feed" can invigorate you. However, if you are exhausted from changing time zones and being "on the go" for 14 hours or more, you might be better off getting some sleep. With even a little exercise experience, you should be able to judge whether exercise will invigorate or deplete you.

Eating and Drinking Tips for Travel

Part of the pleasure of travel is experiencing food that is different. But that does not mean you have to abandon nutrition. Remember this word: *M O D E R A T I O N*. You can enjoy and experience many wonderful foods without having to gorge yourself. If you visit someplace famous for their "deep-fried-saturated-fat-artery-blocker a la mode" and you really want to experience it, then do so, but moderately—not every day or in large quantities.

Depending upon the type of travel, the most difficult elements to control are what, when, and where you will eat and drink. As with exercise, a flexible approach is a valuable tool. As best you can, use the following ideas for eating and hydrating appropriately when traveling.

Plan Ahead

1. Pre-pack. If you are unsure of what, when, and where you will be eating and drinking, pack a water bottle and some nonperishable food items. With the plethora of zipper-style plastic bags, you can pack along dry cereal, dried fruit, and other nonperishable items. With a small plastic bowl, plastic spoon, and hermetically sealed single-serve boxes of rice or soy milk and a box/bag of raisins, you can enjoy a quiet breakfast in your hotel/motel room.

If you are traveling by car or motor vehicle, take along a cooler and an ice brick and pack fresh fruit and vegetables for snacking. Baby carrots, cherry tomatoes, bananas, nonsugary cereals, crackers, and raisins are nutritious in-between meal snacks.

Adjusting F-I-T-T Principles During Travel

- **Frequency:** Be flexible; cut back when necessary.

- **Intensity:** Using the RPE Scale, exercise at level 10 to 11, "fairly light," or use your heart rate monitor to exercise at lower than normal Heart Rate Zones.

- **Time:** Even 10 minutes can make you feel better.

- **Type:** Be creative, flexible, and focus on what you can do under the circumstances.

2. Hydration. Your all-day meeting just finished. Hurriedly, you rush to return the rental car, rush to catch the plane, dart into the office, and then finally you get to go home. Sound familiar? Proper hydration is often sacrificed when traveling, the time when you need it the most. Talking, changes in altitude, changes in environment, stressful situations, and physical activity all cause the body to lose fluid. Combine this with a hectic, on-the-go travel schedule where you may forget your fluid/hydration routine, and you can lose fluids quickly, contributing to dehydration. Take along a water bottle and refill it as often as possible, especially during travel, meetings, or when you exercise. High altitude environments (airplane travel, skiing, hiking) can cause a dehydrating effect, so stick to your hydration plan for timely fluid consumption. Consume a minimum of 64 ounces per day of hydrating fluids. Remember that alcohol and carbonated beverages dehydrate the body.

3. Use service businesses to your advantage. Hotels are service businesses. Use their services to help you to eat healthfully. If you spot nutritious items (fish, vegetables, fruit, etc.) on the menu that are prepared in an unhealthy way, ask them to prepare the item for you without the deep fry, cream sauce, or butter. Another idea is to order your next day's lunch/meal "to go" from the hotel restaurant (or from the restaurant where you are having dinner) the night before and ask them to hold it in their refrigerator for you to pick up in the morning.

4. A Family Visit? Share your desire. Before arriving, share with your family members your desire to eat nutritiously. Many family members will support and welcome your showing them how to do so. Share your knowledge. Bring any special foods along with you, especially morning grains, cereals, and so on. Inquire about local farmer's markets that you could visit; make it a shared outing.

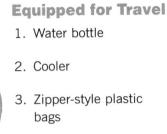

Equipped for Travel

1. Water bottle

2. Cooler

3. Zipper-style plastic bags

4. Plastic trash bag

5. Nonperishable foods when necessary

6. Fresh fruit and vegetables in addition to nonperishables when possible

Travel Tip

1. With travel, there is a tendency toward dehydration; compensate.

2. When air travel is involved, increase water consumption *while flying*.

3. Take your bottle(s) with you on the plane/train/bus or buy bottled water.

4. *Consume a minimum of 64 ounces* per day and try for more.

5. Remember, *alcohol dehydrates the body*.

5. Yellow Pages. Use the Yellow Pages to find restaurants that give you options. Especially in the United States we have plenty of options! For example, Mexican restaurant food is typically high in fat and salt. Call before going or ask before ordering for healthier options. Tell them you are looking to eat a good meal without heavy uses of salt, cheese, or fat and that you want to order sauces and dressings on the side. Or ask if they would be willing to prepare something per your requests. It is not much more difficult to make a tostada on a soft shell tortilla as on one that is crispy, deep fried. If they wince, or seem like they don't know what you're talking about, or make you feel like you're asking for too much, you're better off trying a different restaurant.

6. Be inclusive—be respectful of differences. Some will see you as a healthy example and ask you to share your healthy experiences. Others may not be ready or interested. Don't make people feel bad about the way they eat or exercise, just as you would want them to respect your healthy choices. You can respect differences without sacrificing your health.

Conclusion—Special Needs and Populations

Attitude is a tremendous factor when it comes to exercising and eating appropriately. If you replace "I can't" thinking with "how to" thinking, you will reap the benefits. Whatever your special needs might be, remember that appropriate exercise and nutrition can enhance just about every special need.

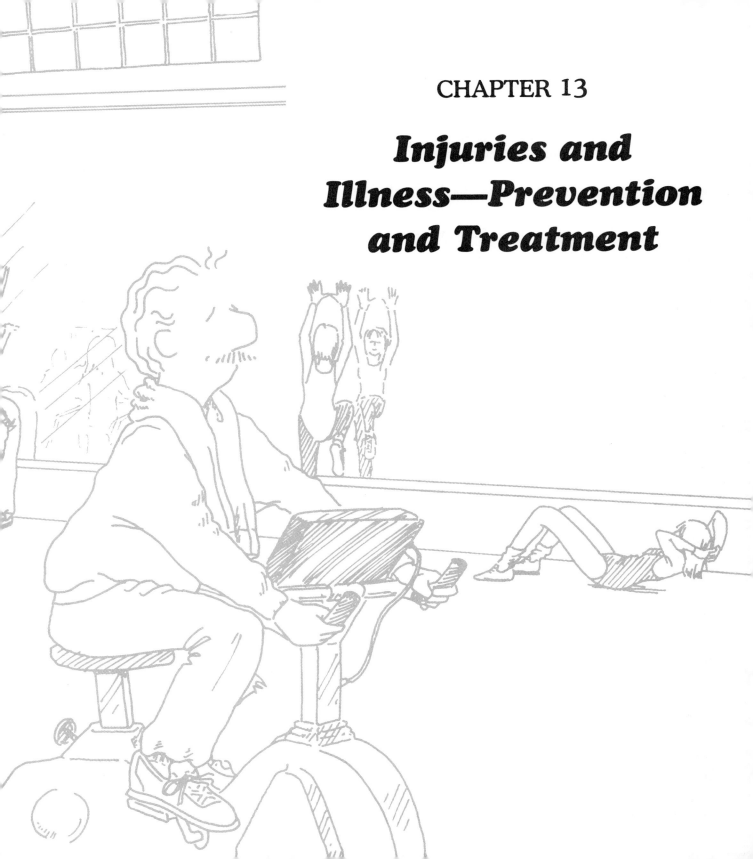

CHAPTER 13

Injuries and Illness—Prevention and Treatment

W hat is the best way to avoid the risk of injury and illness? The answer is, Prevention. By planning for rest and recovery time and adequate equipment and/or facilities, selecting appropriate activities, applying the F-I-T-T Principles (see Chapter 4), and following recommended advice and procedures for certain diseases, you can greatly reduce the risk of injury and serious illness.

Two common myths to dispel are "no pain no gain" and "more is better." These are outdated, old-school proverbs, and they are dangerous. They threaten your overall fitness because they can cause injury that can lead to inactivity. The healthy performance goal is "train, don't strain." Fitness activities should be incorporated *gradually* into your life, especially when you have previously been sedentary.

Rest and Recovery

During exercise, muscle fibers are actually torn down. During rest and nutrition periods, these fibers recover and are rebuilt even stronger than before. However, if the ratio of exercise to rest is intensified without adequate time for recovery, the body has a difficult time rebuilding. The result is "feeling tired." This is a sure signal that rest is needed.

What is rest specifically? And how much do you need? Although highly subjective, rest can be a planned "sleep in" and abstention from a regular workout; rest can be taking an afternoon nap, having a massage, or total abstinence from activity. If you typically exercise 7 days a week at a low intensity, for a short time then rest might mean abstaining from exercise for an entire day. Or rest could be a reduction of the intensity level or amount of time you normally exercise. For an athlete who trains at high intensity levels for performance, a rest day might be total abstinence for a few days, even weeks, or rest might be an activity at a very low level of intensity. The amount and type of rest is very individual, but the need for it is universal.

The American College of Sports Medicine (ACSM) guidelines specify regular exercise three to four times per week, up to seven times per week, depending on intensity. Exercising at lower intensity levels puts less stress on the body, and therefore, the amount of time needed for rest is minimal. But when the frequency, intensity, and time of exercise is high, the need for rest and recovery time is heightened and important to sustaining good health.

Tip

Create your own rating scale for how you feel (on a scale of 1 to 10, 1 = feeling very, very poorly; 10 = feeling tremendous). If you are frequently below level 5, you may need to adjust your exercise program. Or adapt and use the RPE Scale and apply it to how sore, tired, or energized and flexible you feel.

Recovery as Indicator

Recovery is an important yet easily overlooked indicator of your fitness. The more fit you become, the quicker and more thorough your recovery will be. Pay attention to how your body feels the day/morning *after* completing your fitness activity and adjust your plan accordingly. If you hurt or feel pain, your body needs rest. If you describe your soreness as "light" or as "I can feel that I did something" but you are not experiencing pain, then you can probably continue with your program (include some flexibility exercises!). If you do not experience any negative effects from the session, then you are probably within your current limits and can continue; you can even adjust your "overload" (see Chapter 4) if you desire. Recovery is an insightful message from the body to be used to your benefit; be attentive to yours.

Overexercising and the Credit Card Theory

One way to remember to exercise within reasonable limits is to think of overexercising as exceeding your physical credit card limit. If you exceed your limits, you will be denied the activity (no approval) with an acute injury, or you will pay later (you still pay, plus interest accrues) with a chronic injury. Exercising beyond your capabilities (that includes your ability to recover) can be costly, and you will pay for overexercising in some way. Overexercising comes in two forms: overexerting yourself during the activity and overtraining, which is doing too much without enough rest in between. If you treat fitness activities with respect, you will spend within your budget, and your gains will be many.

Symptoms of Overtraining— Too Much Is Not Good!

Too much of even something good is not good, and this holds true for exercise. Your body needs that fourth component of a complete exercise program (see Chapter 2)—rest. If you have some of the symptoms listed in the overtraining chart, look at your workout calendar and check for signs of overtraining. Overtraining is a completely individual phenomenon that can change from time to time. Even if you are in better shape now than you were 3 months ago, if you are pushing with

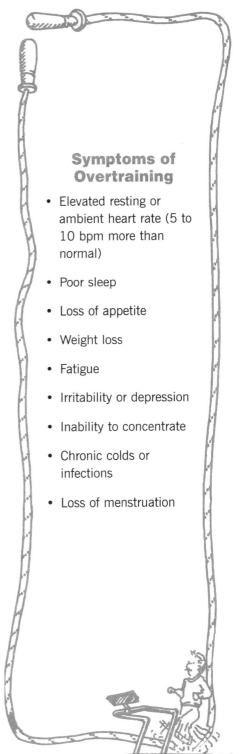

Symptoms of Overtraining

- Elevated resting or ambient heart rate (5 to 10 bpm more than normal)

- Poor sleep

- Loss of appetite

- Weight loss

- Fatigue

- Irritability or depression

- Inability to concentrate

- Chronic colds or infections

- Loss of menstruation

Common Soft Tissue Injuries That Need PRICE Treatment

- Sprains—stretching or tearing of ligaments
- Strain—stretching or tearing of muscle or tendons
- Contusion—an impact force that causes bleeding to underlying tissues
- Wounds—lacerations, incisions, abrasions (Clean with antiseptic solutions such as hydrogen pyroxide; follow with soap and water cleansing; apply a petroleum-based anti-septic agent to keep the wound moist; apply non-stick gauze over the injury.)
- Punctures—a hole, wound, or perforation made by puncturing (If the object is imbedded deeply, refer to a physician for removal and treatment; otherwise, follow the same treatment as for other wounds.)

greater intensity, your need for rest could be greater than before. Of course, having some of these symptoms doesn't necessarily mean you are overtraining; you could have other factors in your life causing them. But check your exercise calendar to rule it out, and if you have an inkling that you could be overtraining, work in some extra rest days. Enter them in your calendar as "rest days," and mentally include them as the vital part of your fitness program that they truly are.

Soft Tissue Injuries— the P-R-I-C-E Is Right

Even with the best planning and prudent practices, injuries can happen. The most common soft tissue injuries are sprains, strains, and, no, not automobiles, contusions. These injuries call for an immediate treatment procedure best remembered by the acronym P-R-I-C-E (**P**rotection, **R**est, **I**ce, **C**ompression, **E**levation). **P**rotect or support the injured area from further injury. **R**est the injured area. Do not use it. **I**ce the injured area to reduce inflammation for 20 to 30 minutes when possible. **C**ompress the area firmly but not tightly with a stretch-type bandage. **E**levate the injured area above the level of the heart to reduce bleeding and compensate for gravity, which can increase bleeding. If injury is severe, seek medical treatment.

Orthopedic Injuries

Remember the credit card theory as related to overexercising? Just as you can overextend yourself with your credit card, so too can you bring about orthopedic injuries. Many common orthopedic injuries are a result of overextending oneself, overuse, overexertion, or chronic irritation of a problem. In the beginning, these injuries do not keep you from participating completely. But if ignored or left untreated, they can become more serious and debilitating.

If you have a nagging condition, consult with a knowledgeable fitness professional or medical doctor about your symptoms. The source of your problem may be your technique, the fit of your equipment, clothing, or shoes, the conditions in which you exercise, or improper application of the F-I-T-T Principles. For acute injuries, sharing an accurate account of what happened can be valuable to the professional in helping to determine the appropriate treatment. This problem-solving approach is more effective than ignoring the problem and trying to "exercise through it." With an attitude of "I'll exercise through it," the only thing that will be through will be you!

Bursitis, tendinitis, plantar fasciitis, and epicondylitis are common orthopedic conditions. They can be caused by overuse, improper joint mechanics, improper technique, pathology (disease), trauma, and infection. Symptoms include redness, swelling, pain, and increased skin temperature.

Stress fractures are caused by overuse, abrupt changes in training, in training surface, and in mechanics/gait. Symptoms include pain.

Causes of shin splints include overuse, muscular imbalance, and improper shoes, skills, or technique. Symptoms include pain between the knee and ankle.

NSAIDS—Non-steroidal Anti-inflammatory Drugs

Generic (common names) for NSAIDS include ibuprofen and acetaminophen. These drugs, when used properly, can ease the pain often associated with fitness activities. As their name implies, they are steroid-free and work against inflammatory responses in the body that can cause discomfort or pain. The marketing efforts of drug companies have made these powerful little pills; they are as prevalent as candy. And some people take them as such. Yet they can have very powerful effects upon your kidneys, liver, and stomach lining and should not be taken like candy. They can reduce inflammation that may occur, especially in fitness activities, and help to reduce discomfort and pain. If taken improperly, either too frequently or in too high a dosage, they can be very harmful.

A word of caution about taking pain-relieving medication: Pain is an indication that something in the body is wrong or out of balance. If you trace the source of your pain, you have a better chance of learning how to heal it. Medication can ease a painful situation, providing rest, recovery, and healing. But medicating a painful condition for the purpose of quickly returning to activity before healing has occurred puts you at risk for further pain and injury. Listen to your pain, go to the source, and seek a healthy solution. And if you need pain-relieving

High Heels and Osteoarthritis of the Knee

If the cartilage that cushions the bones in the knee gets worn down, it can cause a painful condition known as osteoarthritis. Twice as many women as men suffer from osteoarthritis of the knee, and 87 percent of all foot surgery is performed on women. In a small sample of women, researchers found that when they wore 2-inch heels, the rotational force upon their knees was 23 percent greater than when they were barefoot. That is enough to damage cartilage over time and cause arthritis. The bottom line is this: High heels cause foot deformities and backache.

Advice for high heel wearers: Wear flat or athletic shoes to and from work, wear low-heeled or flat dress shoes, and if you must wear high heels, wear them for short durations.

medication, use it to improve the condition, not to push it deeper toward serious injury.

Exercise and Heat

Exercising in a hot environment can cause the body to lose fluid at an unusually high rate. Anyone at any level of fitness can suffer a heat-related illness. If not treated, this can result in serious illness and death. The evaporation of sweat is the body's most common cooling mechanism. Sweating excessively is one indication of rapid fluid loss, though not the best indicator. For instance, when exercising in dry climates, your sweat may evaporate so quickly that you do not feel your body sweating much. However, you can still experience rapid fluid loss and heat-related complications.

The Heat Index

The heat index is the number that tells you how hot it really feels and takes into account air temperature, humidity, and radiant heat. The local weather service and many radio and television stations will broadcast the heat index on hot days. When the heat index is above 90 degrees, exercising outside should be approached with caution. For temperatures below 90 degrees, add the humidity; if the sum is between 130 and 150, outdoor exercise should be reconsidered. If you plan to exercise in hot and/or humid conditions, wear appropriate clothing and consume cool fluids regularly to combat some of the potentially harmful effects of extreme heat exercise.

Clothing

The clothes you wear will impact how efficiently evaporation can take place. Wear clothing that enhances evaporation, such as CoolMax, Supplex, and other "wick" style fabrics. Cotton blended fabrics are also okay. Dark colored clothing absorbs more heat than light colored clothing and can exacerbate an already heated condition, so dress in light colors when possible (see Chapter 6, Exercise Clothing).

Health Cues for When Not to Exercise

- Headache: Sometimes exercise can help, but not if pain is intense.

- Allergy, hay fever: Do mild *indoor* exercise.

- Mild sore throat: Do mild exercise only. Do not exercise if soreness is intense.

- Coughing: Do not exercise.

- Bronchitis, pneumonia: Exercise only when symptoms are gone.

Fluids

Running for as little as 15 minutes in the heat can raise your core body temperature to an unhealthy 104 degrees F. Frequently drinking water and electrolyte fluids during exercise in hot and/or humid conditions can help keep your body hydrated.

Pay attention to the symptoms of dehydration and heat illness and keep those fluids flowing regularly. Remember that you should be urinating clear and copious fluids; if you are not, drink until you do.

These guidelines should prevent heat injury:

1. Acclimatize to heat and humidity by training over a 7- to 12-day period.
2. Hydrate prior to and frequently during activity—6 to 8 ounces every 15 to 20 minutes during exercise.
3. Decrease intensity (how hard, how fast, etc.) of exercise if the temperature or humidity is high.
4. Monitor weight loss by weighing before and after workouts. If more than 3 percent of body weight is lost, force fluids and minimize participation until weight is within the 3 percent range.
5. Consume high water content carbohydrates (fruit, vegetables) to help maintain fluid balance.
6. Wear appropriate clothing for hot and humid conditions. Avoid plastic, painted screens, or other nonbreathable fabrics that prevent evaporation of sweat.

Sunny Exposures

Exercising outdoors is a treat for the senses as well as for the body. Pure pleasure can be derived from a walk along a beautiful path, seeing tall striking trees, hearing the sounds of a rushing river or creaky creek, feeling the dirt beneath your feet, and smelling the scent of pine, eucalyptus, or other fragrant trees and flowers. Your entire soul is lifted.

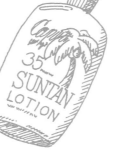

Unfortunately, the effects of direct sunny exposure on skin can be seriously damaging to your health. In 1998, more than one million new cases of skin cancer were diagnosed. We need to protect our skin from

Symptoms of Heat Illnesses (Overheating)

Symptoms include headache, nausea, vomiting, chills, extreme dry or "cotton" mouth, dizziness, muscle cramping, and hair standing on end at chest or upper arms.

What to do: Stop the activity. Get out of direct sun and heat (find shade). Ingest cold fluids (fluids at 41 to 59 degrees F are absorbed faster than fluids at other temperatures).

the damaging rays. When used in conjunction with limited exposure, sunscreen lotions can reduce the risk of developing skin cancer. But a recent study showed that while sunscreen is effective in blocking many of the sun's harmful rays, the overall sunscreen effect can be negative, since people are using it to stay out in the sun for longer periods of time.

Read and follow the recommendations of the American Academy of Dermatology. The American Academy of Dermatology recommends the following sun exposure guidelines:

1. Limit your exposure to the sun. Morning sun is the best; avoid exposure between 10 A.M. and 4 P.M.
2. Cover body parts with a hat (a 4-inch brim is good), long-sleeved shirt, and pants.
3. Apply sunscreen* at least 20 minutes before going outside to allow time for the active ingredients to soak into your skin.
4. Sunscreen lotions that contain zinc oxide or titanium dioxide are very effective.
5. Wear protective clothing with high SPF (sun protection factor) ratings. You can now buy clothing made from fabrics that have been specially treated to protect against the harmful rays of the sun. They have been laboratory-tested and rated as providing SPF 30. (See Appendix for source.) Untreated fabrics that are tightly woven (some cottons) block some of the harmful rays and offer a sun protection factor of 8.
6. Recognize the ABCDs of melanoma:
   A—asymmetry—one half unlike the other half
   B—border irregular; scalloped or poorly circumscribed border
   C—color varied from one area to another; shades of tan and brown, black; sometimes white, red, or blue
   D—diameter larger than 6 millimeters (the diameter of a pencil eraser)

*SPF—sun protection factor: use 25 minimum.

Prevention, Early Detection

Being committed to and taking an active role in your health through regular physical activity and solid nutrition can boost your immune system. Healthy behavioral practices, such as getting regular exercise,

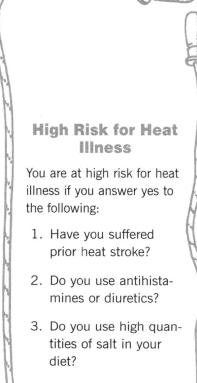

High Risk for Heat Illness

You are at high risk for heat illness if you answer yes to the following:

1. Have you suffered prior heat stroke?

2. Do you use antihistamines or diuretics?

3. Do you use high quantities of salt in your diet?

4. Do you use salt tablets?

5. Do you use alcohol in large quantities?

6. Do you have a fever?

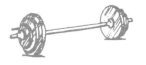 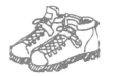 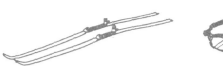

Exercising While Sick—Yes or No?

We know that exercise is good for your health and that it boosts your immune system. However, there are times, such as when your immune system is already working hard, that not exercising is better. Use the following guide to help you make healthy choices about whether or not to exercise.

Do you know the difference between a cold and flu symptoms?

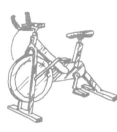

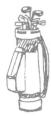

	COLD SYMPTOMS	FLU SYMPTOMS
Fever	None or low (99 to 100 degrees F/ 37.5 to 38 degrees C	High (102 to 104/39 to 40); lasts 3 to 4 days
Headache	Rare	Common
Body ache	Slight	Usually, often severe
Fatigue and weakness	Mild	Common; can last up to 3 weeks
Extreme exhaustion	Never	Common; soon after onset of sickness
Congested nose	Common	Sometimes
Sneezing	Common	Sometimes
Exercise: Yes or no?	Yes, but mildly	No

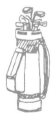

  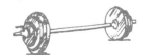 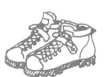

eating nutritiously, and getting enough sleep, are choices you make and are some of the best preventive measures you can take to guard against certain conditions. And although that does not necessarily make you immune from some illnesses, it has been demonstrated to have a powerful effect upon recovery.

In the case of two high profile diseases, breast cancer and prostate cancer, early detection is a critical factor in survival and recovery. Regular and timely examination is strongly recommended. So include the following prevention recommendations as part of your regular maintenance by making time for them. Even though they won't make you fit, they just might save your life and, therefore, are worthy of your attention. Your loved ones will love you for it too.

Breast Cancer

More women in the United States are diagnosed with breast cancer every year than with any other cancer. This year approximately 180,000 cases will be diagnosed, and 44,000 women will die of the disease. Many of these lives could have been saved by early diagnosis.

At Risk

Most women who get breast cancer have no family history of the disease or other risk factors. Although some women are at slightly higher risk (women whose mothers or sisters had breast cancer, who have never had children, and who had their first child after age 30), the biggest risk factor for breast cancer is being a woman.

Breast Self-Exam

All women over age 20 should practice regular monthly breast self-examinations (BSE). It can help you find changes in your breasts that occur between clinical breast examinations by a health professional and mammograms. The American Cancer Society has a pamphlet called "Breast Self Examination—A New Approach" (see the Appendix for contacting the American Cancer Society).

Best Defense Against Breast Cancer

Ages 20 to 39
Perform a breast self-exam each month. Have a clinical breast exam by a health care professional every 3 years.

Ages 40 and over
Have a mammogram every year. Have a clinical breast exam by a health care professional every year. Perform a breast self-exam each month.

Prostate Cancer

The prostate, a collection of male sex glands, is a pea-sized, tiny organ at birth and reaches full growth when a man reaches his 20s. The prostate may continue to grow slowly, which can create problems for men after they reach age 40 or 50. Up to 80 percent of men will develop an enlarged prostate, but not all will develop symptoms of cancer. The best action a man can take is prevention.

These are the symptoms of prostate cancer:

1. Frequent urination, especially at night
2. Difficulty controlling the flow of urine
3. Inability to urinate
4. Urgency to urinate
5. Frequent pain or stiffness in the lower back, hips, or upper thighs

These symptoms may not necessarily indicate prostate cancer; they are also common indicators of other prostate problems.

Prevention

After the age of 40, every man should have an annual physical exam and testing to monitor any signs of prostate cancer. A diet high in fiber and low in fat is highly recommended. Fruits and vegetables rich in antioxidants are also recommended.

A recent study found that men who ate more than ten servings a week of tomatoes, tomato sauce, tomato juice, and even pizza had significantly lower rates of prostate cancer. Tomatoes contain the antioxidant lycopene, which helps support the suspicion that a diet high in antioxidants can play a role in preventing prostate cancer.

Irrational Thinking

The belief that "if I wear sunscreen, I can stay in the sun far longer" is akin to the "if I eat only low-fat food, I can eat as much as I want" attitude. Both are irrational and incorrect. Low-fat foods have calories, which in excess cause weight gain; exposure to the sun for long periods of time increases risk for skin cancer.

• • •

Antioxidants

Antioxidant-rich foods include the following:

- Broccoli
- Cauliflower
- Dark green leafy vegetables
- Citrus fruits

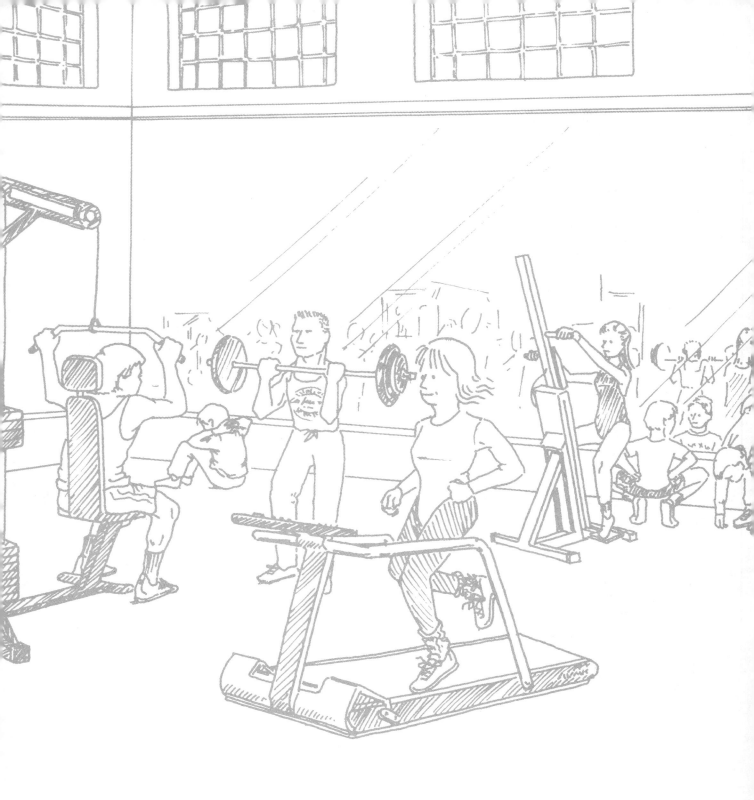

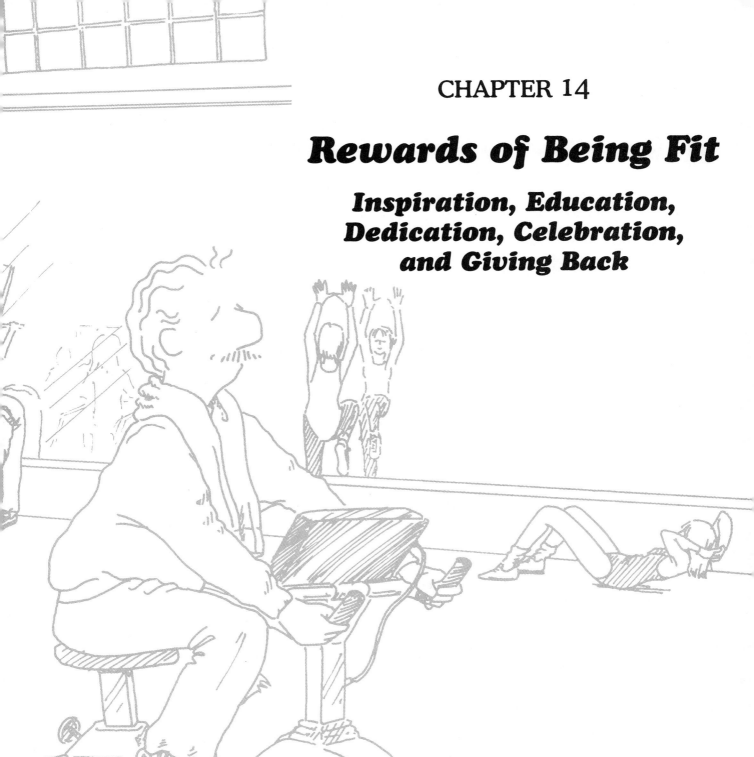

CHAPTER 14

Rewards of Being Fit

Inspiration, Education, Dedication, Celebration, and Giving Back

Nearly 10 years ago a man went to Hawaii to watch a friend swim 2.4 miles in the ocean, to bike ride 112 miles in the lava fields, and then to run 26.2 miles in the race known as the Ironman Triathlon Championship. Although the man enjoyed exercise, it was not something he included in his daily life. His responsibilities of being an active husband and father of two young children, plus having a full-time career, left him little time for consistent exercise.

But on that day his self-perspective as a spectator changed. He was impressed by the difficulty of the event, by the athletes' fitness and attitudes, by their commitment, and by their accomplishment. But he was even more struck when he read in the program that (aside from a very small percentage of professional athletes) most of the athletes were regular working folk, just like him. He began to wonder, "If they can work and have families and do all of this, can't I at least get fit? And, wow, wouldn't that be awesome if I could do an Ironman triathlon?"

He thought about how he might manage his time and responsibilities to exercise and become fit. And he wondered if he could become fit enough to do the Ironman. He left that experience inspired and motivated. Many seeds had been planted in his mind. Although it seemed like just a dream, he held onto the idea that maybe he could do it. When he returned home, he turned his inspiration to dedication.

He made a plan for including exercise a minimum of three times a week. He started with the exercise he enjoyed most, swimming. As he became fit, he "dabbled" at bike riding. Then occasionally he ran a couple of miles. He began to talk to others who did those same things and learned more about how to train. He started reading and talking to others about how to improve his nutrition and how to exercise appropriately. His entire family noticed that as his fitness improved so did his joy and appreciation for life. He was happier than before. He celebrated his accomplishments, his newly developed fitness, and his reward was great health and happiness. As he got more involved, so did his children. Seeing Dad having fun swimming, biking, and running was inspiring. They too began participating in triathlons.

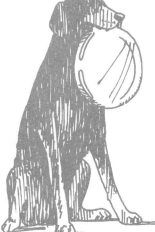

Within 4 years, he ran his first marathon. Two years after that he completed his first century (100-mile) bike ride and then several short triathlons. He continued to train, to get fitter, and to feel happier than ever before. Nine years after his original inspiration, he and his family traveled to Lake Placid, New York, to celebrate his dream come true. He completed the 2.4-mile swim, 112-mile bike ride, and 26.2-mile race at the Ironman USA Triathlon.

Inspiration, Education, Dedication, and Celebration

You can achieve your fitness goal by applying the same methods. Committing to regular exercise could be your Ironman. But as the man above demonstrated, seek inspiration and education, channel your dedication, and make time for celebration. This is how you can achieve your fitness goals.

See Your Possibilities

Luckily, there is neither an exclusive nor a quota on who and how many people can be fit. Although there are already many fit people, you can be one too. Allow yourself to see your fitness possibilities. Start small, start slowly, and start today. Start with the things that you can see yourself doing. As you do them, you will gain momentum. There are many simple "I can do's" that will launch you into healthy improvements. "I can . . . eat breakfast, eat a midmorning snack, drink water, go for a walk, invite a friend to exercise with me, buy or borrow that piece of exercise equipment." Go for it!

Forget Perfection!

Fitness is not an all-or-none proposition; it is a work in progress. We are human with ever-changing conditions. You do not have to eat "the perfect meal" or do "the perfect exercise" to get fit. Think of fitness as your lifelong companion who will enhance your life experience. Every little bit contributes toward a healthier you. Even daily physical activity accumulated in shorter bouts of 10 minutes can yield fitness improvements. And every little bit you do gives you success and momentum to continue and build on.

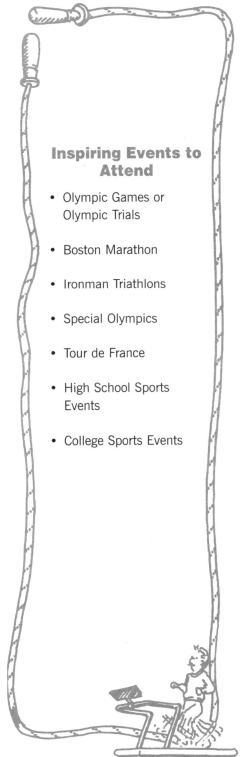

Inspiring Events to Attend

- Olympic Games or Olympic Trials

- Boston Marathon

- Ironman Triathlons

- Special Olympics

- Tour de France

- High School Sports Events

- College Sports Events

Social Rewards

Being fit opens your life up to new interests and experiences. In addition to the physiological rewards, there are unlimited social rewards. There is a whole world of activities open to those who are fit, those who can do.

Giving Back
Holidays and Charitable Causes

Holidays are perfect target dates for socializing and achieving your goals. You can also receive great satisfaction by running a 10k and raising funds for a charity. Many communities and charities hold their activity-based fundraising events on holidays. Participating with others is a fun way to celebrate your blessings of good health. Look for events in your area around holidays and recruit your family and friends to participate too. If there is a cause, there is likely to be an event. Some of the better known organizations and holidays with events are listed below. Many cities have a monthly activity-based newspaper/magazine with a thorough listing of events, information, and entry forms.

Holidays and causes with themed fitness events include the following: AIDS, American Heart Association, American Lung Association, breast cancer, campaigns against domestic violence, Christmas, Easter Seal Society, Father's Day, Halloween, Humane Society (bring your dog!), Independence Day, Mother's Day, New Year's Day, St. Patrick's Day, SPCA, Thanksgiving, Valentine's Day, and more.

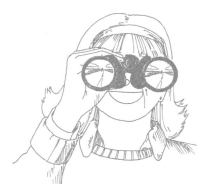

Be a Humanitarian Hero

Another blessing of being fit is the ability to give and help others. Consider how many lives you affect when you are one of the humanitarian heroes who donates blood (to the American Red Cross at local hospitals and organizations) or signs up to be an organ donor (sign the donor card on the back of your driver's license). Giving and receiving are the complete life cycle, and when you give, you will receive. Consider the ultimate gifts of life you could give to others.

Organized Events and Vacations

Traveling to a new destination coupled with achieving a fitness goal is an exciting combination. How about running a 10k event in Hawaii or Florida? What about bicycling across your favorite state or European country? What about playing in a special soccer tournament or dance-a-thon? As more people are enjoying the travel plus physical activity combination, there are more and more organized events and companies offering planned courses and official support. These events offer you the opportunity to go and see places you have never seen before, to be active in the great outdoors, and to meet new people while having fun.

Here are just a few destination events:

- Bay to Breakers, San Francisco, California
- Peachtree Road Race, Atlanta, Georgia
- Gasparilla Distance Classic, Tampa, Florida
- Bike Ride Around Lake Tahoe, Lake Tahoe, California
- Run to the Far Side, San Francisco, California

Inspiration

Feed your inspiration by participating or attending events that may inspire you. They do not even have to be sport-activity specific. Seeing others striving to do and be their best is inspiring no matter what the medium. Television broadcasts of many inspiring events can be just the thing to get you going. Pick up or subscribe to a new magazine, visit a related Web site, attend an equipment demonstration, a fitness or sporting event, or a conference or workshop. Feed your interest, and as you do, you will continue to inspire yourself.

Fitness Goals

Just like the man in the story at the beginning of this chapter, you too can dream of an accomplishment that will get your attention and motivate you to get or stay fit. Choose something impressive but within your reach. Stay away from goals that are too lofty and will overwhelm or intimidate you. Make a plan about how you will attain your goal. Put it down on your calendar and chart out your journey.

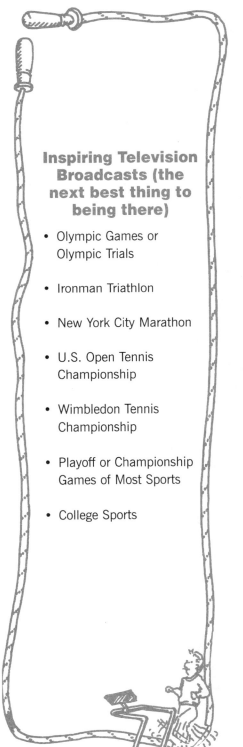

Inspiring Television Broadcasts (the next best thing to being there)

- Olympic Games or Olympic Trials

- Ironman Triathlon

- New York City Marathon

- U.S. Open Tennis Championship

- Wimbledon Tennis Championship

- Playoff or Championship Games of Most Sports

- College Sports

Goals

Here are a few sample fitness goals:

- Walk for 30 minutes without stopping.

- Walk in a 5 kilometer event. Run in a 5 kilometer event.

- Bike ride to and from work 1 day a week.

- Canoe or kayak to the end of the lake and back.

- Hike to the top of the hill and back.

- Climb or hike Mt. Whitney, part of the Appalachian, or the Pacific Crest Trails.

Celebrate Your Health

Being fit just feels good. It improves the quality of your day-to-day life as well as your outlook for the future. Do you want to feel better? Do you want to feel your best? You have a choice every day. And now you have many ideas about how to improve the quality and quantity of your life through fitness.

Being fit is another way of putting yourself in the best possible condition to meet life's challenges. It does not mean that your life will be void of stress or difficulties. It does mean that you will be better able to handle stress and difficulties. It does mean you will recover more quickly from illnesses. It also means you will be better able to experience and appreciate the joy and simple pleasures of life. Look at the fun and energy that await you!

Appendix

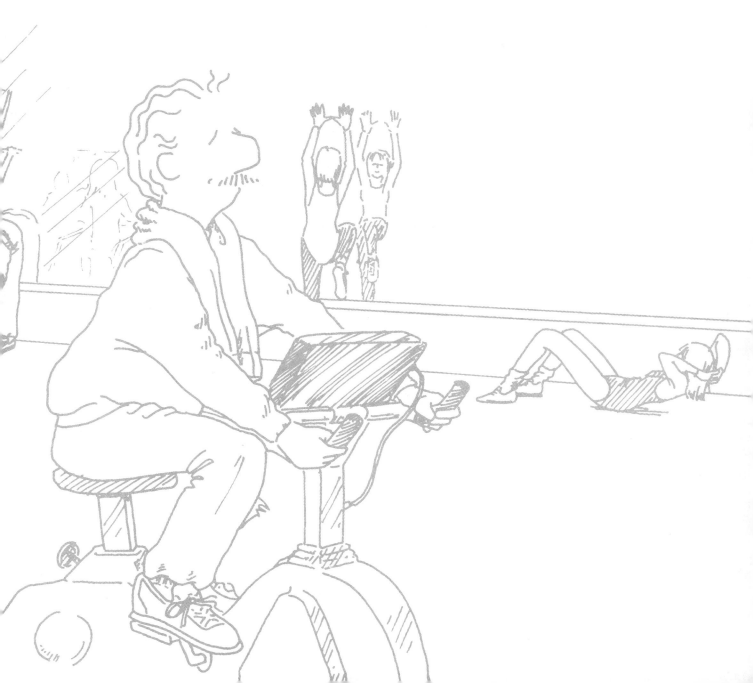

Suppliers of Fitness Essentials

Men's and Women's Apparel

adidas—www.adidas.com

Asics— www.asics.co.jp

Bike Nashbar—www.bikenashbar.com

California Best (800) 225-2378 www.californiabest.com

Champion—www.championsports.com

Fleet Feet Sports—www.fleetfeet.com

Hind—www.hind.com

Insport—www.insport.com

New Balance—www.newbalance.com

Nike—www.nike.com

Pearl izumi—www.Pearlizumi.com

Reebok—www.reebok.com

Performance Bicycle—www.performancebike.com (800) 727-2453

Road Runner Sports—www.roadrunnersports.com

Women's Apparel

Athleta—sports apparel. Toll free (888)322-5515
www.athleta.com

Champion sport bras—www.championjogbra.com

Moving Comfort—www.movingcomfort.com

Title Nine Sports—(800) 609-0092 www.title9sports.com

Terry Precision Cycling for Women—(800) 289-8379
www.terrybicycles.com

General Fitness Equipment

Aerobics, Inc. / Pacemaster Treadmills www.pacemaster.com

Concept II, Inc. (Rowing Machines) (800) 245-5676 www.conceptII.com

Cybex International (800) 677-6544 www.ecybex.com or
www.cybexintl.com

DynaBand—Fitness Wholesale (800) 537-5512—
www.fwonline.com

Fischer Ski Equipment—www.skifischer.com

Just Balls—www.justballs.com

Life Fitness—(800) 735-3867 www.lifefitness.com

Lifeline International (800) 553-6633 www.lifeline-usa.com

Monark (arm ergometers)—see Stairmaster

Nautilus—see Life Fitness
Nordic Equipment, Inc. (801) 655-7225
    www.nordicequipment.com
NordicTrack/Icon Health and Fitness, Inc. (800) 727-9777
    www.nordictrack.com
Performance Bicycle—www.performancebike.com
Precor—(800) 4PRECOR www.precor.com
Quinton Instrument Co.—see StairMaster
Reebok—www.reebok.com
Schwinn Cycling and Fitness (800) SCHWINN www.schwinn.com
SPRI Products, Inc. (800) 222-7774
Stairmaster Sports Medical Products—(800) 635-2936
    www.stairmaster.com
Stretch Cordz—NZ Mfg., Inc. (800) 886-6621
The Step Co. (800) SAY-STEP
Tectrix Fitness Equipment—see Cybex International
Tunturi—www.tunturi.com
Trotter—see Cybex International
Versaclimber—Heart Rate Inc., (800) 237-2271 www.heartrateinc.com

Hands-Free Hydration System Specialists
CamelBak—www.camelbak.com
Platypus—(800) 531-9531 www.cascadedesigns.com
Ultimate—(800) 426-7229 www.ultdir.com

Heart Rate Monitor Specialists
Cardiosport—www.cardiosport.com
Heart Monitor—www.heartmonitor.com
Heart Zone—www.heartzone.com
Polar—www.polar.com

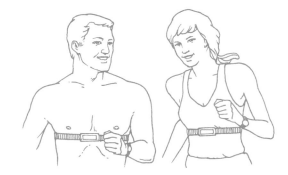

In-Line Skating
Rollerblade, Inc. (800) 328-0171 www.Rollerblade.com

Pilates™ and Pilates-based Exercise
The Pilates Studio/ NY and CA (800) 474-5283 www.pilatesstudio.com
Physicalmind Institute, Santa Fe, NM (800) 505-1990

Stott Equipment Sales—(800) 901-0001
www.stottconditioning.com (Pilates type)

Snow Shoes
Red Feather—www.redfeather.com
Tubbs—www.tubbs.com
Yuba Snowshoe Company—www.yubashoes.com

Special Innovative Stuff
BodyGlide—anti-chafing petroleum-free lubrication (888) 263-9454
www.sternoff.com
The E3 Grip—(hands grips for body alignment). www.biogrip.com
SPF (sun protection factor) clothing available through TravelSmith (800)
950-1600 www.travelsmith.com
60 Leveroni Ct., Novato, CA 95959

Sport Watch Specialists
Timex Ironman—www.timex.com
Casio—www.casio.com

Swimming Specific
Endless Pools, Inc.—(a treadmill for swimming) (800) 233-0741, ext. 853
www.endlesspools.com
Speedo (swimming)—www.speedo.com
Tyr—(800) 252-7878 www.tyr.com
USA Aquatics—usaaquatics.com (800) 445-8721
The Victor—www.swimming.com (800) 356-5132
Zoggs—www.zoggs.com

Wetsuits
Ironman Wetsuits—www.ironmanwetsuits.com
Quintana Roo—www.QuintanaRoo.com

Vacations (Active)
Backroads www.backroads.com

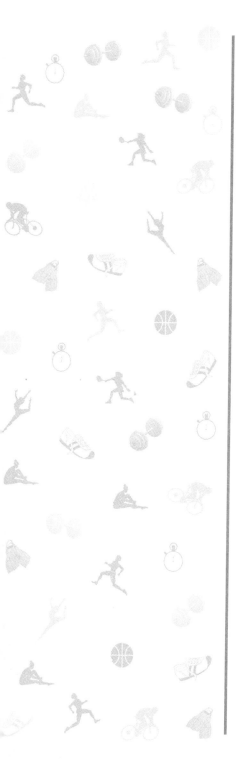

Instructional and Informational

Complete Guide to Exercise Videos Collage Video Specialties
   (800) 433-6769 www.collagevideo.com
Comprehensive Fitness Consulting (Pre and Post Natal Exercise)
   (608) 831-8173 compfc@aol.com
Healthy Learning (videos), P.O. Box 1828, Monterey, CA (888) 229-5745
Medicine Ball Exercise Cycles by Lineaus H. Lorette
Plyometric Exercises by Donald Chu (use of medicine ball)
Weight Training Made Easy, Joyce L. Vedral, Ph.D. Warner Books,
   New York, 1997.

Associations and Organizations

American Academy of Dermatology, (888) 462-DERM www.aad.org/
American Cancer Society, (800) ACS-2345, www.cancer.org
American College of Sports Medicine (ACSM), (317) 637-9200
   www.acsm.org/sportsmed
American Diabetes Association, (800) 232-3472,
   www.diabetes.org
American Dietetic Association, (800) 232-3472, www.eatright.org
American Medical Association, www.ama-assn.org
The Cooper Institute for Aerobics Research (800) 444-5764,
   www.cooperaerobics.com
International In-Line Skating Association, Kensington, MD, (301) 942-9770
Leukemia Society of America—Team in Training,
   (800) 482-TEAM
   www.lsa-teamintraining.org
United States Masters Swimming Inc., (603)
   537-0203, www.usms.org

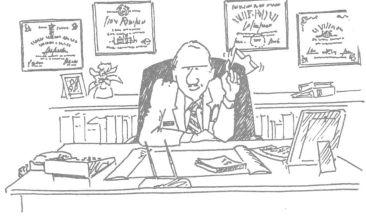

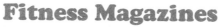

Fitness Magazines

Bicycling—www.bicycling.com
Rodale Press—rodalepress.com
Runner's World—www.runnersworld.com
Triathlete—www.triathletemag.com (800) 778-4852

General Health Web Sites

www.drkoop.com
www.healthfinder.gov

Journals and Newsletters

American Journal of Public Health, www.apha.org
University of California, Berkeley Wellness Letter, P.O. Box 420148, Palm
    Coast, Florida 32142
The Fitness Monitor—www.heartzone.com (916) 481-7283
Harvard Heart Letter, P.O. Box 420378, Palm Coast, Florida 32142-0378
    www.countway.harvard.edu/publications/
    Health_Publications
IMPACT—HealthInvest, Inc. (888) 743-4555
    impact@healthinvest.org
Journal of the American Medical Association,
    www.ama-assn.org
New England Journal of Medicine, www.nejm.org
Nutrition Action Newsletter, Center for Science in the Public Interest,
    (202) 332-9110

Nutrition and Related Resources

Basal Metabolic Testing (BMT), Cooper Wellness Program, (800) 444-
    5192
Food Finder, Food Sources of Vitamins & Minerals, third edition, by
    Elizabeth S. Hands, ESHA Research, Salem, Oregon.
International Food Information Council Foundation—
    www.ificinfo.health.org

Recommended Reading and Reference

ACSM's Guidelines for Exercise Testing and Prescription, Fifth Edition. Lippincott, Williams & Wilkins, Inc., 1995.

Advanced Nutritional Therapies by Dr. Kenneth H. Cooper, 1996, Thomas Nelson, Inc.

Aerobics by Dr. Kenneth H. Cooper, 1968, Bantam Books.

Creative Visualization by Shakti Gawain, Bantam Books, 1982.

Fit Kids! by Dr. Kenneth H. Cooper, Broadman & Holman Publishers, Nashville, 1999.

Fit or Fat by Covert Bailey, Houghton Mifflin Co., Boston, 1978.

The Heart Rate Monitor Book by Sally Edwards, Polar Electro Oy, Port Washington, NY 1993.

Nancy Clark's Sports Nutrition Guidebook by Nancy Clark, Second Edition, Human Kinetics, 1997.

One Minute for Myself by Spencer Johnson, M.D., Avon Publishers, 1985.

Outsmarting the Female Fat Cell by Debra Waterhouse, Warner Books, 1993.

Power Eating by Susan Kleiner with Maggie Greenwood-Robinson, Human Kinetics, 1998.

Sally Edwards' Heart Zone Training by Sally Edwards, Adams Media, 1996.

The Ultimate Fit or Fat by Covert Bailey, Houghton Mifflin Co., Boston, 1999.

The Ultimate Guide to Marathons, Second Edition, by Craythorn and Hanna, Marathon Publishers, Inc. Sacramento, California.

What to Expect When You're Expecting by Eisenberg, Murkoff, and Hathaway, Workman Publishing, New York, 1996.

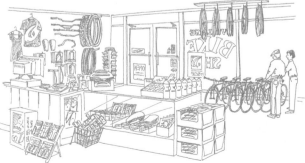

Push-up Norms—Men

%ile	20-29	30-39	40-49	50-59	60+	
			AGE			
99	≥100	≥86	≥64	≥51	≥39	
95	62	52	40	39	28	S
90	57	46	36	30	26	
85	51	41	34	28	24	
80	47	39	30	25	23	E
75	44	36	29	24	22	
70	41	34	26	21	21	
65	39	31	25	20	20	
60	37	30	24	19	18	G
55	35	29	22	17	16	
50	33	27	21	15	15	
45	31	25	19	14	12	
40	29	24	18	13	10	F
35	27	21	16	11	9	
30	26	20	15	10	8	
25	24	19	13	9.5	7	
20	22	17	11	9	6	P
15	19	15	10	7	5	
10	18	13	9	6	4	
5	≤13	≤9	≤5	≤3	≤2	VP
N	1045	790	364	172	26	

Total N = 2397

S, superior; E, excellent; G, good; F, fair; P, poor; VP, very poor. N = number

Source: *The Physical Fitness Specialist Manual*, The Cooper Institute for Aerobics Research, Dallas, Texas, revised 1999; reprinted with permission.

Modified Push-up Norms
(or Women)

%ile	AGE 20-29	30-39	40-49	50-59	60+	
99	≥70	≥56	≥60	≥31	>20	
95	45	39	33	28	20	S
90	42	36	28	25	17	
85	39	33	26	23	15	
80	36	31	24	21	15	E
75	34	29	21	20	15	
70	32	28	20	19	14	
65	31	26	19	18	13	
60	30	24	18	17	12	G
55	29	23	17	15	12	
50	26	21	15	13	8	
45	25	20	14	13	6	
40	23	19	13	12	5	F
35	22	17	11	10	4	
30	20	15	10	9	3	
25	19	14	9	8	2	
20	17	11	6	6	2	P
15	15	9	4	4	1	
10	12	8	2	1	0	
5	≤9	≤4	1	0	0	VP
N =	579	411	246	105	12	

Total N = 1353

S, superior; E, excellent; G, good; F, fair; P, poor; VP, very poor. N = number

Source: *The Physical Fitness Specialist Manual*, The Cooper Institute for Aerobics Research, Dallas, Texas, revised 1999; reprinted with permission.

12 Minute Run Distance (miles)— Women

	AGE					
%ile	20-29	30-39	40-49	50-59	60+	
99	≥1.78	≥1.66	≥1.61	≥1.48	≥1.55	
95	1.61	1.53	1.45	1.33	1.35	S
90	1.54	1.45	1.41	1.29	1.29	
85	1.49	1.43	1.35	1.24	1.21	
80	1.45	1.38	1.32	1.21	1.18	E
75	1.41	1.35	1.29	1.20	1.17	
70	1.37	1.33	1.25	1.17	1.13	
65	1.35	1.29	1.23	1.14	1.09	
60	1.33	1.27	1.21	1.13	1.07	G
55	1.31	1.26	1.19	1.11	1.05	
50	1.29	1.25	1.17	1.10	1.03	
45	1.27	1.22	1.16	1.09	1.01	
40	1.25	1.21	1.13	1.06	.99	F
35	1.22	1.17	1.12	1.04	.98	
30	1.21	1.16	1.10	1.02	.97	
25	1.17	1.13	1.09	1.01	.97	
20	1.16	1.11	1.05	.98	.94	P
15	1.13	1.09	1.02	.97	.93	
10	1.10	1.05	1.01	.93	.89	
5	1.03	1.01	.96	.90	.86	VP
1	≤.94	≤.93	≤.89	≤.83	≤.81	

N = 764   N = 2049   N = 1630 N = 878 N = 202

S, superior; E, excellent; G, good; F, fair; P, poor; VP, very poor. N = number

Source: *The Physical Fitness Specialist Manual*, The Cooper Institute for Aerobics Research, Dallas, Texas, revised 1999; reprinted with permission.

12 Minute Run Distance (miles)— Men

%ile	20-29	30-39	40-49	50-59	60+	
			AGE			
99	≥1.94	≥1.89	≥1.85	≥1.77	≥1.71	
95	1.81	1.77	1.71	1.62	1.57	S
90	1.74	1.71	1.65	1.57	1.49	
85	1.69	1.65	1.57	1.49	1.41	
80	1.65	1.61	1.54	1.45	1.37	E
75	1.62	1.57	1.53	1.41	1.30	
70	1.61	1.55	1.47	1.38	1.29	
65	1.57	1.53	1.45	1.35	1.26	
60	1.54	1.49	1.42	1.33	1.24	G
55	1.53	1.47	1.41	1.31	1.21	
50	1.50	1.45	1.37	1.29	1.19	
45	1.49	1.41	1.35	1.26	1.17	
40	1.45	1.39	1.33	1.25	1.15	F
35	1.43	1.37	1.30	1.22	1.13	
30	1.41	1.35	1.29	1.21	1.11	
25	1.37	1.33	1.25	1.17	1.08	
20	1.34	1.29	1.23	1.15	1.05	P
15	1.33	1.25	1.21	1.13	1.01	
10	1.27	1.21	1.17	1.09	.95	
5	1.19	1.17	1.10	1.01	.89	VP
1	≤1.06	≤1.13	≤.98	≤.92	≤.82	

N = 1675   N = 7094   N = 6837   N = 3808   N = 1005

S, superior; E, excellent; G, good; F, fair; P, poor; VP, very poor.
N = number

Source: *The Physical Fitness Specialist Manual*, The Cooper Institute for Aerobics Research, Dallas, Texas, revised 1999; reprinted with permission.

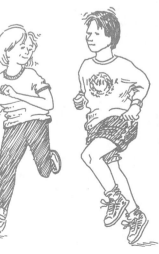

PAR - Q & YOU

(A Questionnaire for People Aged 15 to 69)

Regular physical activity is fun and healthy, and increasingly more people are starting to become more active every day. Being more active is very safe for most people. However, some people should check with their doctor before they start becoming much more physically active.

If you are planning to become much more physically active than you are now, start by answering the seven questions in the box below. If you are between the ages of 15 and 69, the PAR-Q will tell you if you should check with your doctor before you start. If you are over 69 years of age, and you are not used to being very active, check with your doctor.

Common sense is your best guide when you answer these questions. Please read the questions carefully and answer each one honestly: check YES or NO.

YES	NO		
☐	☐	1.	Has your doctor ever said that you have a heart condition <u>and</u> that you should only do physical activity recommended by a doctor?
☐	☐	2.	Do you feel pain in your chest when you do physical activity?
☐	☐	3.	In the past month, have you had chest pain when you were not doing physical activity?
☐	☐	4.	Do you lose your balance because of dizziness or do you ever lose consciousness?
☐	☐	5.	Do you have a bone or joint problem that could be made worse by a change in your physical activity?
☐	☐	6.	Is your doctor currently prescribing drugs (for example, water pills) for your blood pressure or heart condition?
☐	☐	7.	Do you know of <u>any other reason</u> why you should not do physical activity?

If you answered

YES to one or more questions

Talk with your doctor by phone or in person BEFORE you start becoming much more physically active or BEFORE you have a fitness appraisal. Tell your doctor about the PAR-Q and which questions you answered YES.

- You may be able to do any activity you want — as long as you start slowly and build up gradually. Or, you may need to restrict your activities to those which are safe for you. Talk with your doctor about the kinds of activities you wish to participate in and follow his/her advice.
- Find out which community programs are safe and helpful for you.

NO to all questions

If you answered NO honestly to <u>all</u> PAR-Q questions, you can be reasonably sure that you can:

- start becoming much more physically active — begin slowly and build up gradually. This is the safest and easiest way to go.
- take part in a fitness appraisal — this is an excellent way to determine your basic fitness so that you can plan the best way for you to live actively.

DELAY BECOMING MUCH MORE ACTIVE:
- if you are not feeling well because of a temporary illness such as a cold or a fever — wait until you feel better; or
- if you are or may be pregnant — talk to your doctor before you start becoming more active.

Please note: If your health changes so that you then answer YES to any of the above questions, tell your fitness or health professional. Ask whether you should change your physical activity plan.

<u>Informed Use of the PAR-Q</u>: The Canadian Society for Exercise Physiology, Health Canada, and their agents assume no liability for persons who undertake physical activity, and if in doubt after completing this questionnaire, consult your doctor prior to physical activity.

You are encouraged to copy the PAR-Q but only if you use the entire form

Pace versus Miles Per Hour—Converting

Pace refers to the number of minutes it takes to complete each mile; *miles per hour* refers to the number of miles you would cover at that pace in an hour.

Sometimes you want to know your pace and sometimes the miles per hour. Use these steps to convert them back and forth as needed.

Converting pace to miles per hour:

Pace: the number of minutes it takes to complete each mile.

Fractions of a minute are converted to decimal points, for example:

45 secs = .75; 30 secs = .50;
15 seconds = .25; 10 seconds = .166.

Example: A 13:30 pace = 13.5 or 13½ minutes to complete each mile. To convert *pace to miles per hour*, use the following:

1. First, convert pace to a decimal. For example: 13½ minutes per mile = 13.5.
2. Next, divide the pace (in decimal) into the number 60 for the miles per hour. For example: 60 ÷ 13.5 = 4.44 miles per hour.
3. This tells you that at a 13½ minute pace, you would cover 4.44 miles in an hour.

Converting miles per hour to pace:

Miles per hour: the number of miles you would cover in an hour at that pace.

Example: Your treadmill shows that you are walking 4.4 miles per hour. To convert miles per hour to pace, use the following:

1. Divide the miles per hour into the number 60 for the pace in decimal. For example: 60 ÷ 4.44 mph = 13.51 minute pace.
2. This tells you that walking at a speed of 4.4 mph, it takes you 13½ minutes to cover each mile.

Sample Form of a Food Record Analysis

Weekday or Weekend: _____   Date: _____

TIME	MEAL/SNACK	WHERE	ALL SOLIDS AND LIQUIDS	AMOUNT OR SERVING SIZE

Index

THE EVERYTHING SERIES!

BUSINESS

Everything® **Business Planning Book**
Everything® **Coaching and Mentoring Book**
Everything® **Fundraising Book**
Everything® **Home-Based Business Book**
Everything® **Leadership Book**
Everything® **Managing People Book**
Everything® **Network Marketing Book**
Everything® **Online Business Book**
Everything® **Project Management Book**
Everything® **Selling Book**
Everything® **Start Your Own Business Book**
Everything® **Time Management Book**

COMPUTERS

Everything® **Build Your Own Home Page Book**
Everything® **Computer Book**
Everything® **Internet Book**
Everything® **Microsoft® Word 2000 Book**

COOKBOOKS

Everything® **Barbecue Cookbook**
Everything® **Bartender's Book, $9.95**
Everything® **Chinese Cookbook**
Everything® **Chocolate Cookbook**
Everything® **Cookbook**
Everything® **Dessert Cookbook**
Everything® **Diabetes Cookbook**
Everything® **Indian Cookbook**
Everything® **Low-Carb Cookbook**
Everything® **Low-Fat High-Flavor Cookbook**

Everything® **Low-Salt Cookbook**
Everything® **Mediterranean Cookbook**
Everything® **Mexican Cookbook**
Everything® **One-Pot Cookbook**
Everything® **Pasta Book**
Everything® **Quick Meals Cookbook**
Everything® **Slow Cooker Cookbook**
Everything® **Soup Cookbook**
Everything® **Thai Cookbook**
Everything® **Vegetarian Cookbook**
Everything® **Wine Book**

HEALTH

Everything® **Alzheimer's Book**
Everything® **Anti-Aging Book**
Everything® **Diabetes Book**
Everything® **Dieting Book**
Everything® **Herbal Remedies Book**
Everything® **Hypnosis Book**
Everything® **Massage Book**
Everything® **Menopause Book**
Everything® **Nutrition Book**
Everything® **Reflexology Book**
Everything® **Reiki Book**
Everything® **Stress Management Book**
Everything® **Vitamins, Minerals, and Nutritional Supplements Book**

HISTORY

Everything® **American Government Book**
Everything® **American History Book**
Everything® **Civil War Book**
Everything® **Irish History & Heritage Book**

Everything® **Mafia Book**
Everything® **Middle East Book**
Everything® **World War II Book**

HOBBIES & GAMES

Everything® **Bridge Book**
Everything® **Candlemaking Book**
Everything® **Casino Gambling Book**
Everything® **Chess Basics Book**
Everything® **Collectibles Book**
Everything® **Crossword and Puzzle Book**
Everything® **Digital Photography Book**
Everything® **Easy Crosswords Book**
Everything® **Family Tree Book**
Everything® **Games Book**
Everything® **Knitting Book**
Everything® **Magic Book**
Everything® **Motorcycle Book**
Everything® **Online Genealogy Book**
Everything® **Photography Book**
Everything® **Pool & Billiards Book**
Everything® **Quilting Book**
Everything® **Scrapbooking Book**
Everything® **Sewing Book**
Everything® **Soapmaking Book**

HOME IMPROVEMENT

Everything® **Feng Shui Book**
Everything® **Feng Shui Decluttering Book, $9.95 ($15.95 CAN)**
Everything® **Fix-It Book**
Everything® **Gardening Book**
Everything® **Homebuilding Book**

All Everything® books are priced at $12.95 or $14.95, unless otherwise stated. Prices subject to change without notice.
Canadian prices range from $11.95–$31.95, and are subject to change without notice.

Everything® **Home Decorating Book**
Everything® **Landscaping Book**
Everything® **Lawn Care Book**
Everything® **Organize Your Home Book**

EVERYTHING® KIDS' BOOKS

All titles are $6.95
Everything® **Kids' Baseball Book, 3rd Ed.** ($10.95 CAN)
Everything® **Kids' Bible Trivia Book** ($10.95 CAN)
Everything® **Kids' Bugs Book** ($10.95 CAN)
Everything® **Kids' Christmas Puzzle & Activity Book** ($10.95 CAN)
Everything® **Kids' Cookbook** ($10.95 CAN)
Everything® **Kids' Halloween Puzzle & Activity Book** ($10.95 CAN)
Everything® **Kids' Joke Book** ($10.95 CAN)
Everything® **Kids' Math Puzzles Book** ($10.95 CAN)
Everything® **Kids' Mazes Book** ($10.95 CAN)
Everything® **Kids' Money Book** ($11.95 CAN)
Everything® **Kids' Monsters Book** ($10.95 CAN)
Everything® **Kids' Nature Book** ($11.95 CAN)
Everything® **Kids' Puzzle Book** ($10.95 CAN)
Everything® **Kids' Riddles & Brain Teasers Book** ($10.95 CAN)
Everything® **Kids' Science Experiments Book** ($10.95 CAN)
Everything® **Kids' Soccer Book** ($10.95 CAN)
Everything® **Kids' Travel Activity Book** ($10.95 CAN)

KIDS' STORY BOOKS

Everything® **Bedtime Story Book**
Everything® **Bible Stories Book**
Everything® **Fairy Tales Book**
Everything® **Mother Goose Book**

LANGUAGE

Everything® **Inglés Book**
Everything® **Learning French Book**
Everything® **Learning German Book**
Everything® **Learning Italian Book**
Everything® **Learning Latin Book**
Everything® **Learning Spanish Book**
Everything® **Sign Language Book**
Everything® **Spanish Phrase Book,** $9.95 ($15.95 CAN)

MUSIC

Everything® **Drums Book (with CD),** $19.95 ($31.95 CAN)
Everything® **Guitar Book**
Everything® **Playing Piano and Keyboards Book**
Everything® **Rock & Blues Guitar Book (with CD),** $19.95 ($31.95 CAN)
Everything® **Songwriting Book**

NEW AGE

Everything® **Astrology Book**
Everything® **Divining the Future Book**
Everything® **Dreams Book**
Everything® **Ghost Book**
Everything® **Love Signs Book,** $9.95 ($15.95 CAN)
Everything® **Meditation Book**
Everything® **Numerology Book**
Everything® **Palmistry Book**
Everything® **Psychic Book**
Everything® **Spells & Charms Book**
Everything® **Tarot Book**
Everything® **Wicca and Witchcraft Book**

PARENTING

Everything® **Baby Names Book**
Everything® **Baby Shower Book**
Everything® **Baby's First Food Book**
Everything® **Baby's First Year Book**
Everything® **Breastfeeding Book**

Everything® **Father-to-Be Book**
Everything® **Get Ready for Baby Book**
Everything® **Getting Pregnant Book**
Everything® **Homeschooling Book**
Everything® **Parent's Guide to Children with Autism**
Everything® **Parent's Guide to Positive Discipline**
Everything® **Parent's Guide to Raising a Successful Child**
Everything® **Parenting a Teenager Book**
Everything® **Potty Training Book,** $9.95 ($15.95 CAN)
Everything® **Pregnancy Book, 2nd Ed.**
Everything® **Pregnancy Fitness Book**
Everything® **Pregnancy Organizer,** $15.00 ($22.95 CAN)
Everything® **Toddler Book**
Everything® **Tween Book**

PERSONAL FINANCE

Everything® **Budgeting Book**
Everything® **Get Out of Debt Book**
Everything® **Get Rich Book**
Everything® **Homebuying Book, 2nd Ed.**
Everything® **Homeselling Book**
Everything® **Investing Book**
Everything® **Money Book**
Everything® **Mutual Funds Book**
Everything® **Online Investing Book**
Everything® **Personal Finance Book**
Everything® **Personal Finance in Your 20s & 30s Book**
Everything® **Wills & Estate Planning Book**

PETS

Everything® **Cat Book**
Everything® **Dog Book**
Everything® **Dog Training and Tricks Book**
Everything® **Golden Retriever Book**
Everything® **Horse Book**
Everything® **Labrador Retriever Book**
Everything® **Puppy Book**
Everything® **Tropical Fish Book**

All Everything® books are priced at $12.95 or $14.95, unless otherwise stated. Prices subject to change without notice.
Canadian prices range from $11.95–$31.95, and are subject to change without notice.

REFERENCE

Everything® **Astronomy Book**
Everything® **Car Care Book**
Everything® **Christmas Book, $15.00**
  ($21.95 CAN)
Everything® **Classical Mythology Book**
Everything® **Einstein Book**
Everything® **Etiquette Book**
Everything® **Great Thinkers Book**
Everything® **Philosophy Book**
Everything® **Psychology Book**
Everything® **Shakespeare Book**
Everything® **Tall Tales, Legends, &**
  Other Outrageous
  Lies Book
Everything® **Toasts Book**
Everything® **Trivia Book**
Everything® **Weather Book**

RELIGION

Everything® **Angels Book**
Everything® **Bible Book**
Everything® **Buddhism Book**
Everything® **Catholicism Book**
Everything® **Christianity Book**
Everything® **Jewish History &**
  Heritage Book
Everything® **Judaism Book**
Everything® **Prayer Book**
Everything® **Saints Book**
Everything® **Understanding Islam**
  Book
Everything® **World's Religions Book**
Everything® **Zen Book**

SCHOOL & CAREERS

Everything® **After College Book**
Everything® **Alternative Careers Book**
Everything® **College Survival Book**
Everything® **Cover Letter Book**
Everything® **Get-a-Job Book**
Everything® **Hot Careers Book**

Everything® **Job Interview Book**
Everything® **New Teacher Book**
Everything® **Online Job Search Book**
Everything® **Resume Book, 2nd Ed.**
Everything® **Study Book**

SELF-HELP/ RELATIONSHIPS

Everything® **Dating Book**
Everything® **Divorce Book**
Everything® **Great Marriage Book**
Everything® **Great Sex Book**
Everything® **Kama Sutra Book**
Everything® **Romance Book**
Everything® **Self-Esteem Book**
Everything® **Success Book**

SPORTS & FITNESS

Everything® **Body Shaping Book**
Everything® **Fishing Book**
Everything® **Fly-Fishing Book**
Everything® **Golf Book**
Everything® **Golf Instruction Book**
Everything® **Knots Book**
Everything® **Pilates Book**
Everything® **Running Book**
Everything® **Sailing Book, 2nd Ed.**
Everything® **T'ai Chi and QiGong Book**
Everything® **Total Fitness Book**
Everything® **Weight Training Book**
Everything® **Yoga Book**

TRAVEL

Everything® **Family Guide to Hawaii**
Everything® **Guide to Las Vegas**
Everything® **Guide to New England**
Everything® **Guide to New York City**
Everything® **Guide to Washington D.C.**
Everything® **Travel Guide to The**
  Disneyland Resort®,
  California Adventure®,

Universal Studios®, and
the Anaheim Area
Everything® **Travel Guide to the Walt**
  Disney World Resort®,
  Universal Studios®, and
  Greater Orlando, 3rd Ed.

WEDDINGS

Everything® **Bachelorette Party Book,**
  $9.95 ($15.95 CAN)
Everything® **Bridesmaid Book, $9.95**
  ($15.95 CAN)
Everything® **Creative Wedding Ideas**
  Book
Everything® **Elopement Book, $9.95**
  ($15.95 CAN)
Everything® **Groom Book**
Everything® **Jewish Wedding Book**
Everything® **Wedding Book, 2nd Ed.**
Everything® **Wedding Checklist,**
  $7.95 ($11.95 CAN)
Everything® **Wedding Etiquette Book,**
  $7.95 ($11.95 CAN)
Everything® **Wedding Organizer,**
  $15.00 ($22.95 CAN)
Everything® **Wedding Shower Book,**
  $7.95 ($12.95 CAN)
Everything® **Wedding Vows Book,**
  $7.95 ($11.95 CAN)
Everything® **Weddings on a Budget**
  Book, $9.95 ($15.95 CAN)

WRITING

Everything® **Creative Writing Book**
Everything® **Get Published Book**
Everything® **Grammar and Style Book**
Everything® **Grant Writing Book**
Everything® **Guide to Writing**
  Children's Books
Everything® **Screenwriting Book**
Everything® **Writing Well Book**

Available wherever books are sold!
To order, call 800-872-5627, or visit us at everything.com

Everything® and everything.com® are registered trademarks of F+W Publications, Inc.